Dermatoscopic Atlas of Non-Pigmented Lesions

Horacio Cabo • Aimilios Lallas
Editors

Dermatoscopic Atlas of Non-Pigmented Lesions

Case-based Analysis and Management Options

Springer

Editors
Horacio Cabo
Department of Dermatology
University of Buenos Aires
Buenos Aires, Argentina

Aimilios Lallas
First Department of Dermatology
Aristotle University of Thessaloniki
Thessaloniki, Greece

ISBN 978-3-031-34309-4 ISBN 978-3-031-34310-0 (eBook)
https://doi.org/10.1007/978-3-031-34310-0

This Springer imprint is published by the registered company Springer Nature Switzerland AG
The registered company address is: Gewerbestrasse 11, 6330 Cham, Switzerland

Foreword

There has long been a debate about the best way to teach dermoscopy. Some believe that teaching dermoscopy is best done using practical examples. Case-based practical teaching is highly effective and, incidentally, entertaining. According to Kant, "theory without practice is empty and practice without theory is blind"! My recommendation is to study the theory yourself and learn the practice from the best. The authors of this book clearly meet this criterion. Aimilios and Horacio know the pitfalls and challenges, but also the "eureka" moments that dermoscopy offers. And most importantly, they love to share their knowledge. This kind of generosity coupled with eloquence and years of first-hand experience makes them ideal teachers. If ever this enthusiasm for dermoscopy was conveyed in a book, it is in this one. This book is the second best, surpassed only by the pleasure of working with Aimilios and Horacio in person.

Vienna, Austria Harald Kittler

Preface

In 2018, we published the book *Comprehensive Atlas of Dermatoscopy Cases*, and in 2020, another one named *Atlas of Dermatoscopy Cases: Challenging and Complex Clinical Scenarios*, both with Springer.

Today, given the success of this editorial format for the presentation of dermoscopic clinical cases, presented in a similar way AS is observed in our daily medical practice, we decided to carry out a new edition: *Dermatoscopic Atlas of Non-Pigmented Lesions: Case-based Analysis and Management Options*.

Non-pigmented lesions or pink lesions are a diagnosis challenge and require not only training in dermoscopy, but also hybrid dermatoscopes that can be used with or without contact.

We hope this book will be useful for you and represent a new tool to improve your dermoscopy training.

We would like to thank to all the colleagues who have shared with us excellent cases, as well as to Springer for trusting us once again.

Buenos Aires, Argentina
Thessaloniki, Greece

Horacio Cabo
Aimilios Lallas

Contents

How to Examine Vessels: Instruments, Morphology, Distribution and Patterns

Horacio Cabo and Aimilios Lallas

Abstract

Within non pigmented lesions the importance of to know vessels and other non-pigmented structures is very important, since pigmentation is less frequently present in this kind of lesions.

Keywords

Pink lesions • Vessels • White clues

Pink lesions are clinically and dermoscopically challenging.

The first generations of dermatoscopes had only non-polarized light and required the use of an immersion fluid and contact to the skin surface (Fig. 1).

The applied pressure alters the visualization of vessels, causing either their complete disappearance or at least a modified projection. For this reason, the vascular patterns of common skin tumors and the diagnostic significance of different vessel types and distributions remained relatively obscure for several years. The invention and widespread use of polarized non-contact dermoscopy allowed an unimpeded observation of vascular structures a profound investigation of the dermatoscopic morphology of hypopigmented and achromic lesions Fig. 2. In addition, polarized dermoscopy revealed also another group of previously invisible features, the so-called white shiny structures. Several studies have investigated the dermatoscopic pattern and local features of non-pigmented (often referred to as pink) tumors. Later on, dermoscopy started to be applied also in general dermatology, opening a brand new undiscovered morphologic spectrum. During the previous decade, hundreds of studies investigated the dermatoscopic features of numerous inflammatory and infectious dermatoses. In the latter field, the importance of vessels and other non-pigmented structures is even greater, since pigmentation is less frequently present.

Based on the continuously updated knowledge on the dermatoscopic morphology of neoplastic and non-neoplastic skin disorders, we propose an updated categorization of non-pigmented structures as following:

1. ***Vessels***

The 2 main characteristics of vessels that should be assessed are the morphologic type and the distribution.

A. **Types of vessels**: there are 8 types of vessels. Three are globular and five are linear in shape.

- ***Globular vessels***

Three types of vascular structures with a globular shape can be identified: dotted vessels, coiled vessels and lacunas.

1. Dotted vessels: they are small roundish vessels, similar to the head of a pin and red in color (Figs. 3 and 4).
2. Coiled (glomerular) vessels: larger than dotted vascular structures with a roundish outline. In fact, the stem vessel is linear but in a coiled arrangement that mimics the renal glomerulus (glomerular vessels). With hand-held dermatoscope, coiled vessels usually project as large red dots (Figs. 5 and 6).
3. Lacunas: large globular homogeneous areas, often grouped, typically red in color, but occassionaly also milky-red (pink), purple, blue or black (Figs. 7 and 8).

- ***Linear vessels***

This category includes linear stem vessels that might vary in length, thickness and orientation: straight lines, irregular lines, looped lines, curved lines, helical or corkscrew.

H. Cabo (✉)
Clinical Dermatology, University of Buenos Aires, Arenales 1446 1 °C (1061) CABA, Buenos Aires, Argentina
e-mail: cabohoracio@gmail.com

A. Lallas
First Department of Dermatology, Aristotle University, 124 Delfon Street, 54643 Thessaloniki, Greece

H. Cabo and A. Lallas (eds.), *Dermatoscopic Atlas of Non-Pigmented Lesions*,
https://doi.org/10.1007/978-3-031-34310-0_1

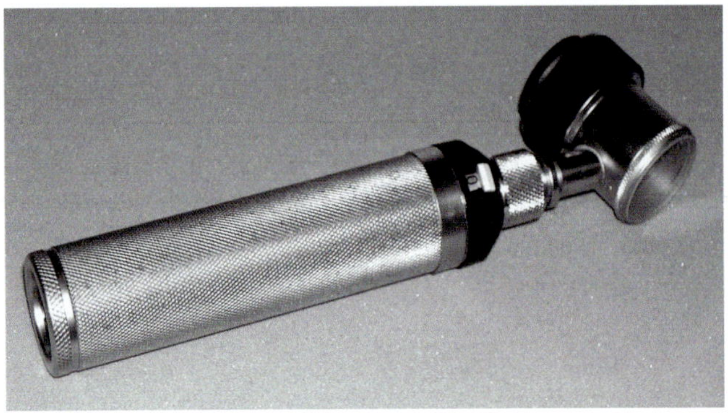

Fig. 1 Dermatoscope with non-polarized light

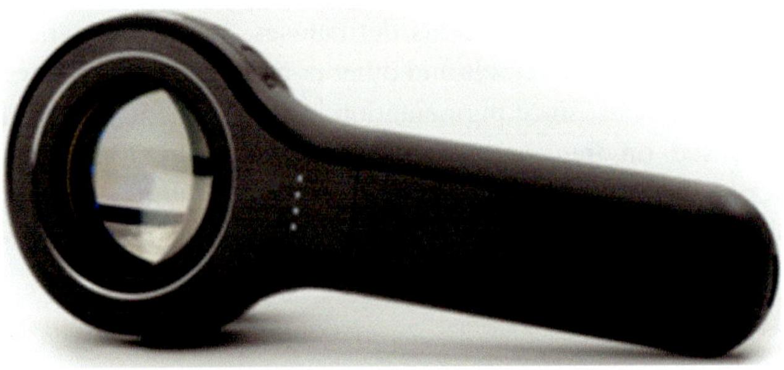

Fig. 2 Hybrid dermatoscope with non-polarized light and polarized light

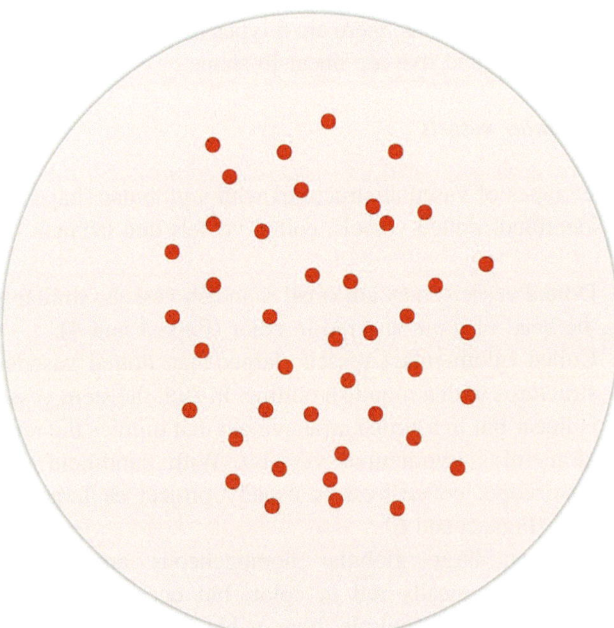

Fig. 3 Schematic drawing of punctate vessels

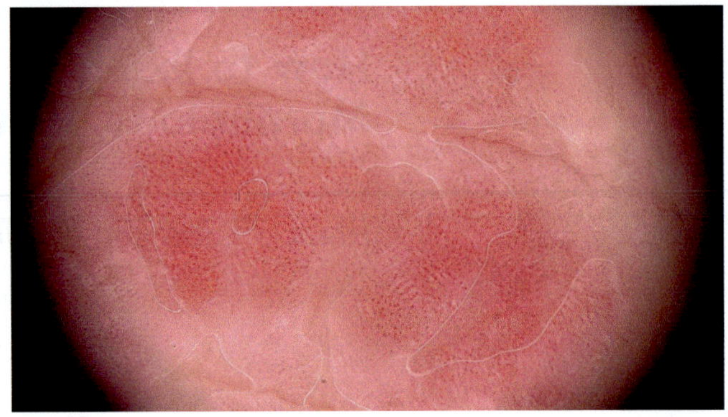

Fig. 4 Dotted vessels (Psoriasis)

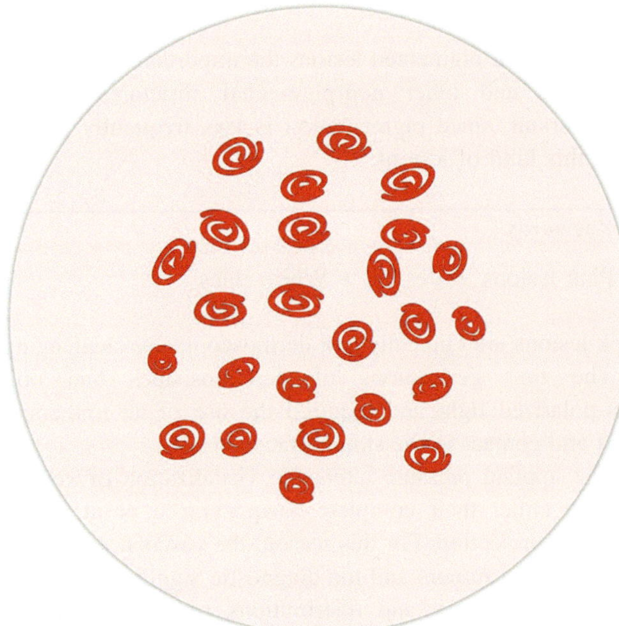

Fig. 5 Schematic drawing of coiled/glomerular vessels

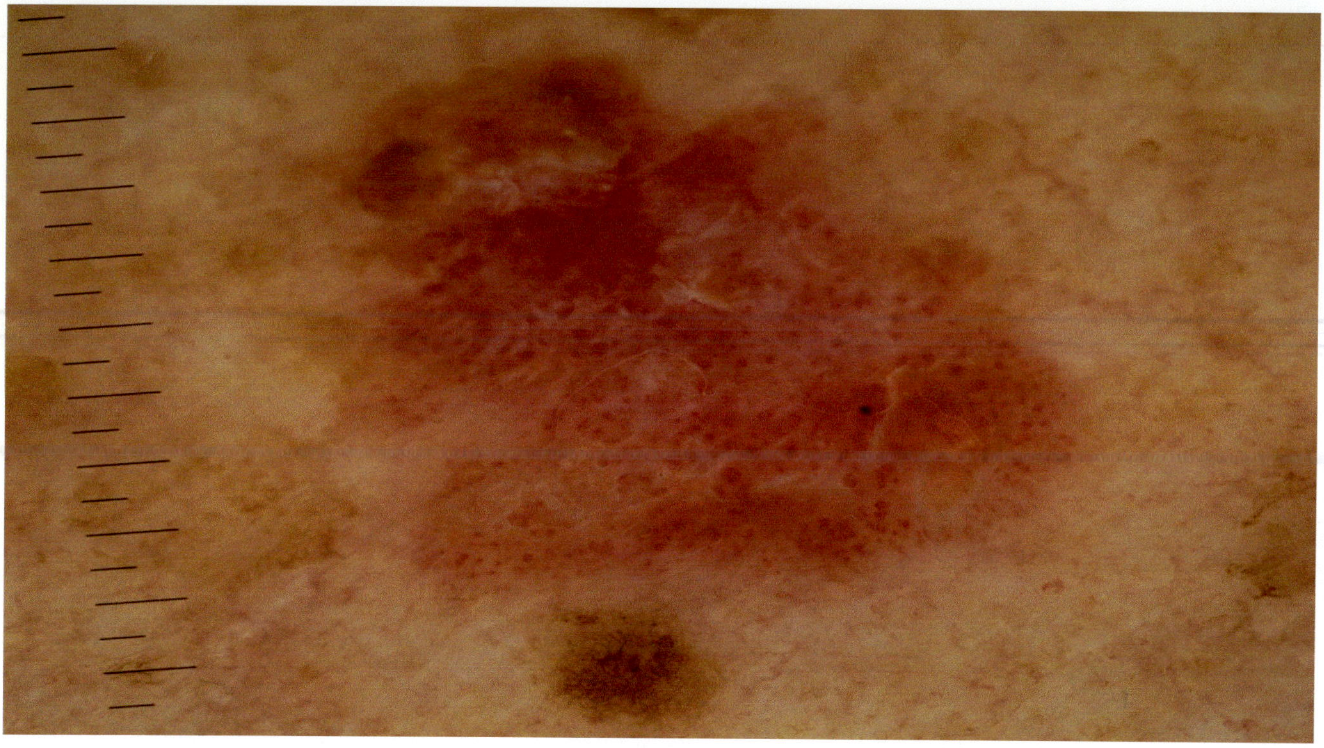

Fig. 6 Coiled/glomerular vessels (Squamous cell carcinoma in situ – Non-pigmented Bowen's disease)

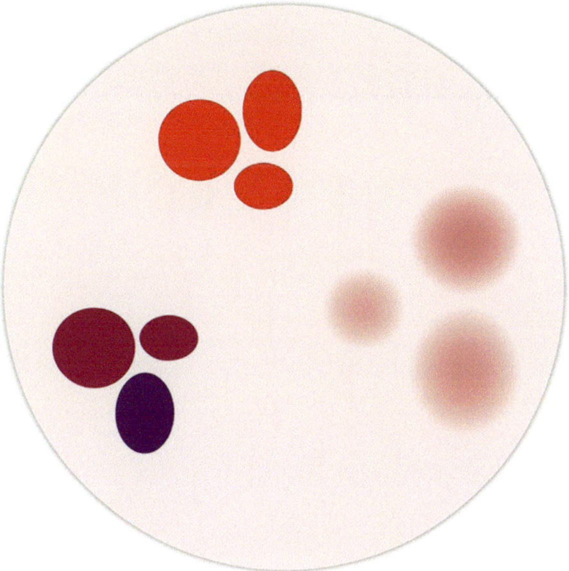

Fig. 7 Schematic drawing of lacunes

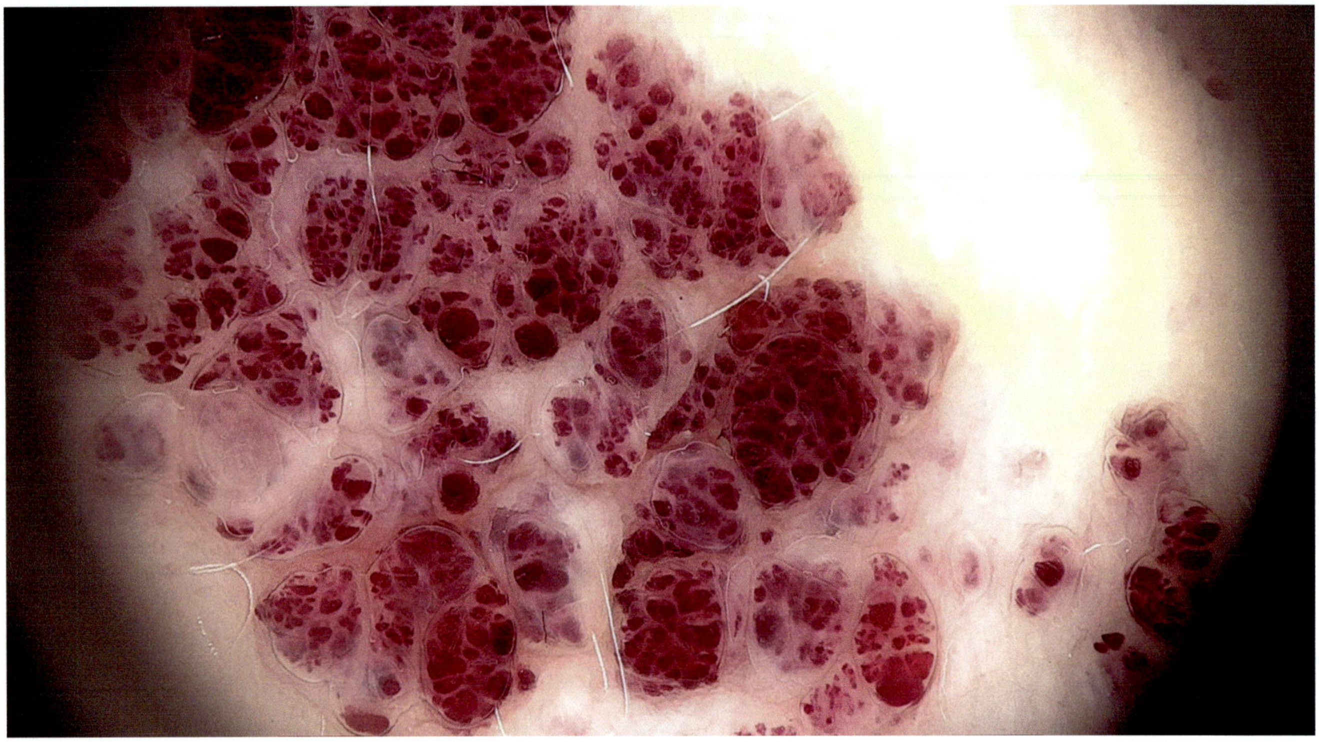

Fig. 8 Multiple red lacunas. Angioma

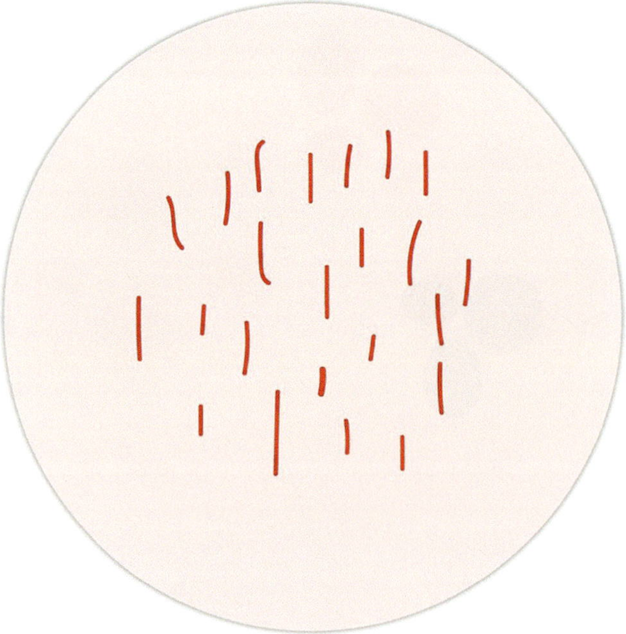

Fig. 9 Schematic drawing of straight linear vessels

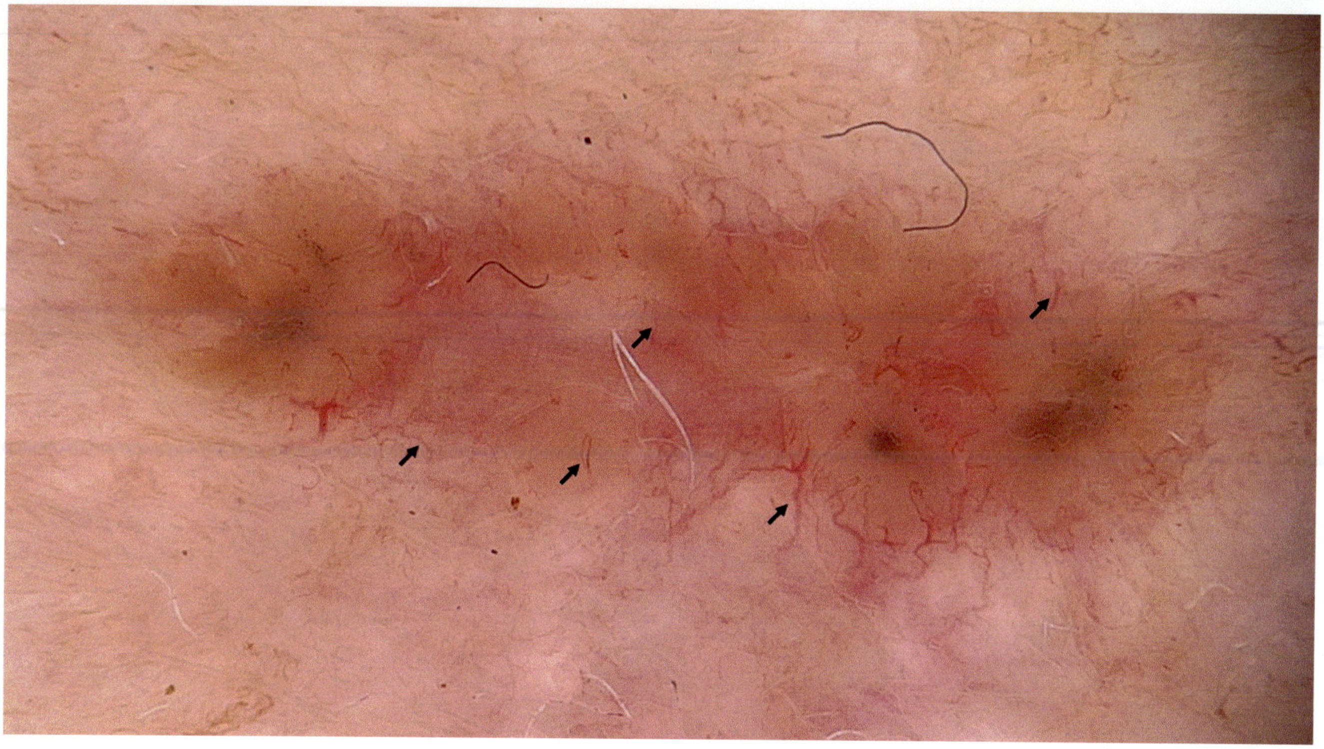

Fig. 10 Straight linear vessels (arrows). Basal cell carcinoma

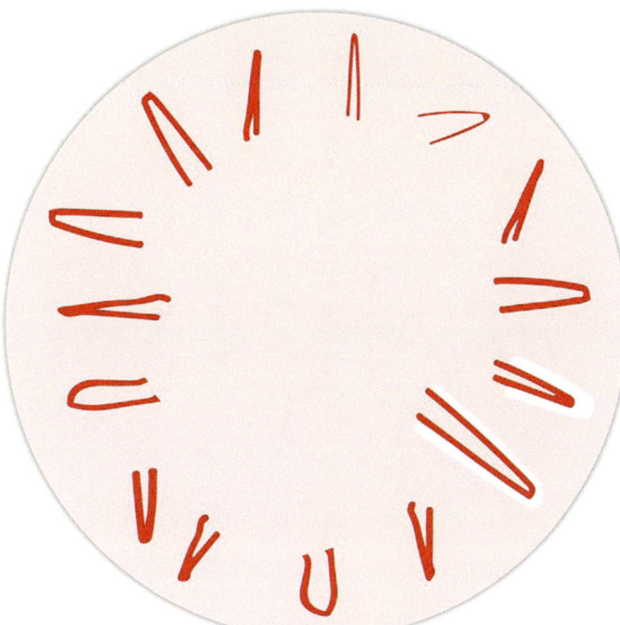

Fig. 11 Schematic drawing of linear hairpin vessels

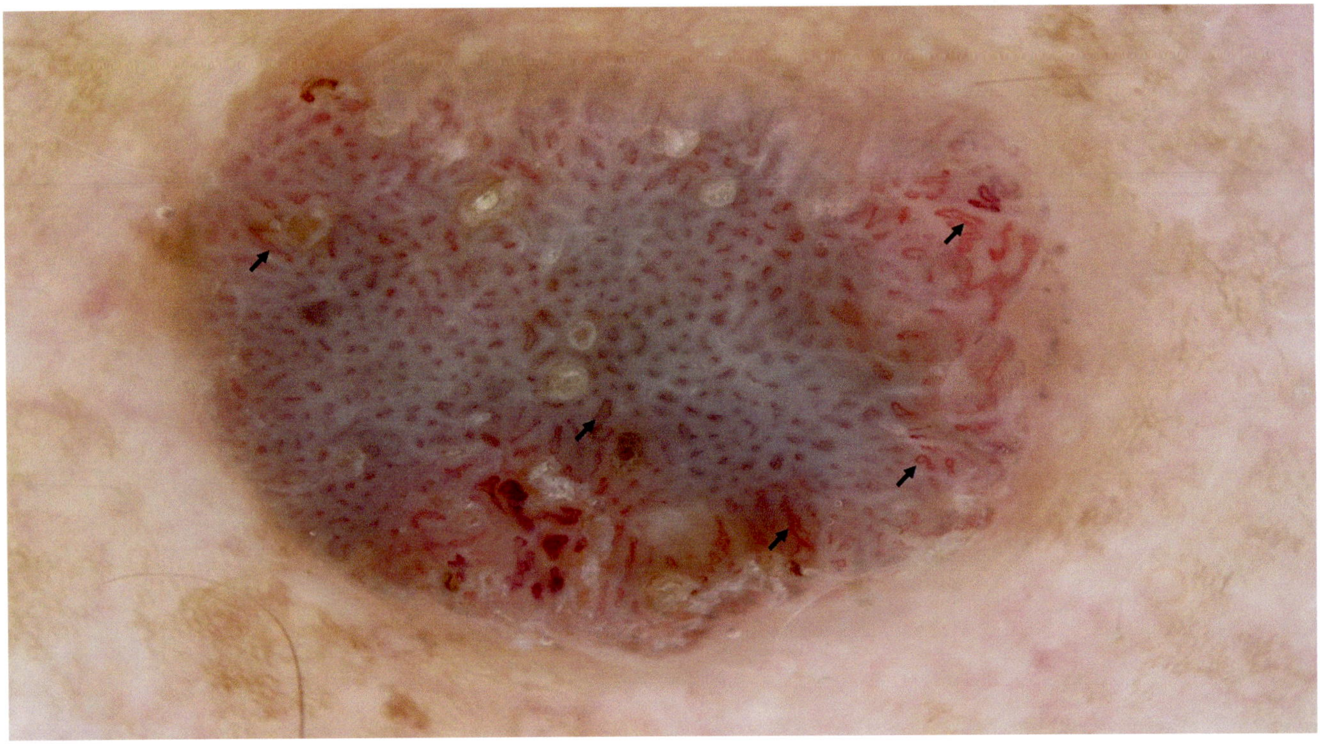

Fig. 12 Linear hairpin vessels (arrows). Seborrheic Keratosis

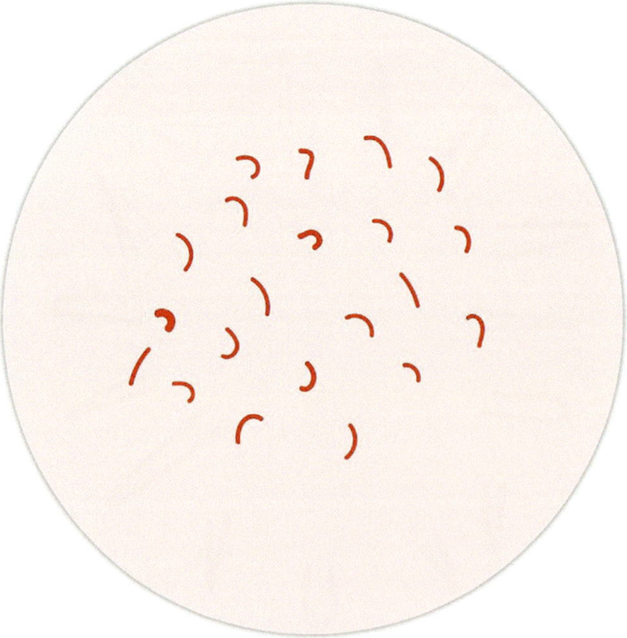

Fig. 13 Schematic drawing of curved or comma-shape

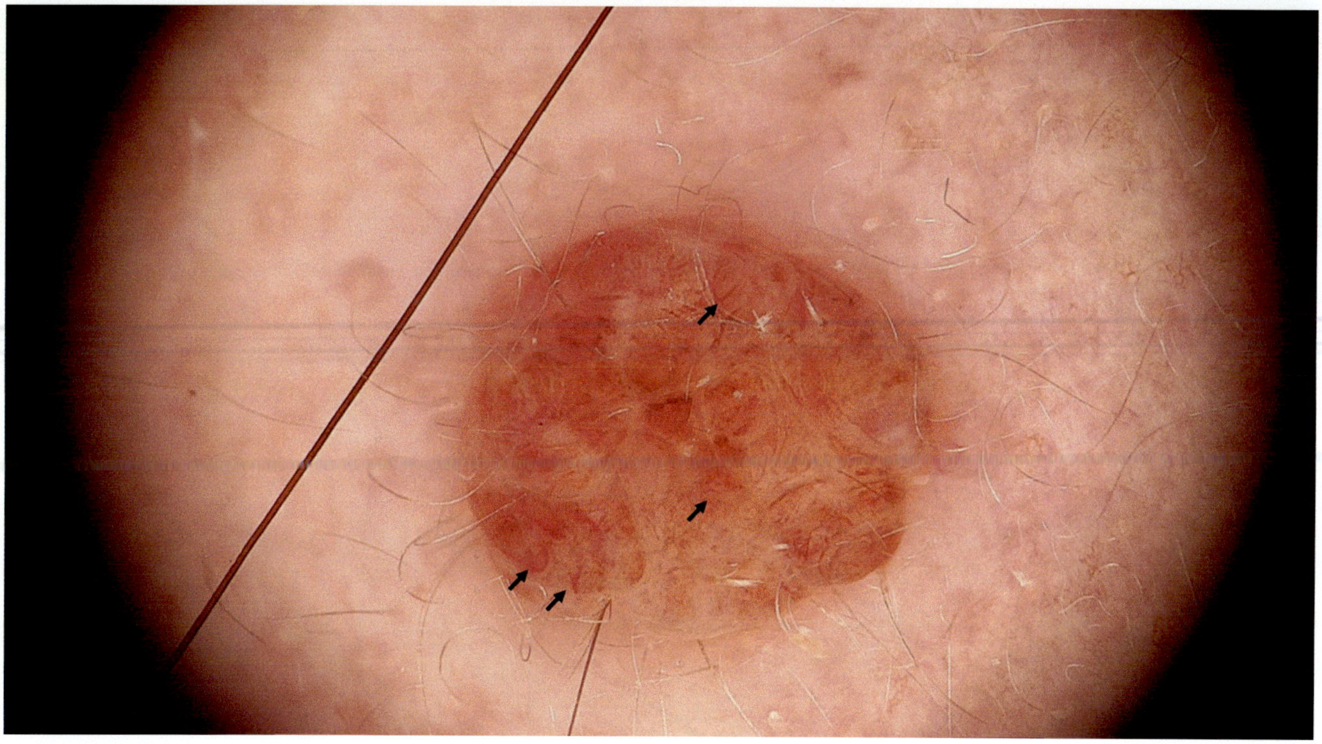

Fig. 14 Curved or comma-shaped vessels (arrows). (Intradermal nevus)

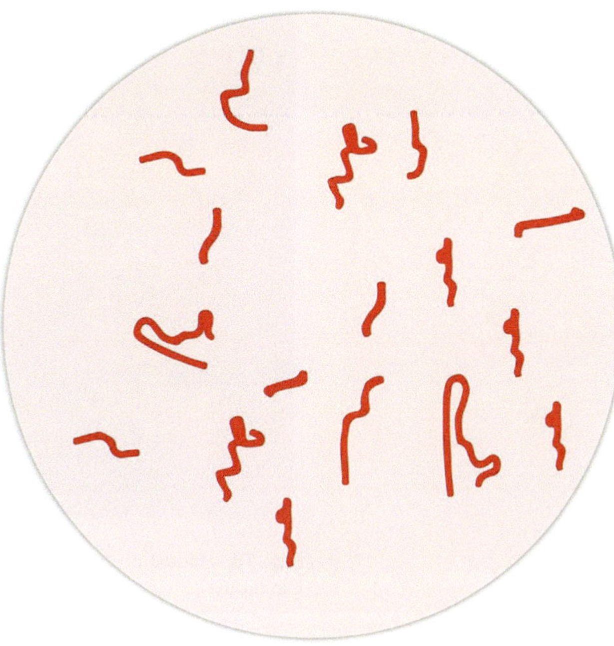

Fig. 15 Schematic drawing of irregular linear vessels

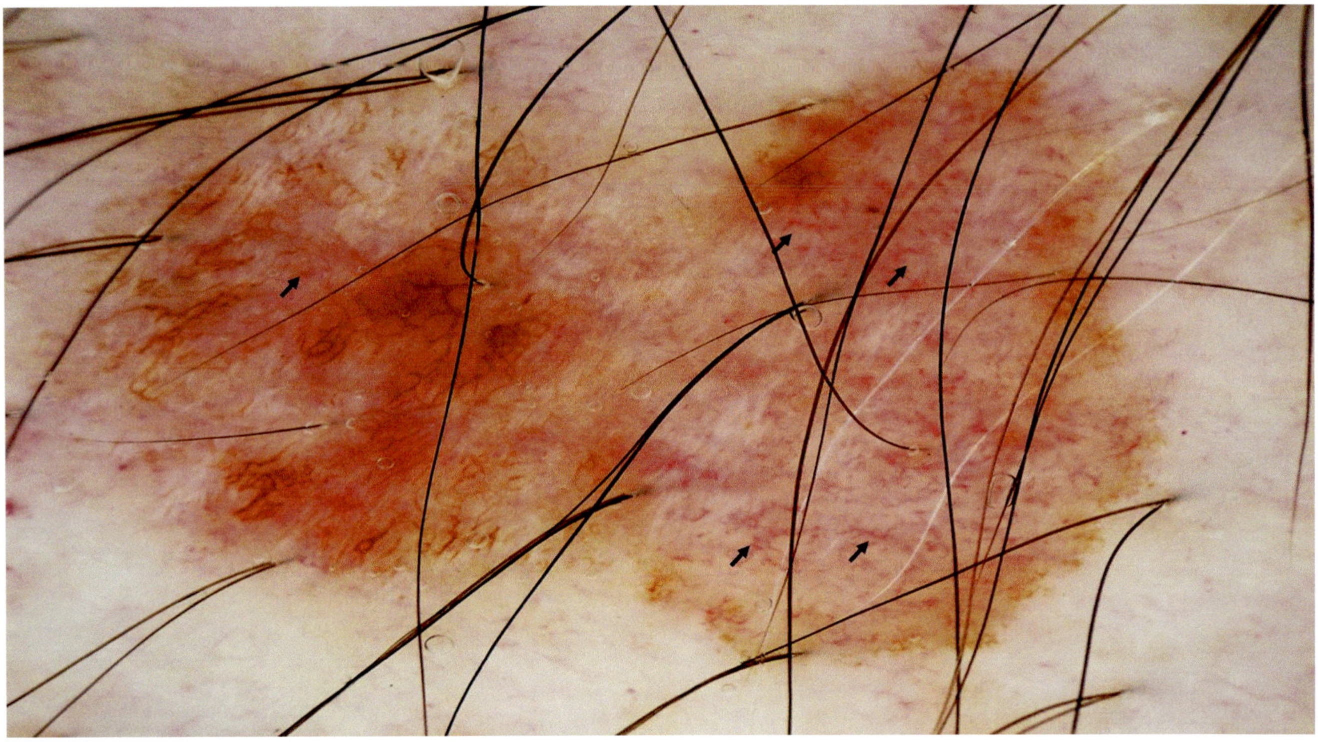

Fig. 16 Irregular linear vessels (arrows). Hypomelanotic melanoma

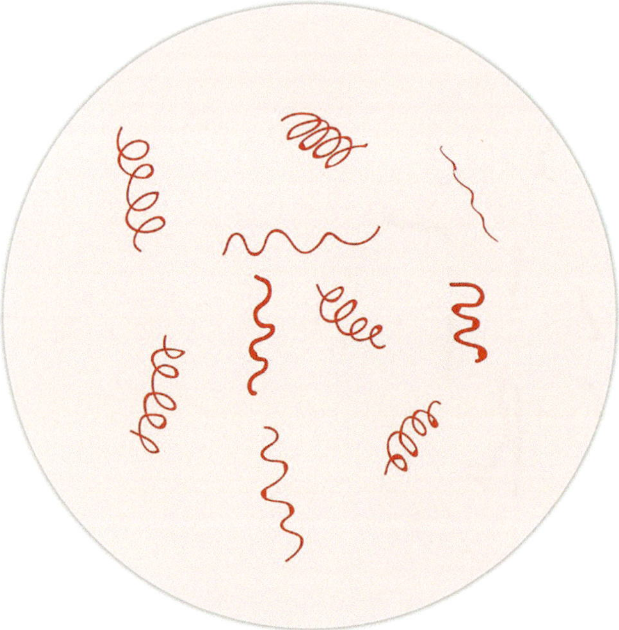

Fig. 17 Schematic drawing of helical or corkscrew linear vessels

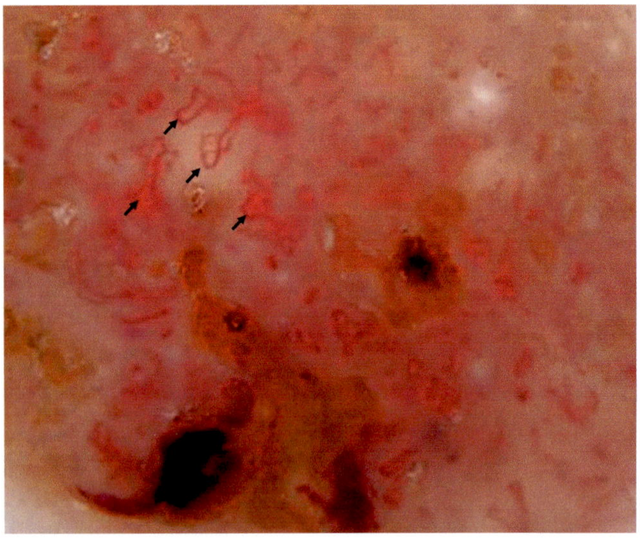

Fig. 18 Helical or corkscrew linear vessels (arrows). Squamous cell carcinoma

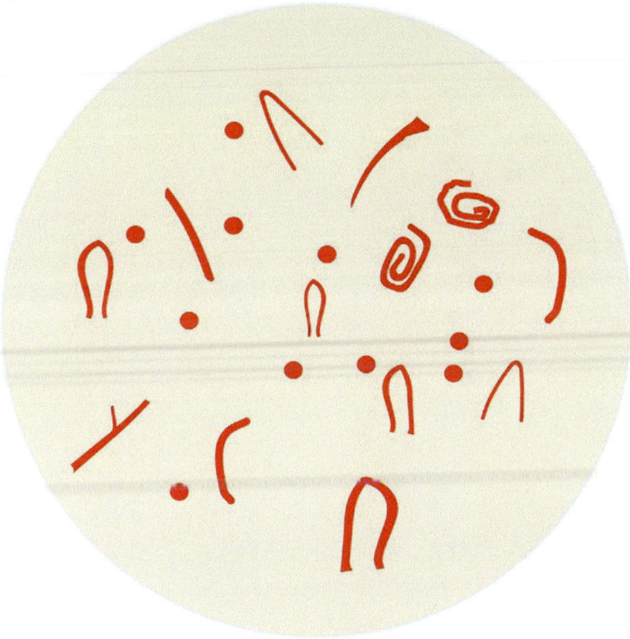

Fig. 19 Schematic drawing of randomly distributed vessels

4. Straight linear vessels: usually short and without significant curves (Figs. 9 and 10).
5. Linear hairpin vessels: they form a loop or a handle (Figs. 11 and 12).
6. Curved or comma-shaped vessels: short, curved vessels with a thicker end (Figs. 13 and 14).
7. Irregular linear vessels: they are short and of variable shape and caliber (Figs. 15 and 16).
8. Helical or corkscrew linear vessels: twisted vessels around themselves in the shape of a corkscrew (Figs. 17 and 18).

Generally, the vascular pattern is characterized monomorphic or polymorphic depending on the presence of only one type of vessels or more than one type of vessels.

B. ***Distribution of vessels***

There are eight possible distributions, one is random, and seven have a specific pattern.

- **Randomly distributed**: it is the most frequent, the vessels are distributed without any specific pattern (Figs. 19 and 20).
- **Specific patterns distribution**

1. In clusters or aggregates: vessels are grouped in some areas of the lesion (Figs. 21, 22 and 23).
2. Serpiginous or pearl necklace: punctate or glomerular vessels distributed in curved lines resembling a necklace or rosary (Figs. 24 and 25).

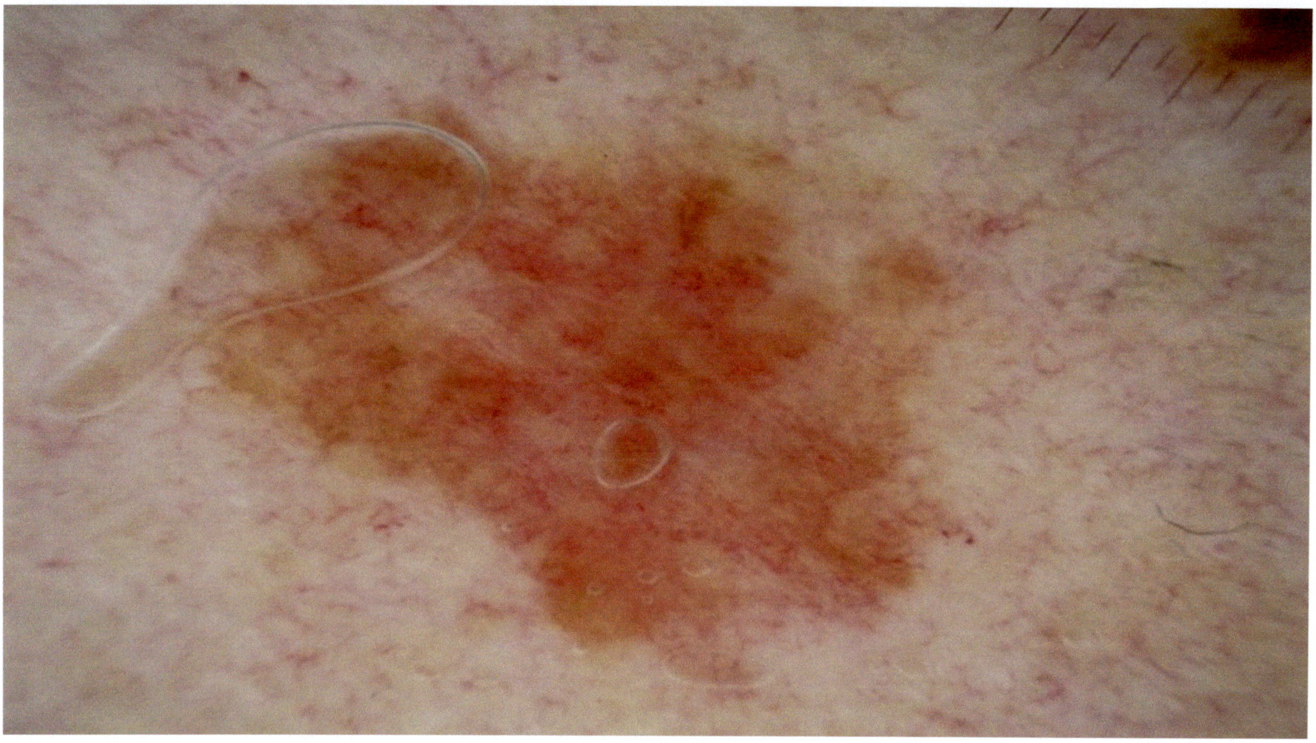

Fig. 20 Randomly distributed vessels. Hypomelanotic melanoma

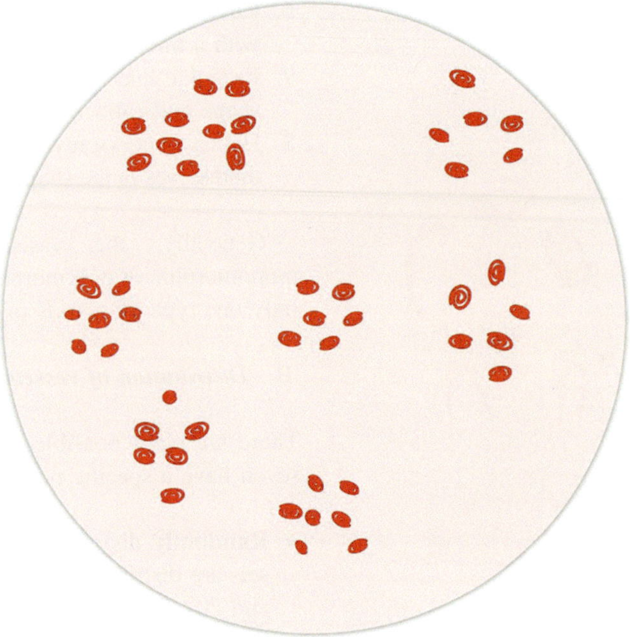

Fig. 21 Schematic drawing of vessels in cluster or aggregates

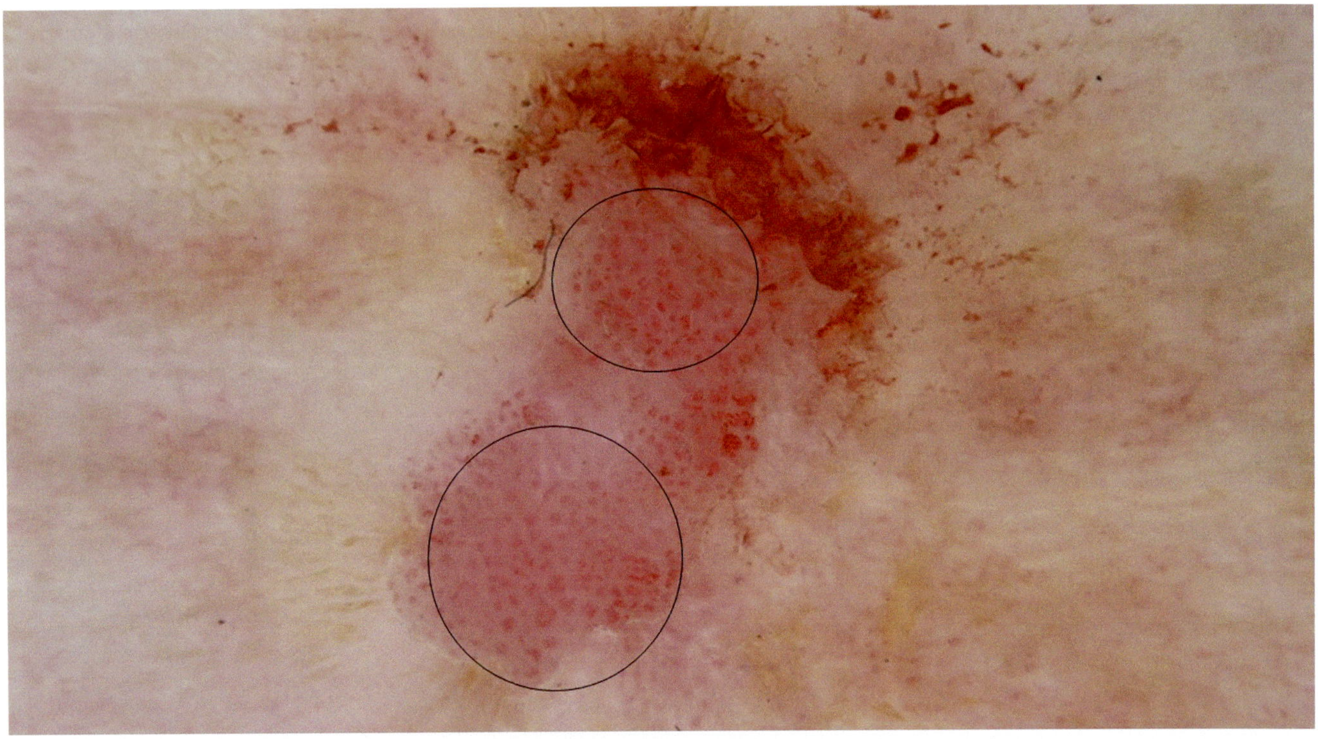

Fig.22 Vessels in cluster or aggregates (black circle). Bowen' disease

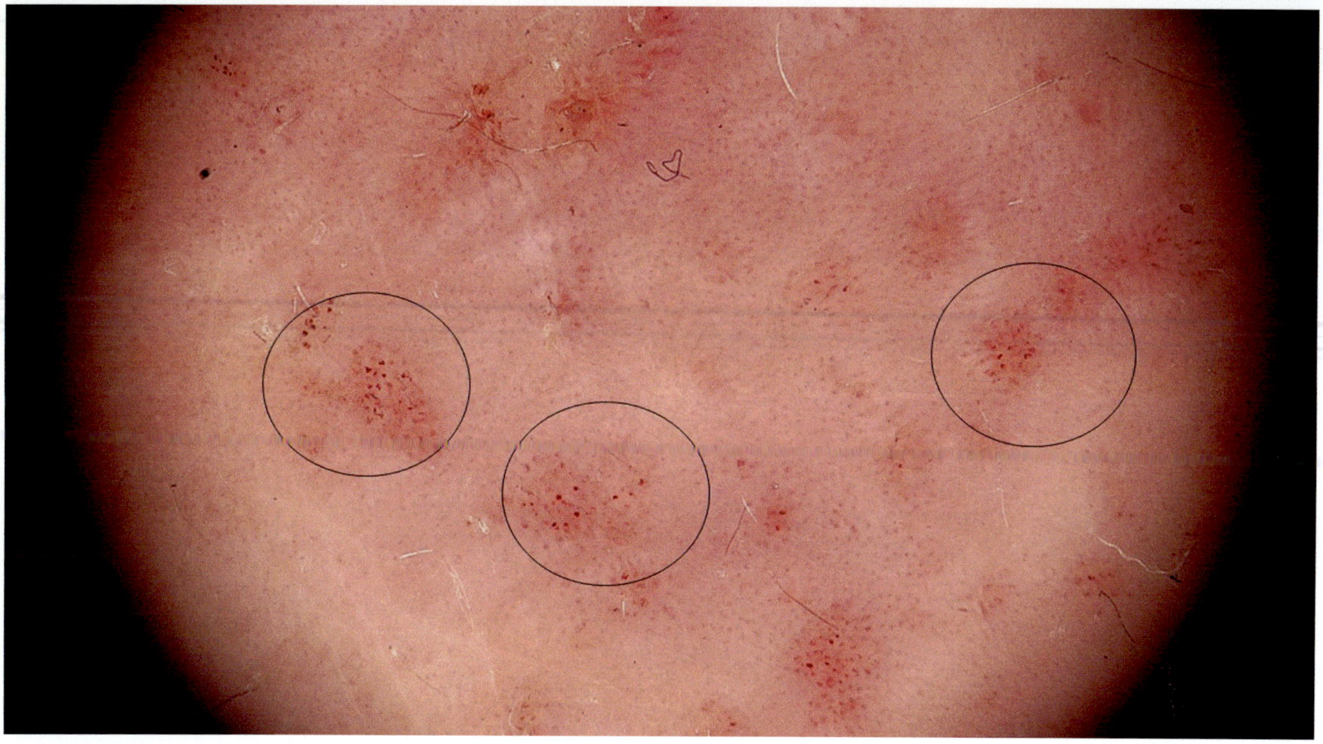

Fig. 23 Vessels in cluster or aggregates (black circle). Dermatitis

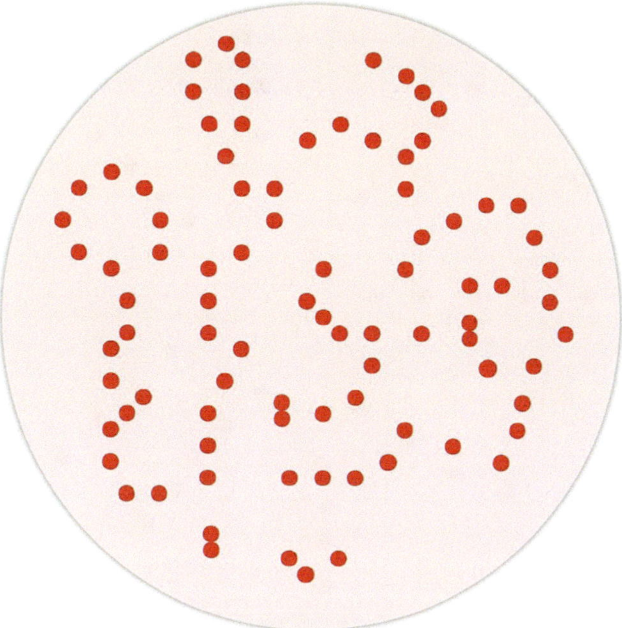

Fig. 24 Schematic drawing of vessels in serpiginous or pearl necklace distribution

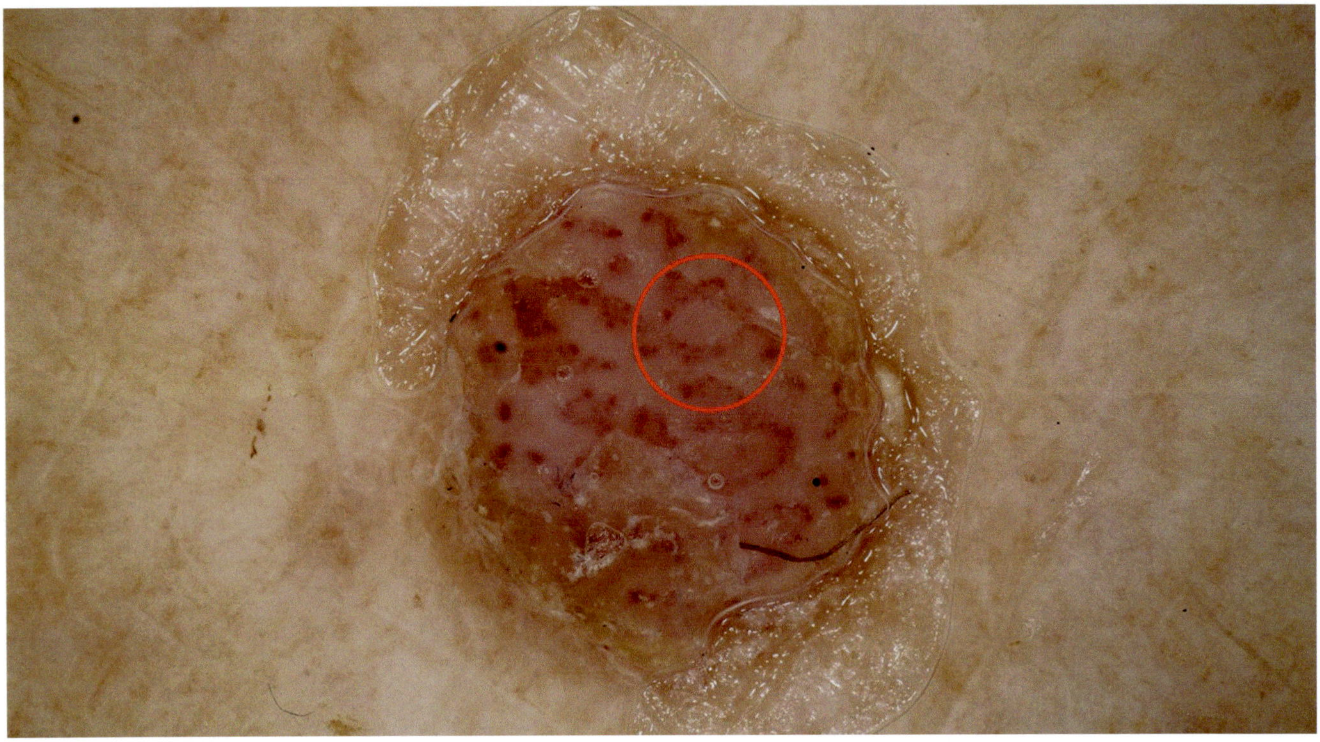

Fig. 25 Vessels in serpiginous or pearl necklace distribution (red circle). Clear cell acanthoma

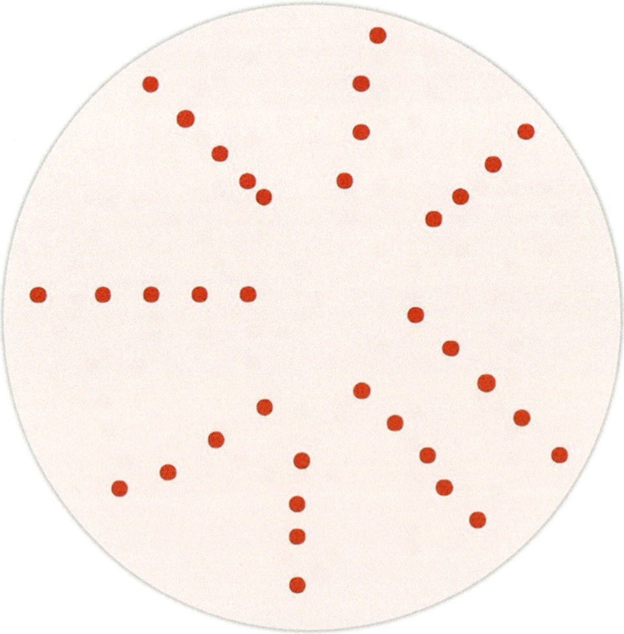

Fig. 26 Schematic drawing of vessels in line

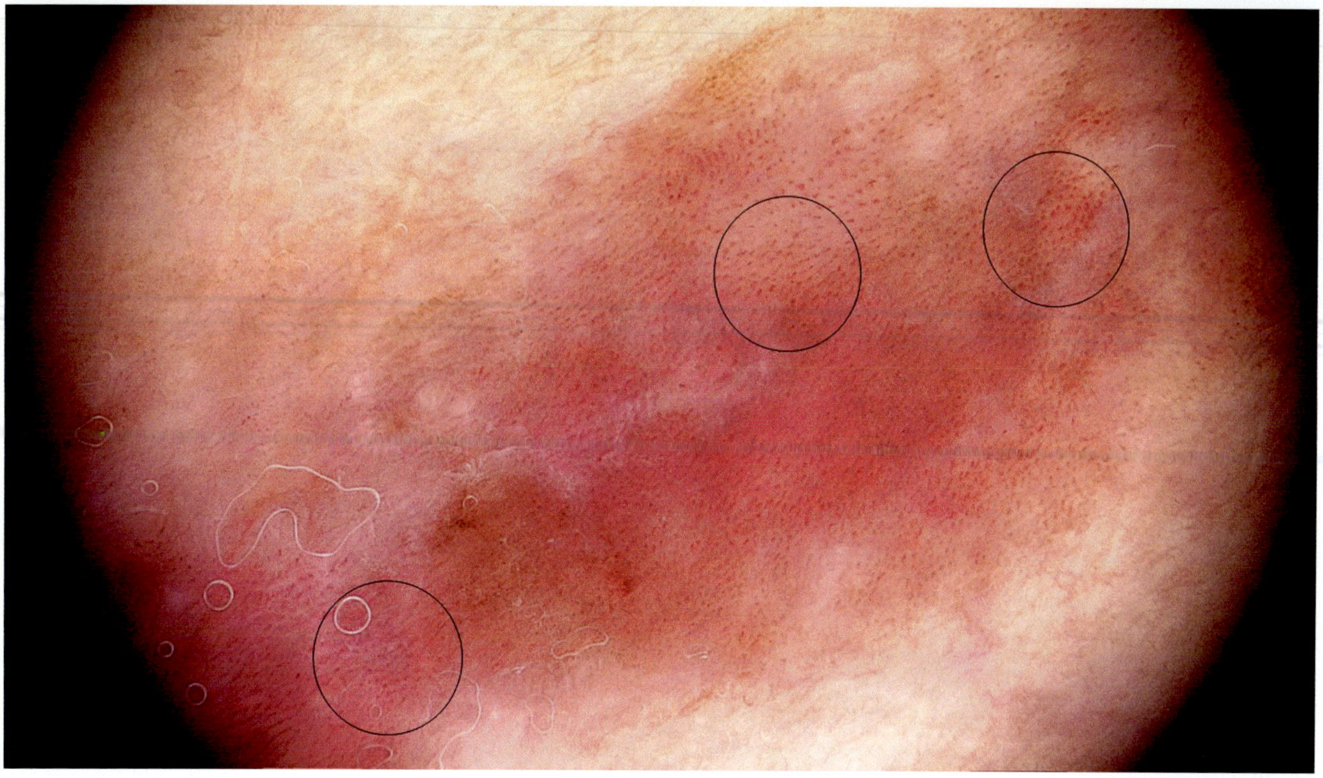

Fig. 27 Vessels in line (black circle). Squamous cell Carcinoma in situ

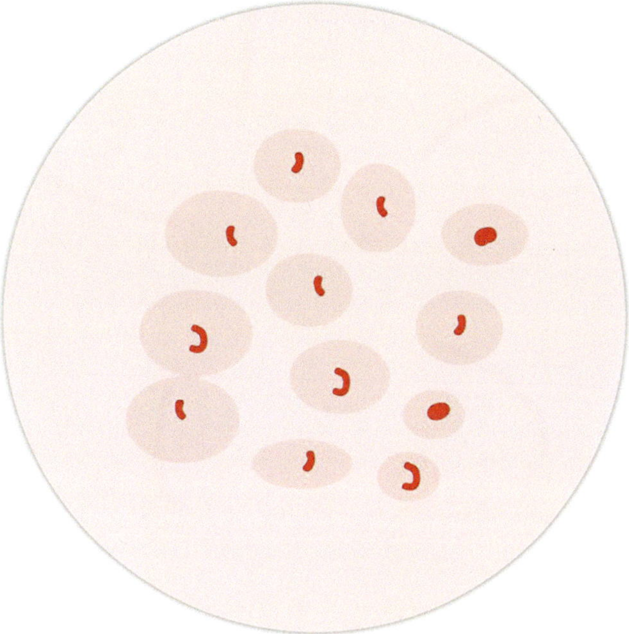

Fig. 28 Schematic drawing of centered vessels

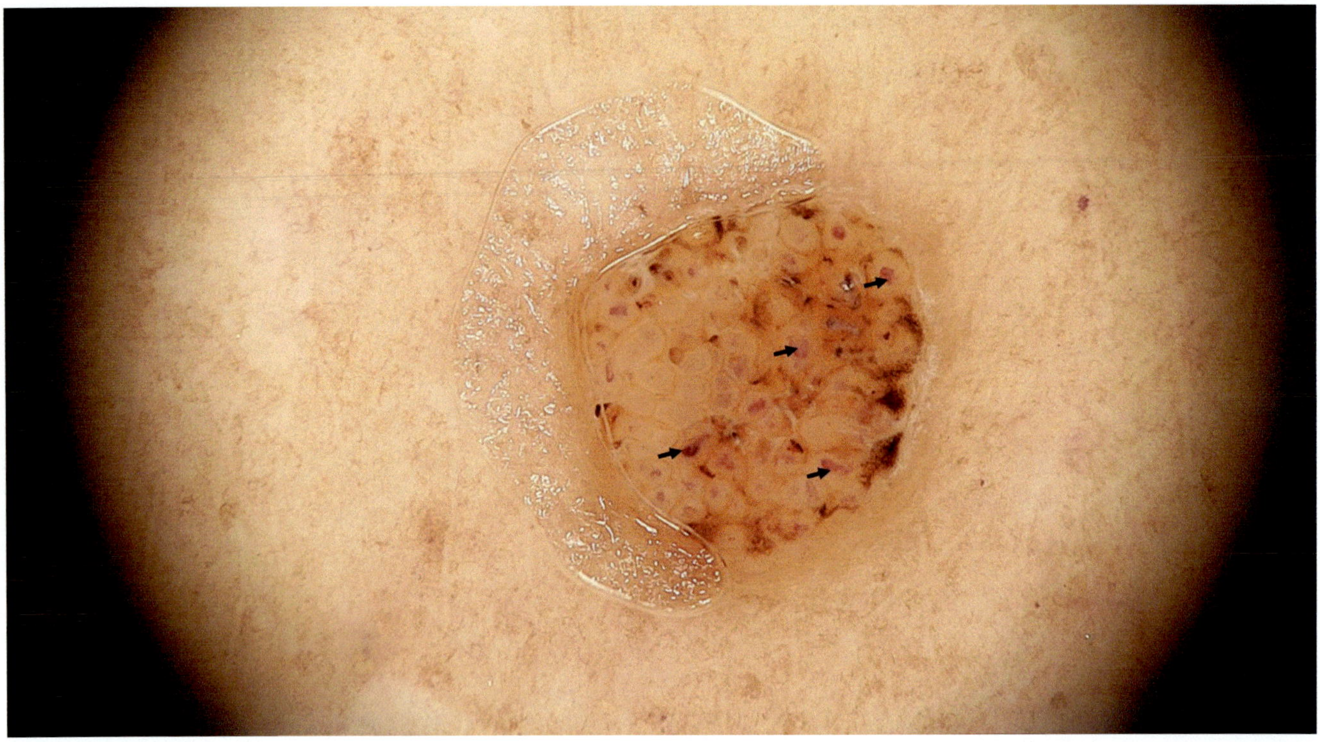

Fig. 29 Centered vessels (arrows). Intradermal nevus

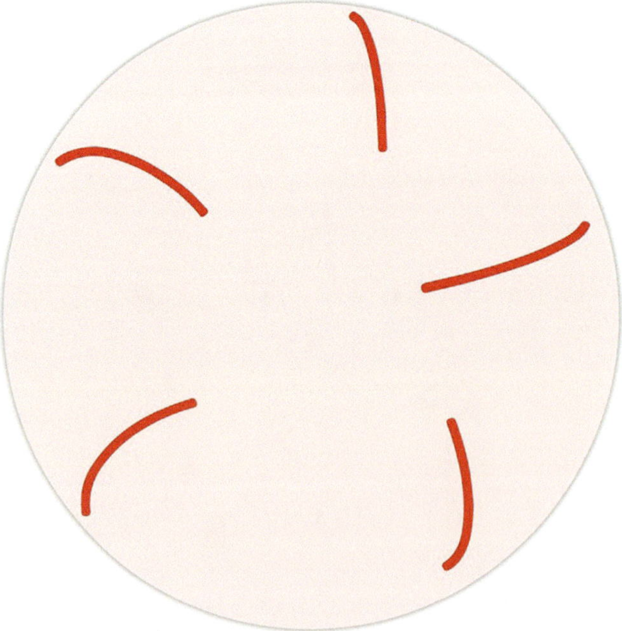

Fig. 30 Schematic drawing of radial vessels

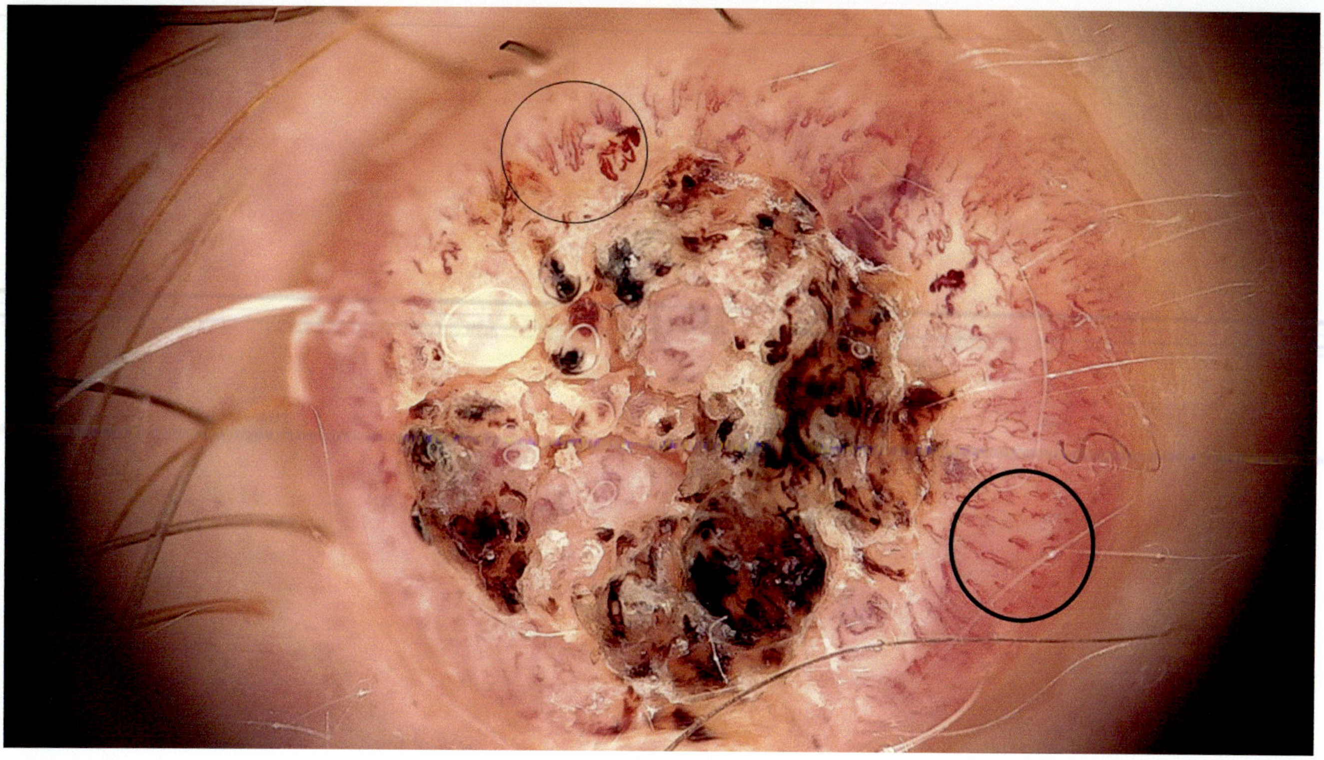

Fig. 31 Radial vessels (black circle). Squamous cell carcinoma

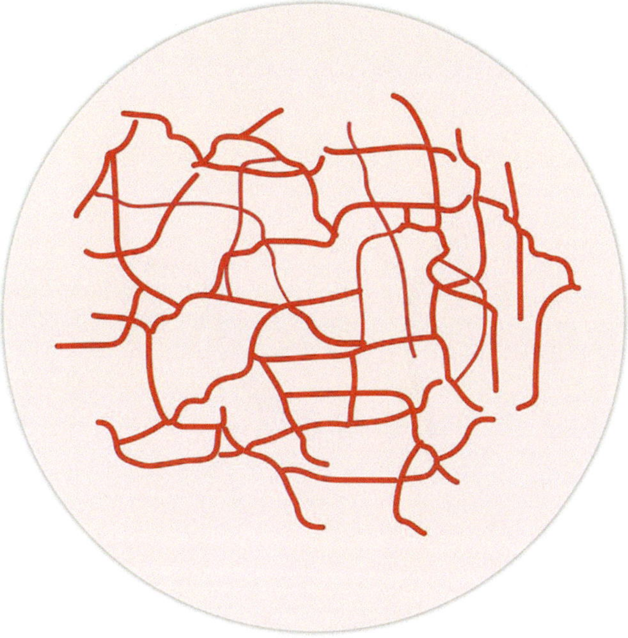

Fig. 32 Schematic drawing of reticular vessels

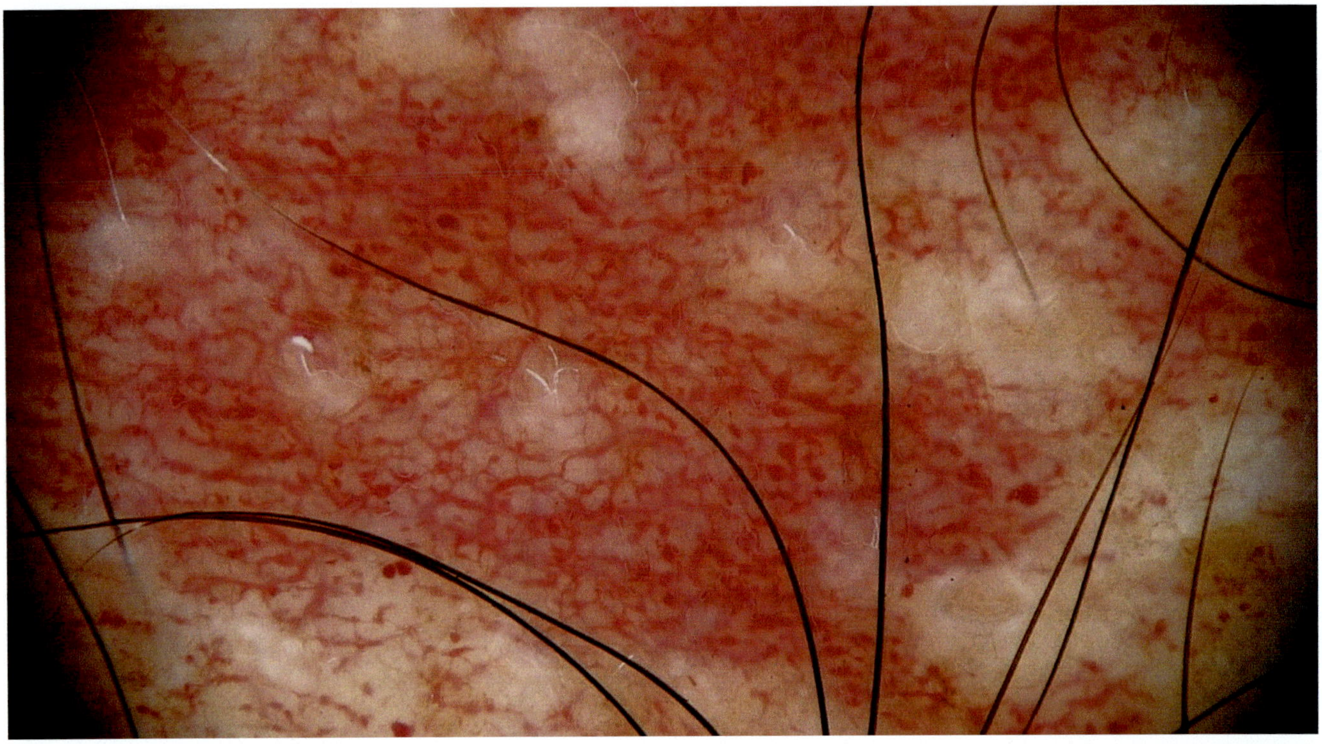

Fig. 33 Reticular vessels on sun damage skin

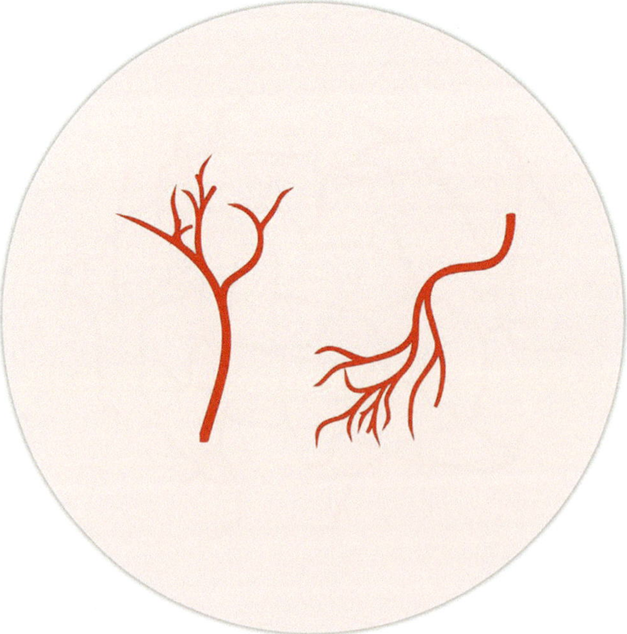

Fig. 34 Schematic drawing of branched or arboriform vessels

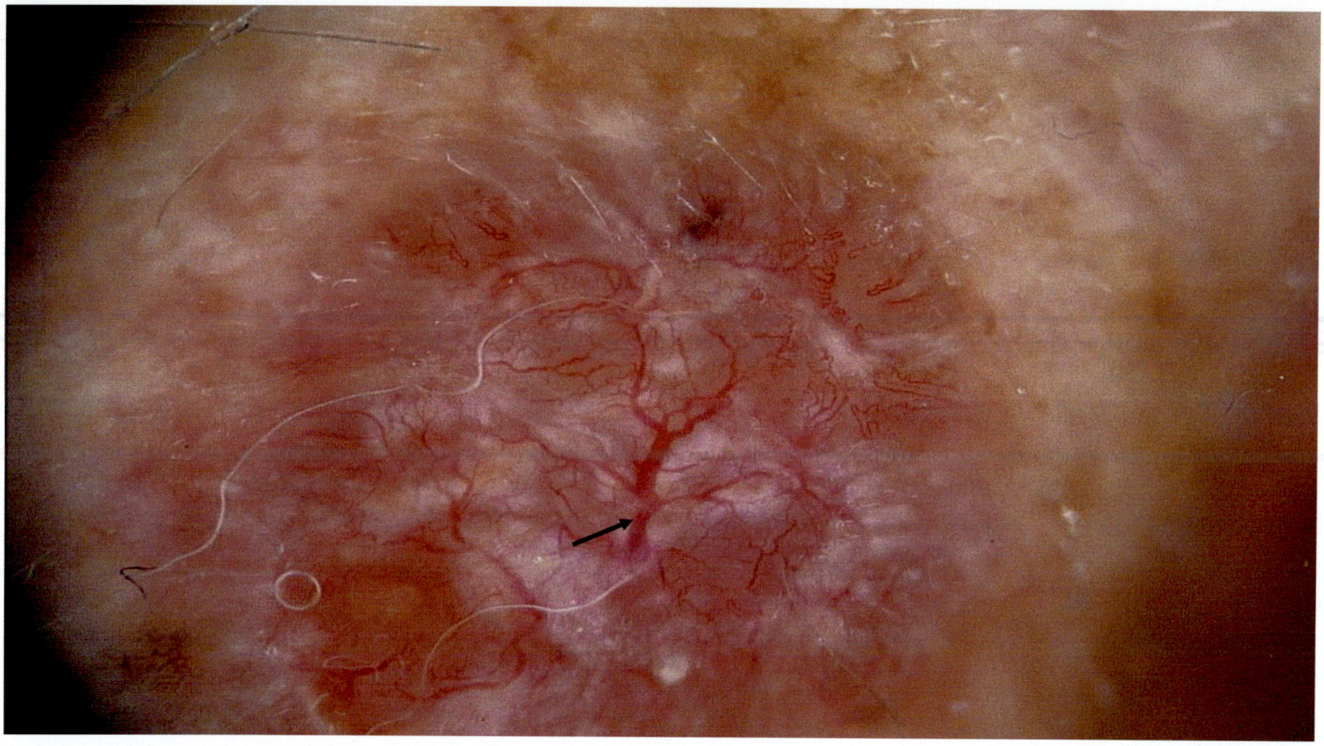

Fig. 35 Arboriform vessels (arrow). Basal cell carcinoma

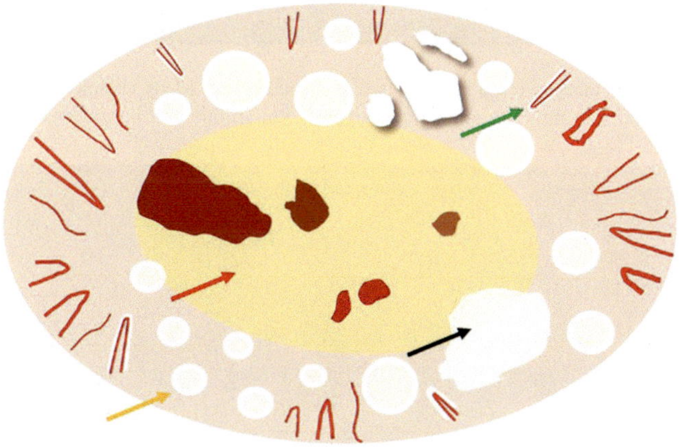

Fig. 36 Schematic drawing of Keratinization Clues**:** white keratin masses (red arrow); white structureless areas (black arrow); white circles surrounding follicular openings (yellow arrow) and white halos surrounding vessels (green arrow)

3. In line: dotted or coiled vessels that follow a linear course, usually at the periphery (Figs. 26 and 27).
4. Centered: vessels distributed in the center of lighter roundish structures (Figs. 28 and 29).
5. Radial: vessels distributed from the periphery to the center of the lesion, but do not cross the center (Figs. 30 and 31).
6. Reticular: fine linear vessels that intersect giving an appearance similar to a network (Figs. 32 and 33).
7. Branched or arboriform: thick linear vessels that branch into thinner, telangiectatic vessels (Figs. 34 and 35).

2. ***White structures***: There are mainly 3 categories of white-colored structures: those associated with keratinization, white or negative network and white shiny structures. The first two can be seen with both light modes, while white shiny structures are visible only with polarized light.

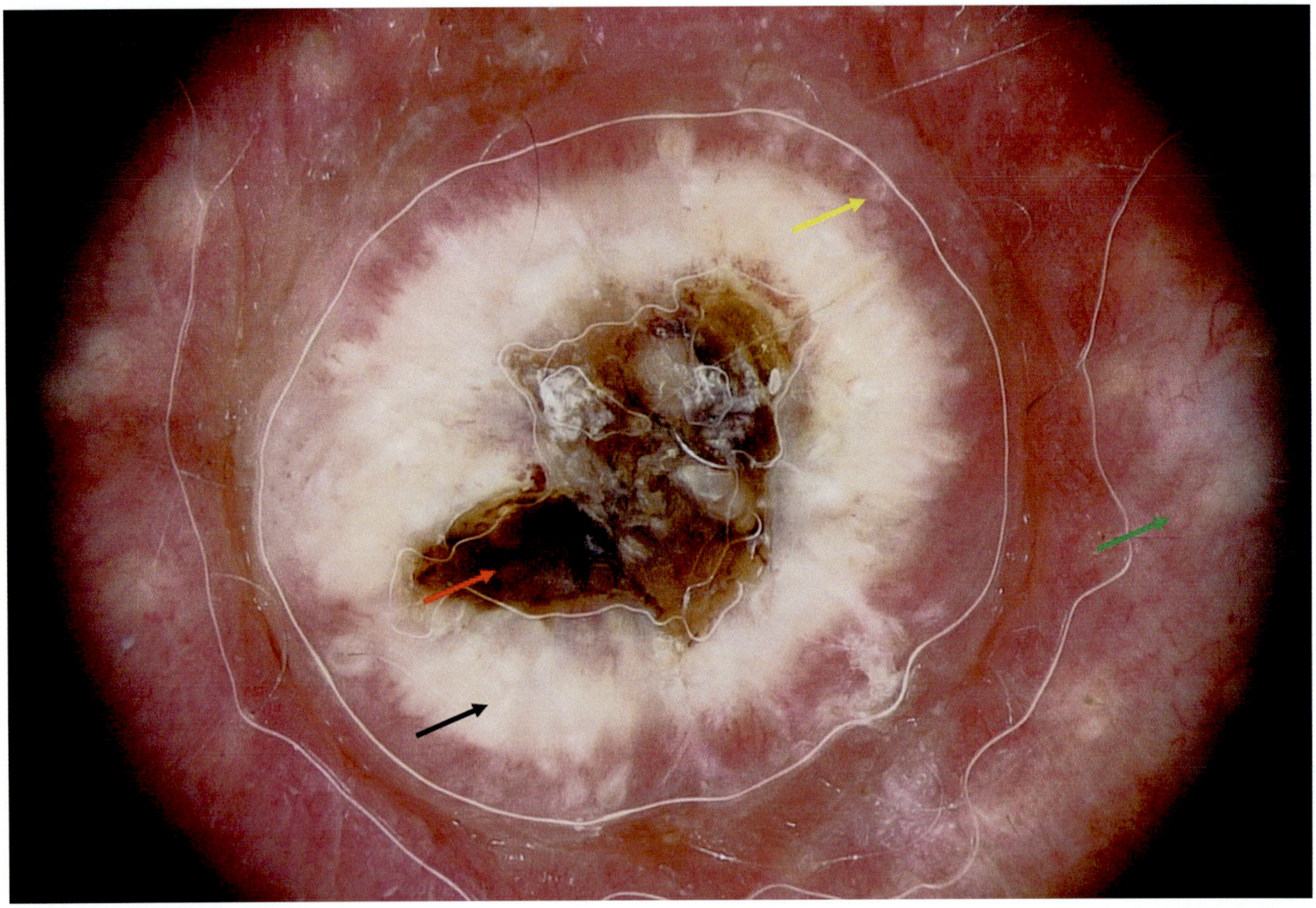

Fig. 37 Keratinization Clues: white keratin masses (red arrow); white structureless areas (black arrow); white circles surrounding follicular openings (yellow arrow) and white halos surrounding vessels (green arrow). Squamous cell carcinoma

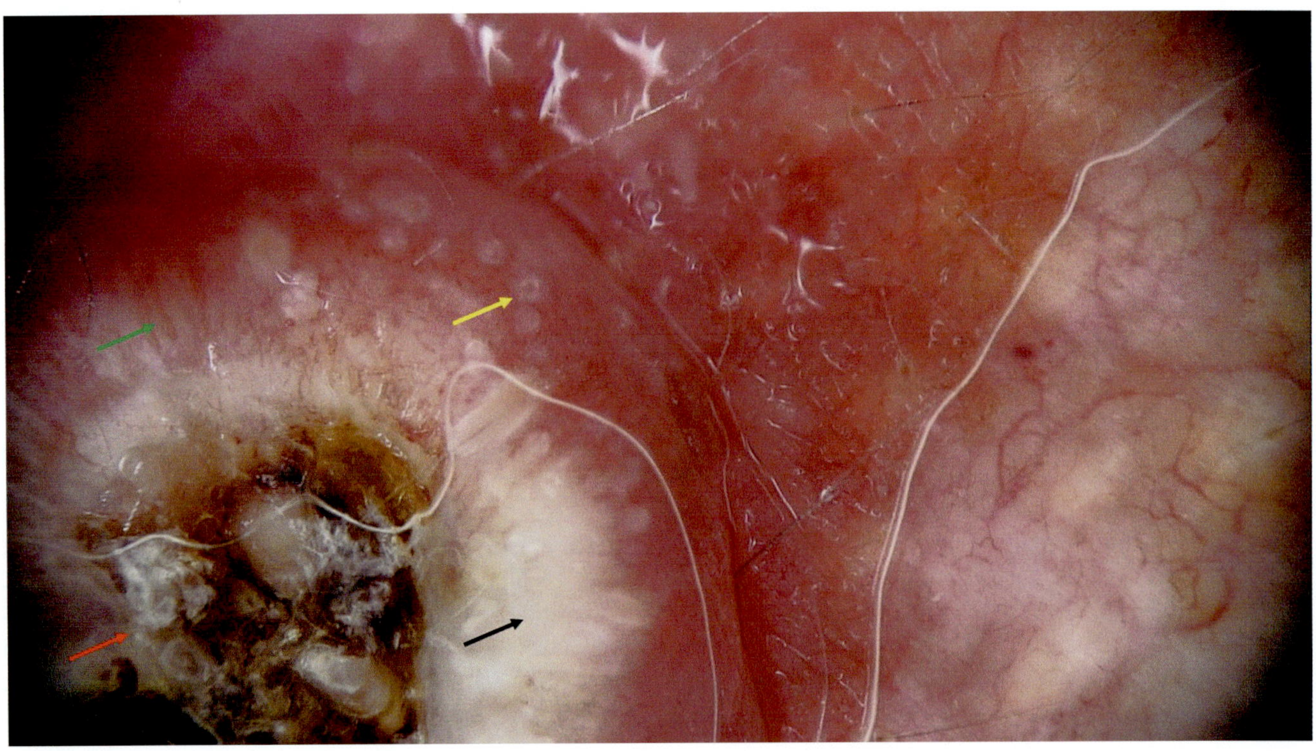

Fig. 38 Keratinization Clues: white keratin masses (red arrow); white structureless areas (black arrow); white circles surrounding follicular openings (yellow arrow) and white halos surrounding vessels (green arrow). Squamous cell carcinoma

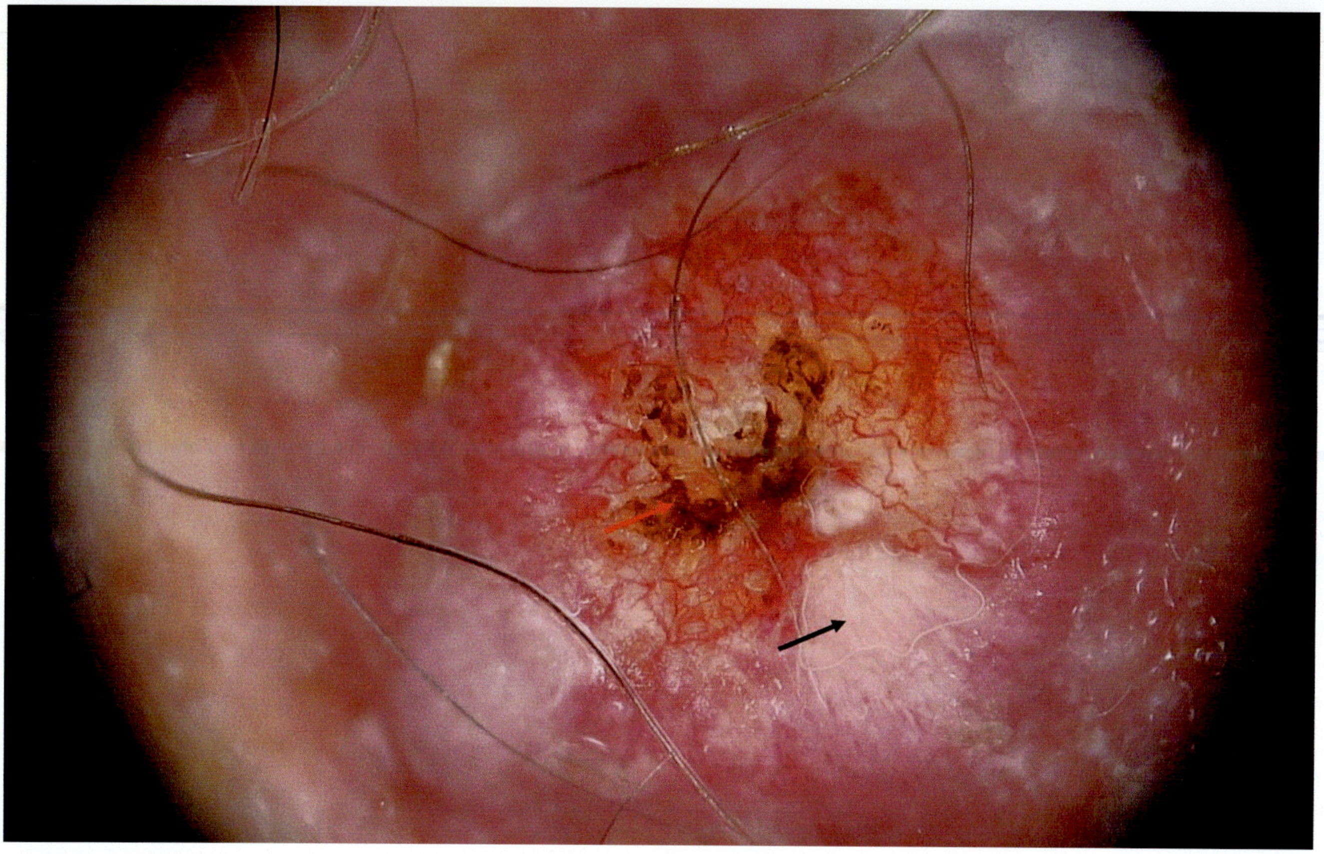

Fig. 39 Keratinization Clues**:** white keratin masses (red arrow); white structureless areas (black arrow); Squamous cell carcinoma

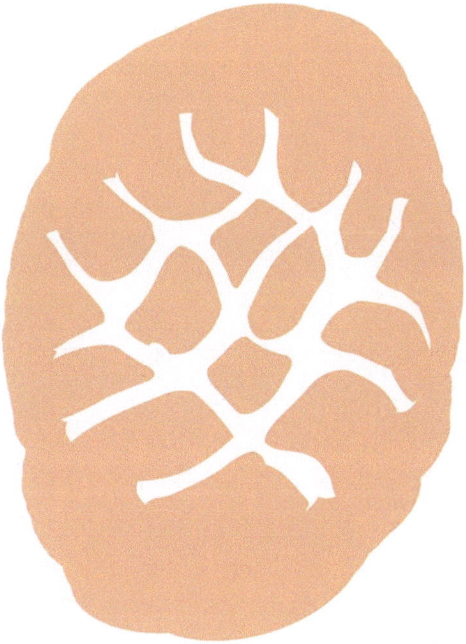

Fig. 40 Schematic drawing of white or negative network

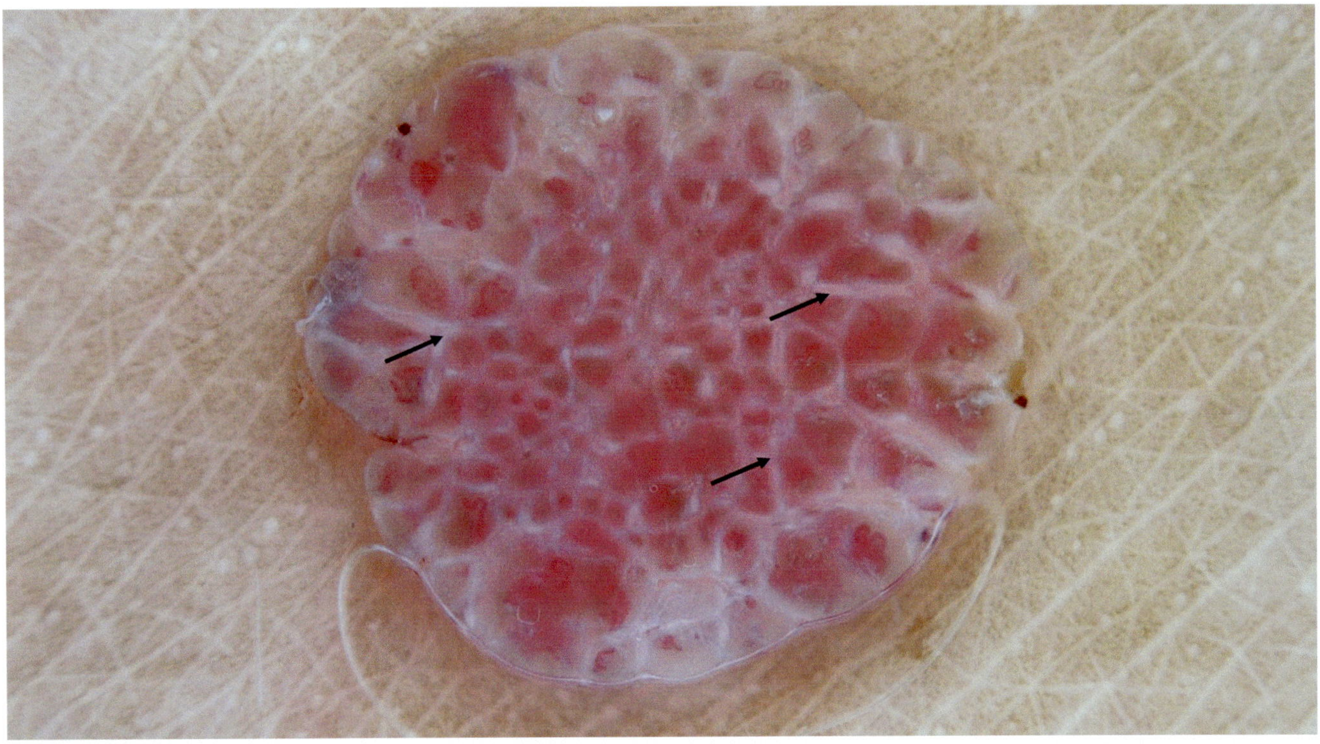

Fig. 41 White or negative network (arrows). Spitz's Nevus

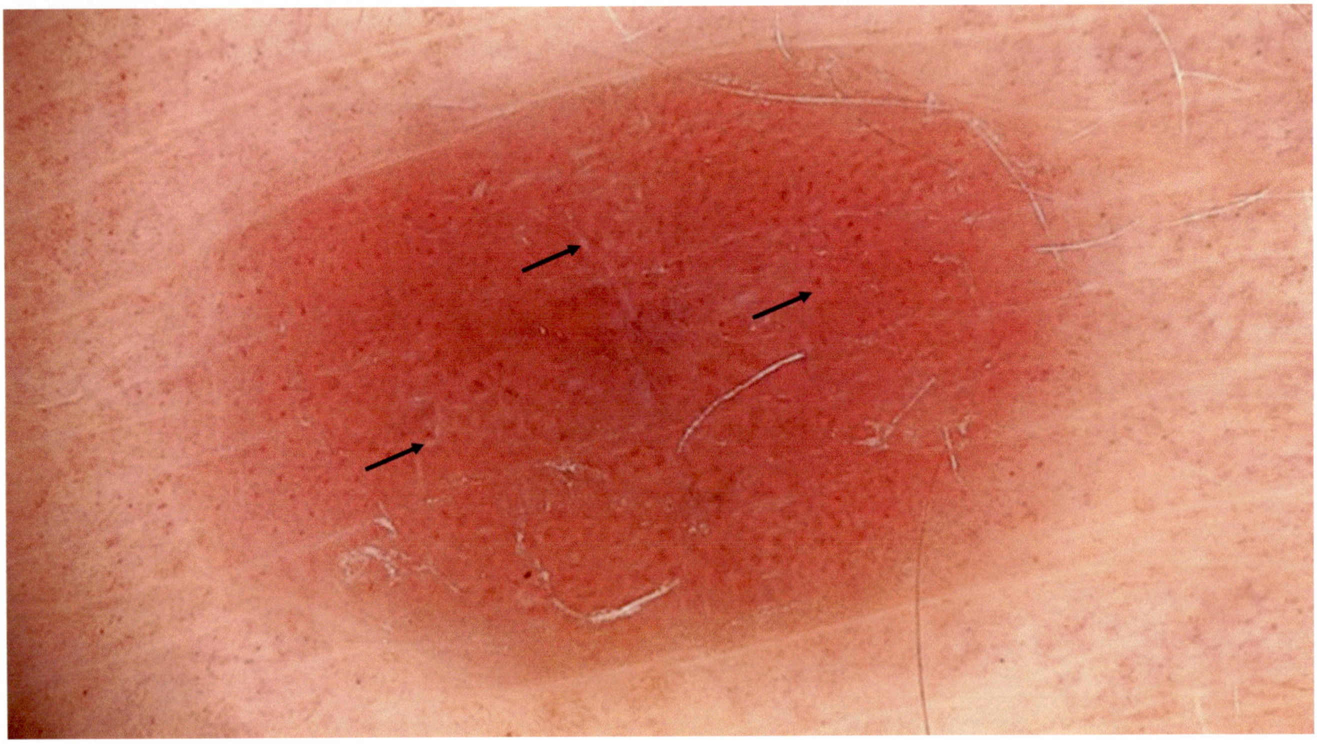

Fig. 42 White or negative network (arrows). Spitz's Nevus

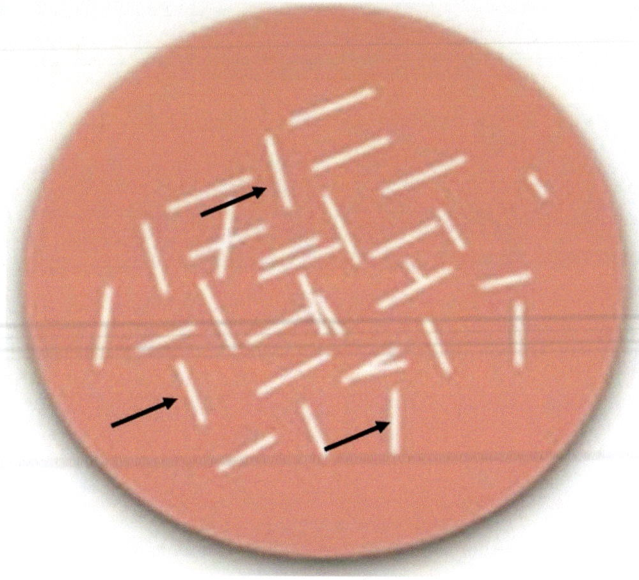

Fig. 43 Schematic drawing of white shiny structures (arrows)

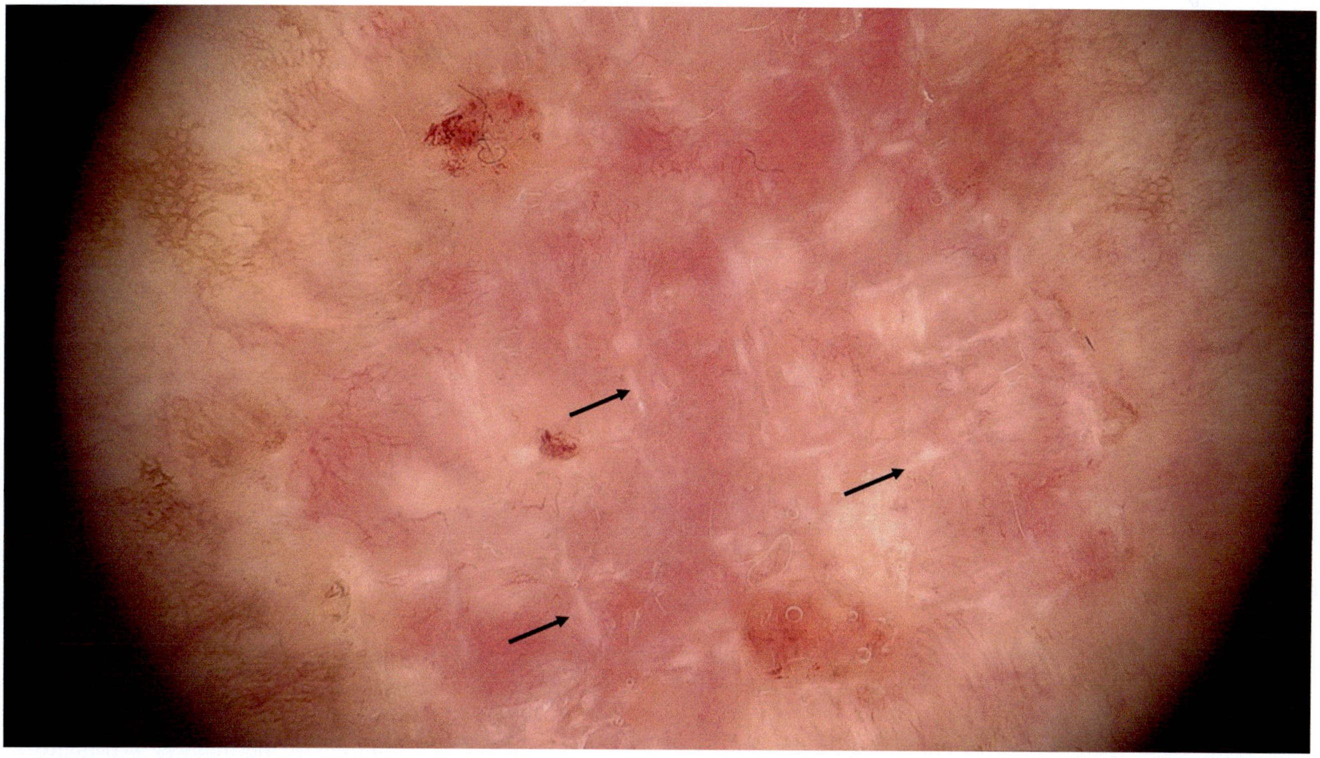

Fig. 44 White shiny structures (arrows). Basal cell carcinoma

- **Keratinization Clues:** (usually on raised lesions) are the white keratin masses, white structureless areas corresponding to epidermal hyperplasia, white circles surrounding follicular openings and white halos surrounding vessels (Figs. 36, 37, 38 and 39).
- **White or negative network:** consists of reticular white lines and can be seen mainly in spitzoid tumors but also in some inflammatory diseases (Figs. 40, 41 and 42).

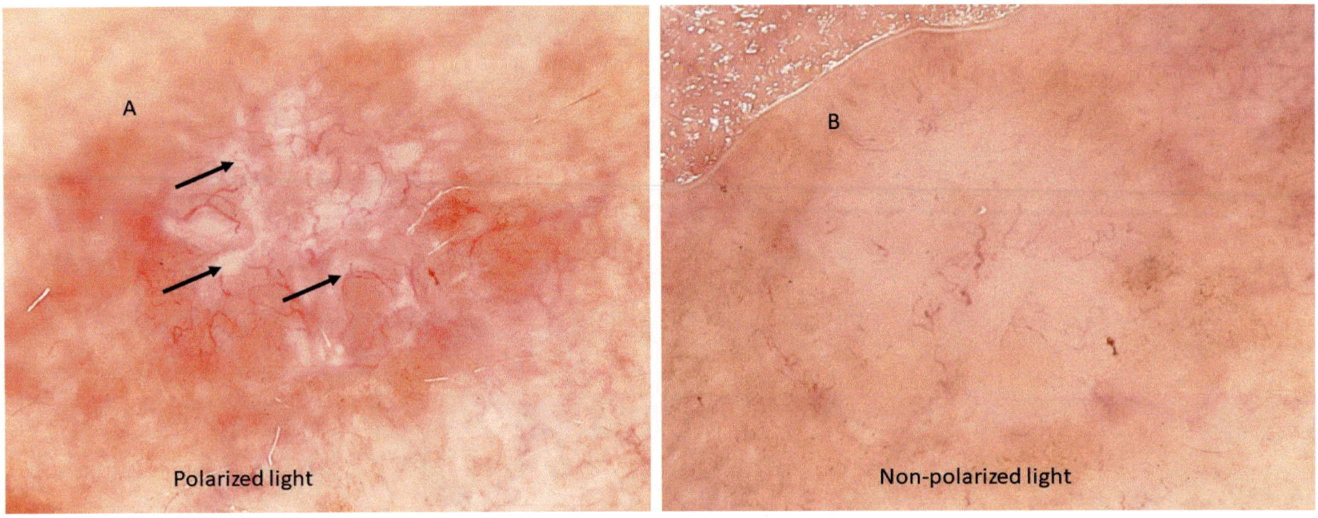

Fig. 45 A: imagen taken with polarized light: white shiny structures (arrows). B: the same imagen with non-polarized light without white shiny structures. Basal cell carcinoma

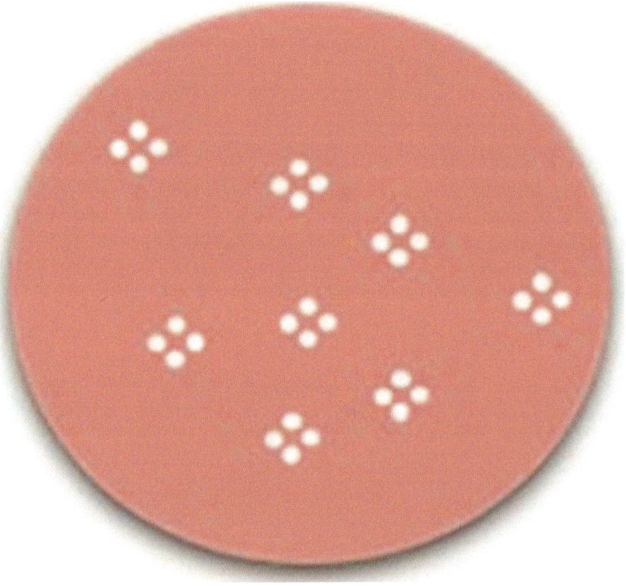

Fig. 46 Schematic drawing of rosettes

- **White shiny structures:** is a category of features seen only under polarized light. They include thin lines or streaks, thick lines or strands, blotches and rosettes. Lines and strands correspond to collagen alterations (thickened collagen bundles in the dermis), and can be present in a variety of benign and malignant neoplasms (Figs. 43, 44 and 45).
  - Rosettes are four white dots located within the follicular openings, corresponding to follicular hyperkeratosis and maybe seen in actinic keratosis and some inflammatory dermatoses especially on sun exposed sites (Figs. 46 and 47).

3. ***Erosions—Ulcerations***

They frequently appear along with the previously described structures, and their presence forces us to rule out malignancy (Figs. 48 and 49).

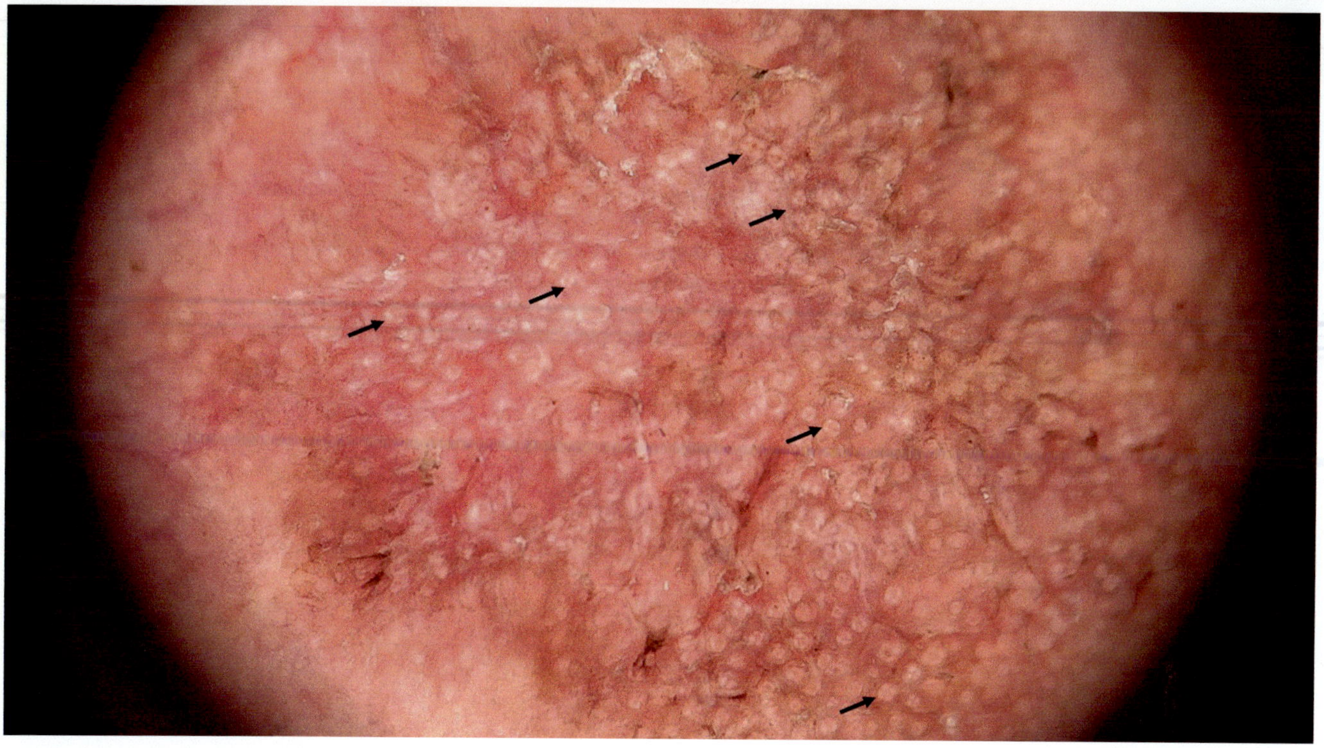

Fig. 47 Rosettes (arrows). Actinic Keratosis

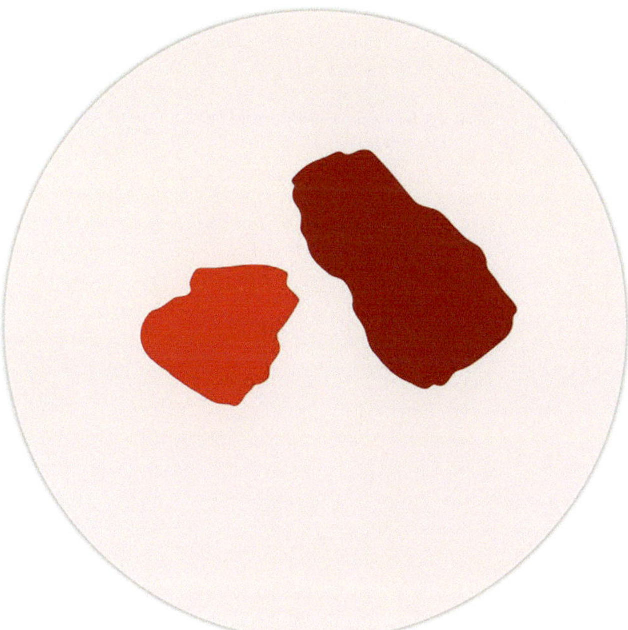

Fig. 48 Schematic drawing of erosion/ulceration

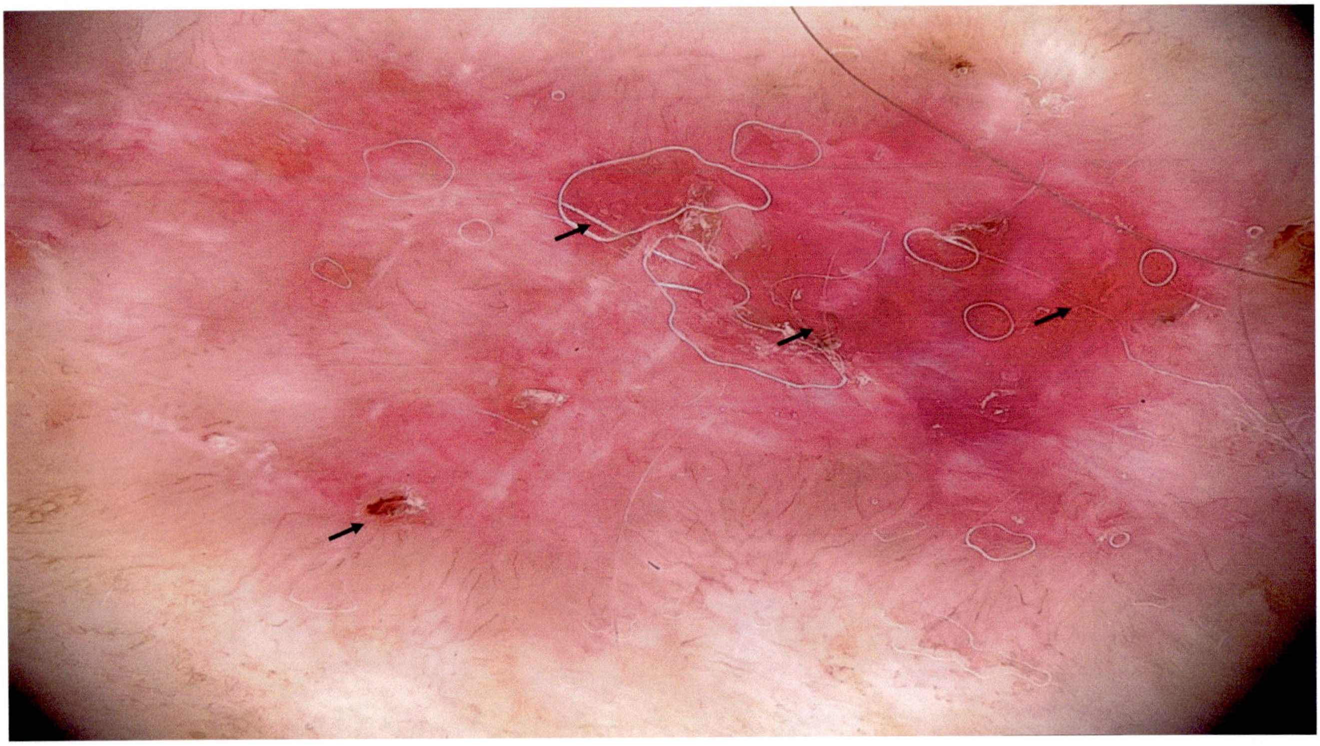

Fig. 49 Multiple erosion (arrows). Basal cell carcinoma

Standardization of Dermoscopic Terminology and Basic Parameters to Evaluate in General Dermatology

Horacio Cabo, Emilia Noemi Cohen Sabban, and Aimilios Lallas

Abstract

In general dermatology five parameters should be assessed when evaluating inflammatory and infectious diseases on dermoscopy: 1-Vessels: morphology and distribution 2-Scales: colours and distribution 3-Follicular abnormalities 4-Other structures (i.e. nonscaling, nonvascular and nonfollicular findings): colour and morphology 5-Specific features or clues.

Keywords

Inflamatoscopy • Scales • Different colors • Vessels distribution • Vessels morphology

During the last years dermoscopy was increasingly gaining appreciation as a supportive tool in the diagnosis of several non-neoplastic dermatological conditions, including inflammatory, infiltrative and infectious diseases.

On behalf of the International Society of Dermoscopy, in 2019 we carried out a study with the aim of standardizing the dermoscopic terminology and identify the basic parameters that should be evaluated in non-neoplastic dermatoses, through a consensus among international experts, which followed the modified Delphi method. In this chapter we will describe them.

We suggest three simple rules to take into account when you are evaluating under dermatoscopy, these non-neoplastic dermatological diseases.

Basic rule 1
Follow standard procedure for acquiering patient´s medical record: history of previous episodes and medication received, physical examination including type and number of the lesions, location, morphology, color, size, durations, etc..

Basic rule 2
Evaluation under dermoscopy will result in dermoscopic findings that should always be interpreted within the overall clinical context of the patient.

Basic rule 3
Selection of the appropriate equipment: second generation hand handle dermatoscopes, with polarized light and and without contact

Five parameters should be assessed when evaluating inflammatory and infectious diseases on dermoscopy:

1-Vessels: morphology and distribution

2-Scales: colours and distribution

3-Follicular abnormalities

4-Other structures (i.e. nonscaling, nonvascular and nonfollicular findings): colour and morphology

5-Specific features or clues

1-Vessels:

Four morphological types of vessels are described:

- Dotted: includes rounded vessels of any size, and they are the most frequent type of vessels found in inflammatory conditions
- Linear: without bends and/or ramifications
- Linear with ramifications: includes arboriform, branched and crown-shaped vessels Fig. 1

H. Cabo (✉)
Clinical Dermatology, University of Buenos Aires, Arenales 1446 1 °C (1061) CABA, Buenos Aires, Argentina
e-mail: cabohoracio@gmail.com

E. N. Cohen Sabban
Dermatology Division of the "Instituto de Investigaciones Médicas A. Lanari", University of Buenos Aires, Arenales 1446 1 ºC, Buenos Aires, Argentina

A. Lallas
First Department of Dermatology, Aristotle University, 124 Delfon Street, 54643 Thessaloniki, Greece

H. Cabo and A. Lallas (eds.), *Dermatoscopic Atlas of Non-Pigmented Lesions*,
https://doi.org/10.1007/978-3-031-34310-0_2

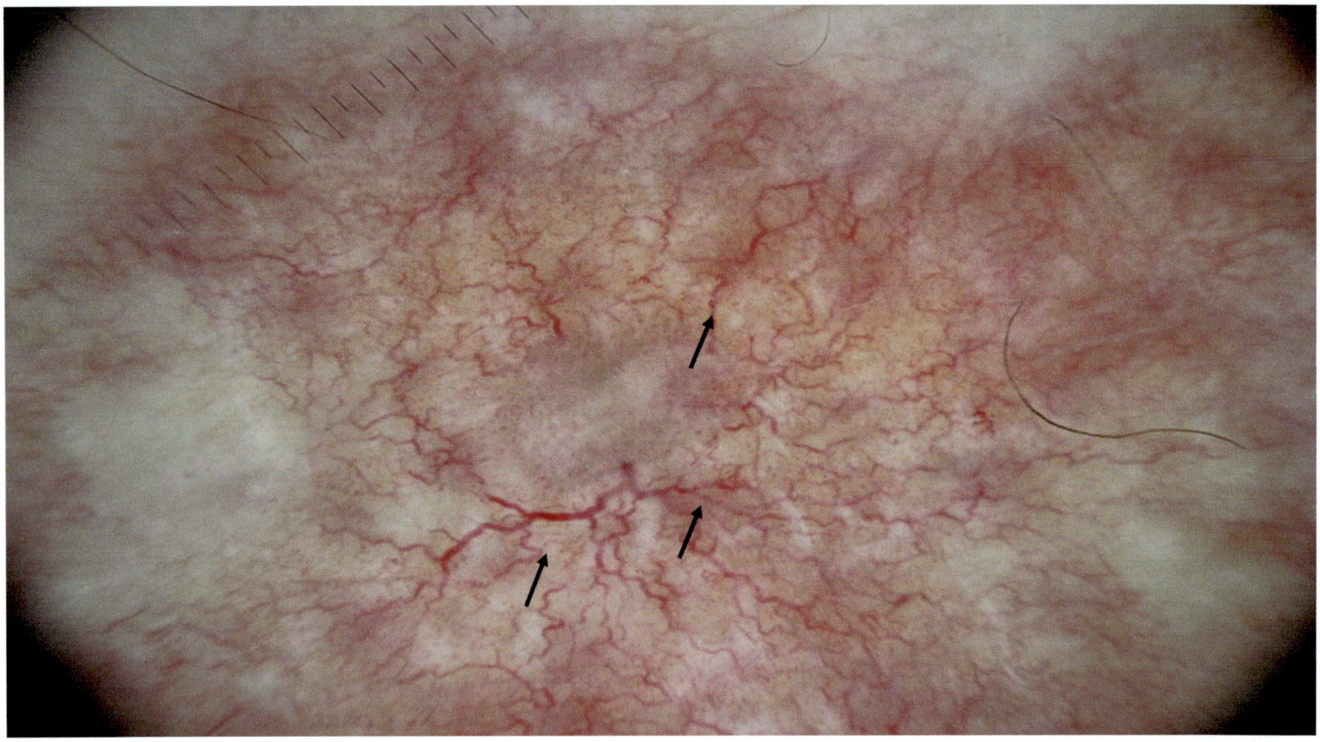

Fig. 1 Linear vessels with ramifications (arrows) Necrobiosis lipoidica diabeticorum

- Linear curved: include comma-shaped, chalice-shaped, hairpin-shaped, and linear-helical vessels

Arrangement of vascular structures

- Uniform: equal and homogeneous distribution over the entire surface of the lesion Fig. 2
- Clustered: distribution in small groups in the lesion Fig. 3
- Peripheral: they are seen at the periphery of lesions characterized by predominant epidermal changes in the central part of them.
- Reticular: form a network or mesh Fig. 4
- Nonspecific (asymmetric or patchy): the vessels are distributed randomly without following any of the other patterns

2-Scales

Colours: the three colours are specifically related to an histologic change

- White: reflect hyperkeratosis (mainly parakeratosis) without serum exudation.
- Yellow: correspond to spongiosis, and they appear as a result of exudation or serum that dries up (scab) or by mixing with keratin (scales)
- Brown: they result from the mixture of keratin with pigment, either endogenous such as melanin, or exogenous as dirt.

Distribution

- Diffuse: they are scattered on the whole surface of the lesion
- Central: in the center of the lesion
- Peripheral: they are distributed at the periphery of the lesion, sparing the centre Fig. 5
- Patchy: which means an irregular distribution of the scales (in random)

3-Follicular abnormalities

- Follicular plugs (the most frequent finding among follicular changes) are related to hypekeratosis and include follicular plugs, yellow "tears", "Demodex tails", "Demodex follicular openings", comedone-like openings, and rosettes (under polarized light) Figs. 6 and 7
- Follicular red dots: represent perifollicular inflammation Fig. 8
- Perifollicular white color: might be associated with different histological changes such as fibrosis, epidermal hyperplasia, or perifollicular depigmentation
- Perifollicular pigmentation

4-Other structures

Previously refer to "background color", is an heterogenous group of structures other than scales, vessels and/or follicular findings, that are evaluated based on their color and morphology.

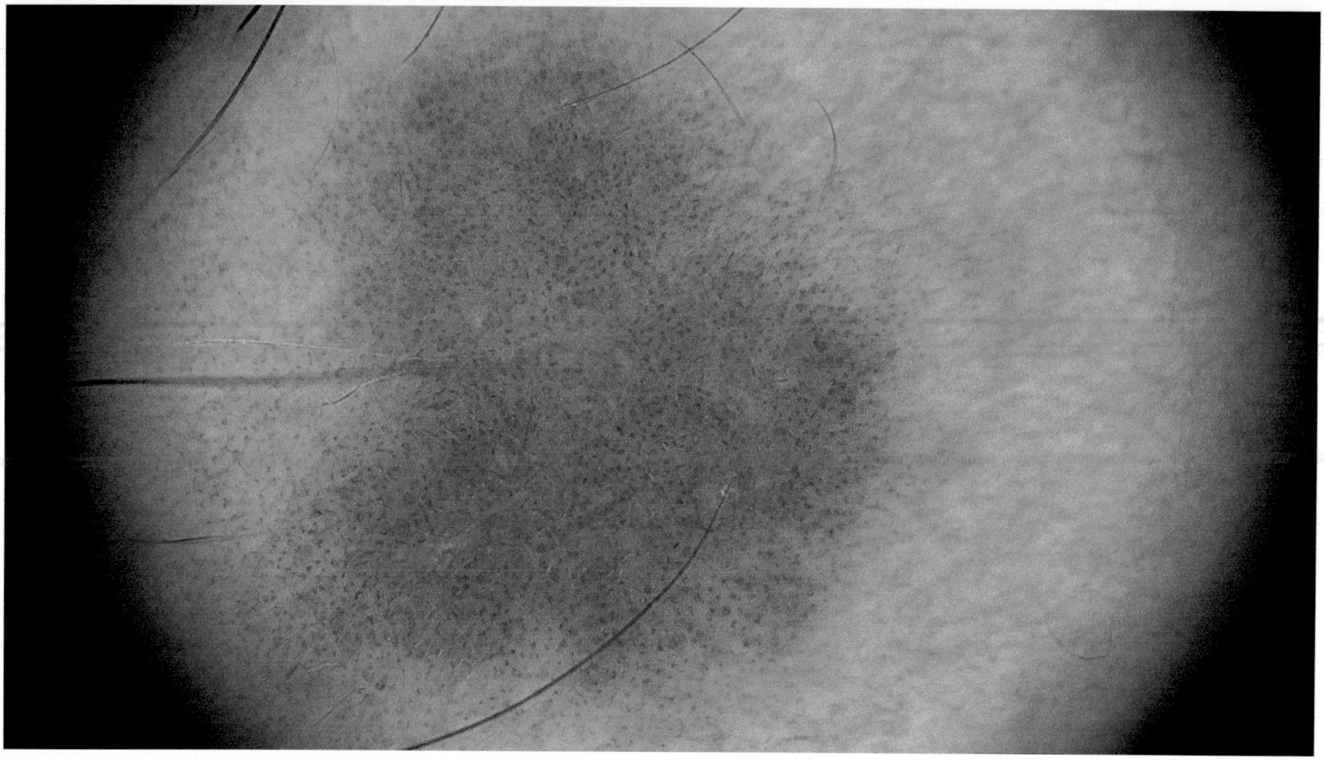

Fig. 2 Dotted vessels with uniform distribution. Psoriasis

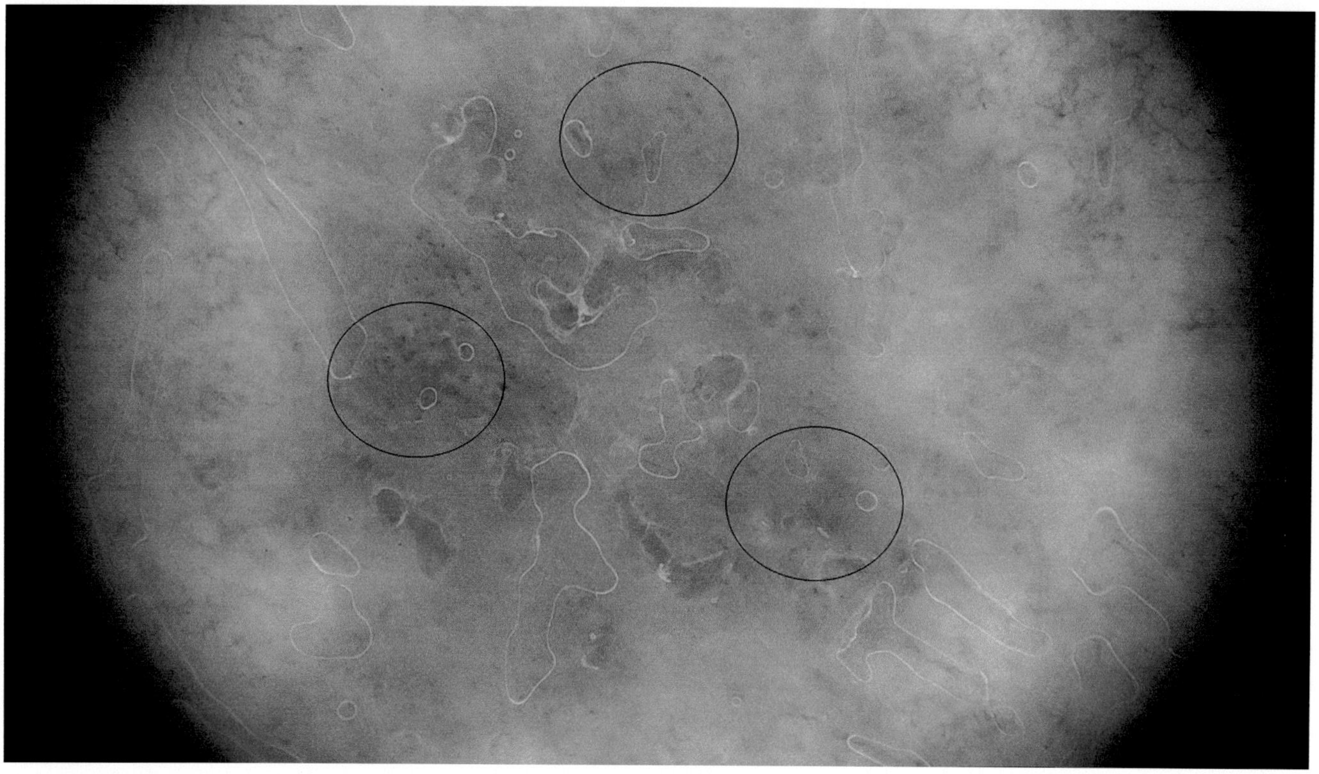

Fig. 3 Dotted vessels with focal distribution, (clustered) (black circles). Dermatitis

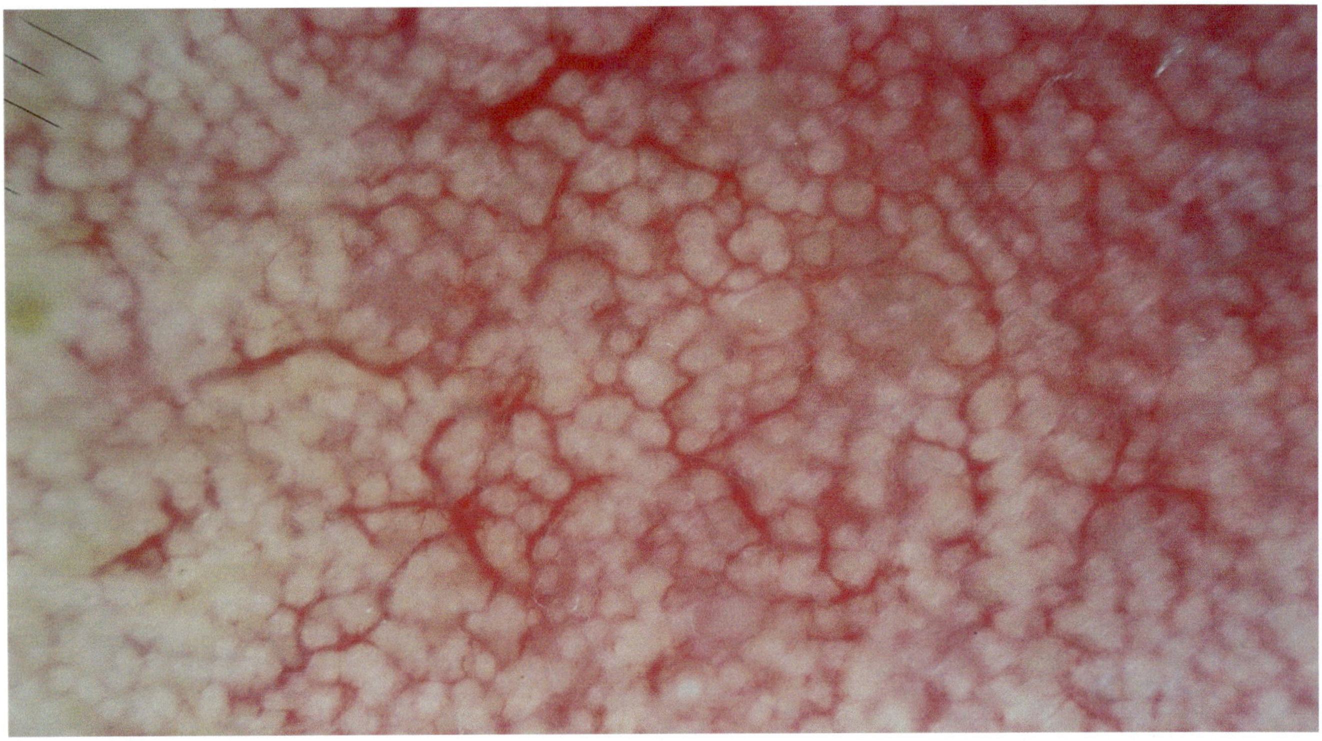

Fig. 4 Reticular arrangement of vascular structures. Rosacea

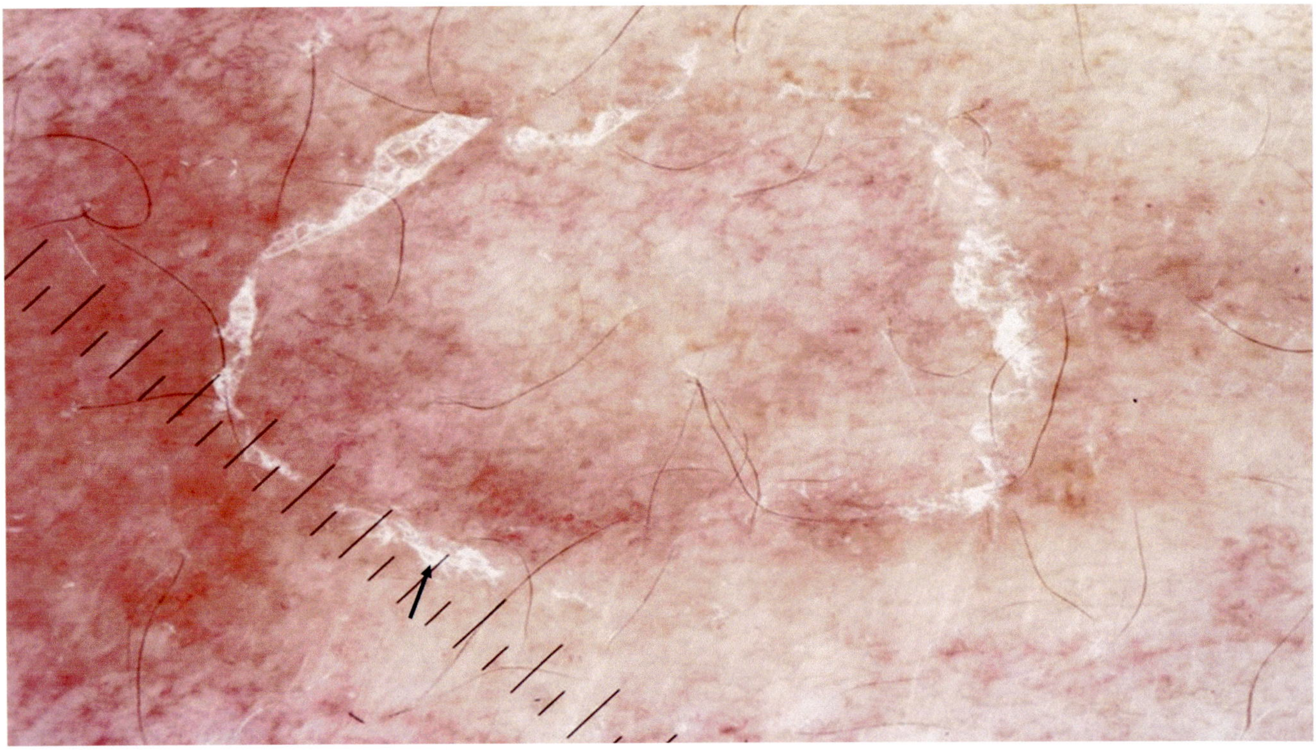

Fig. 5 White peripheral scales in Pityriasis Rosea (arrow)

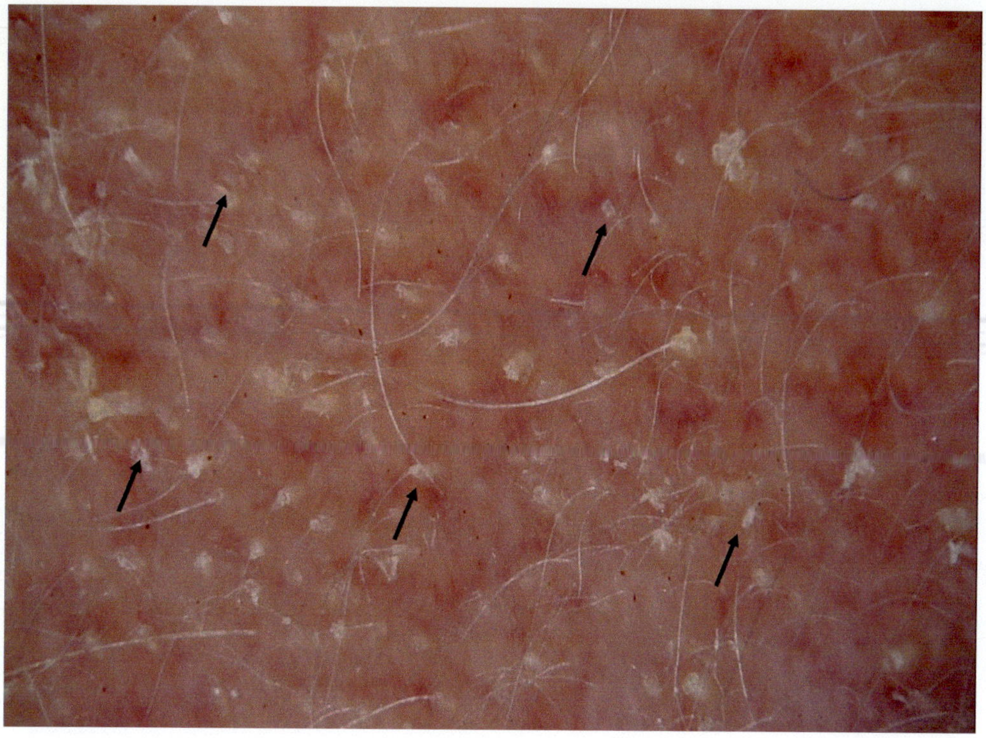

Fig. 6 Demodex tails (arrows)

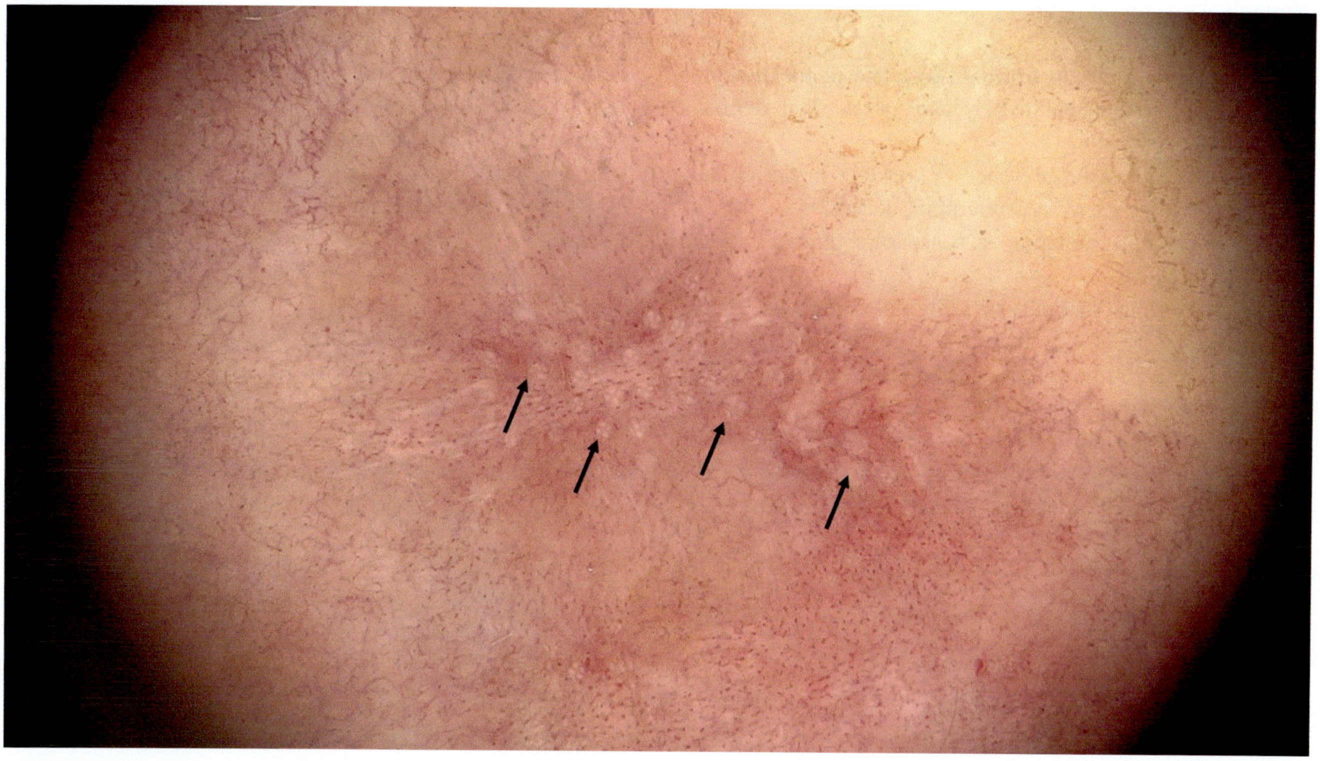

Fig. 7 Rosettes (arrows) Actinic keratosis

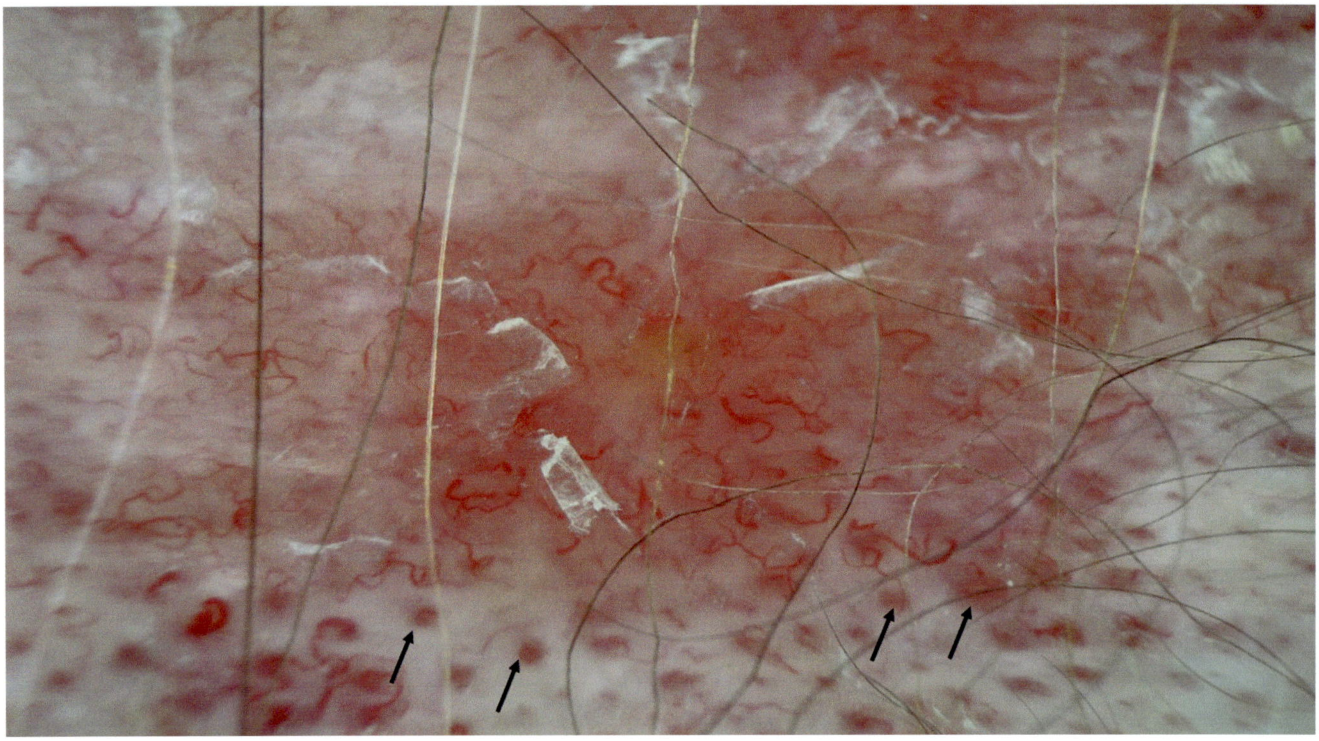

Fig. 8 Follicular red dots (arrows) Discoid lupus on the scalp

7 Colours: again, each of them related to an underlying histological specific alteration

- White: corresponds to fibrosis, decrease in melanocytes or melanin, epidermal hyperplasia or calcium deposits Fig. 9
- Brown: indicates the presence of melanin in the epidermal basal layer or in the superficial dermis
- Grey: represents melanin or ochronotic pigment in the papillary dermis
- Blue: represents melanin or ochronotic pigment in the dermis
- Orange: reflects the presence of a dense granulomatous inflammatory infiltrate in the dermis resulting in a mass effect, or hemosiderin deposits in the dermis Yellow: is due to lipid deposits in the dermis or pustules
- Purple: includes purpura, hemorrhagic areas, and petechiae.

4 Morphologies

- Structureless areas: they can be diffuse or focal zones, but always without any recognizable structure
- Dots o globules
- Lines: distributed in parallel, reticular, angled, or nonspecific way
- Circles: include circles, annular, arcuate and curvilinear shapes

5-Specific clues
Wickham's striae: lichen planus Fig. 10

White keratotic ring with double free edge: cornoid lamella of porokeratosis Fig. 11

Jet with contrail: in scabies—corresponding to the anterior part of the female mite in the gallery Fig. 12

Pediculosis: lice and nits.

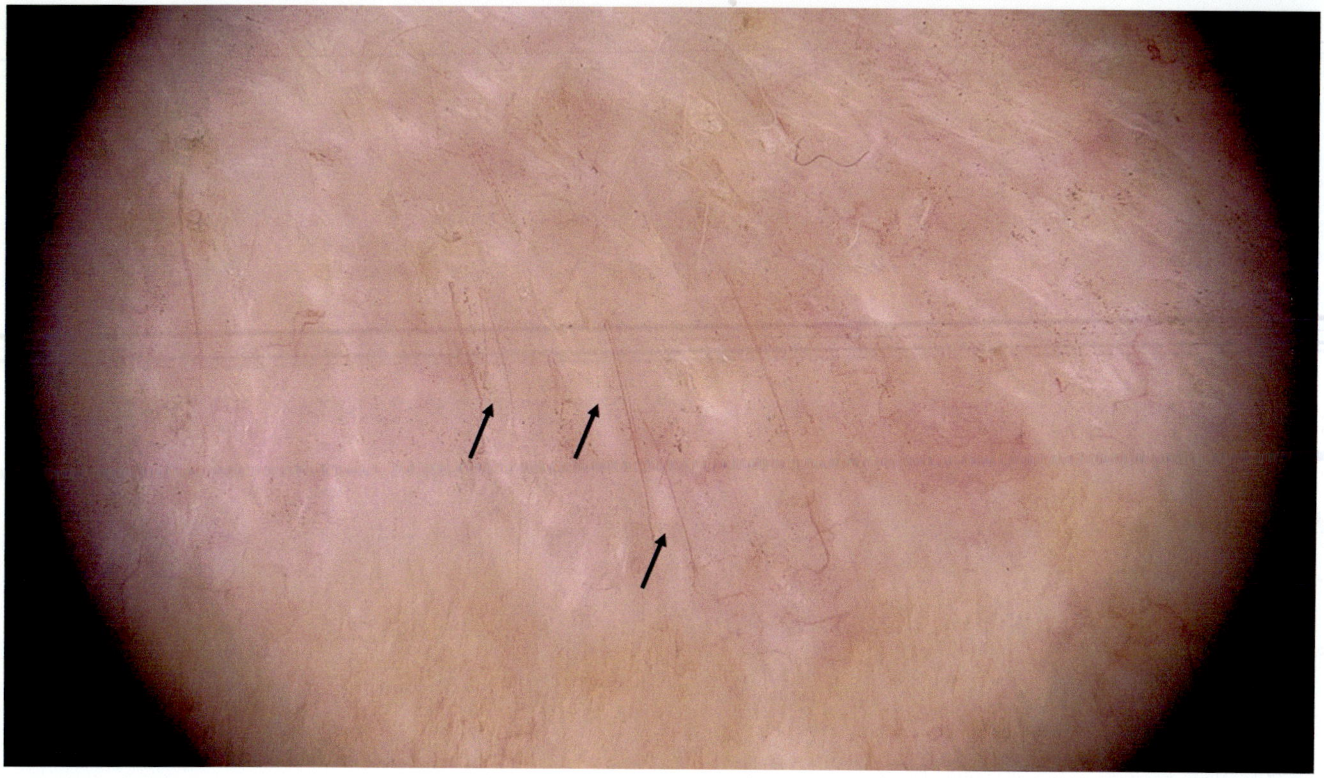

Fig. 9 Whitish fibrotic bands (arrows). Morphea

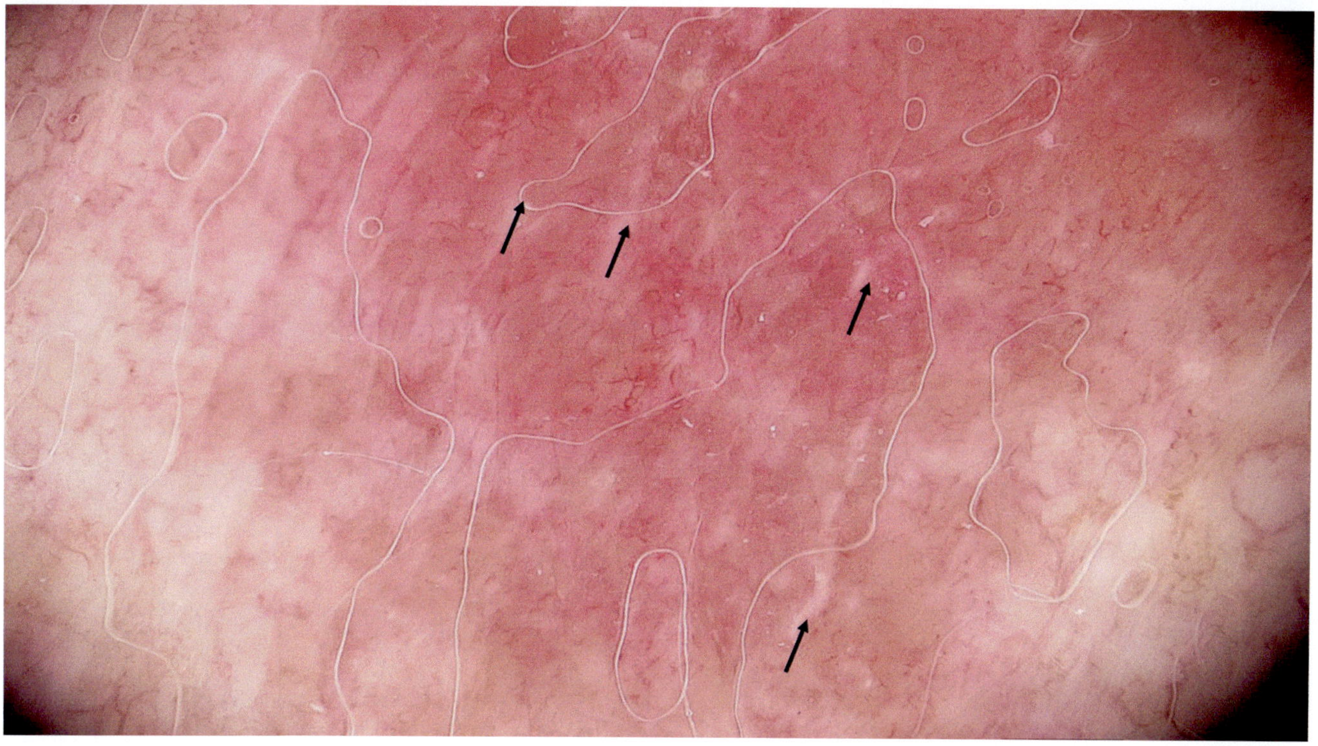

Fig. 10 Wickham's striae (arrows). Lichen planus

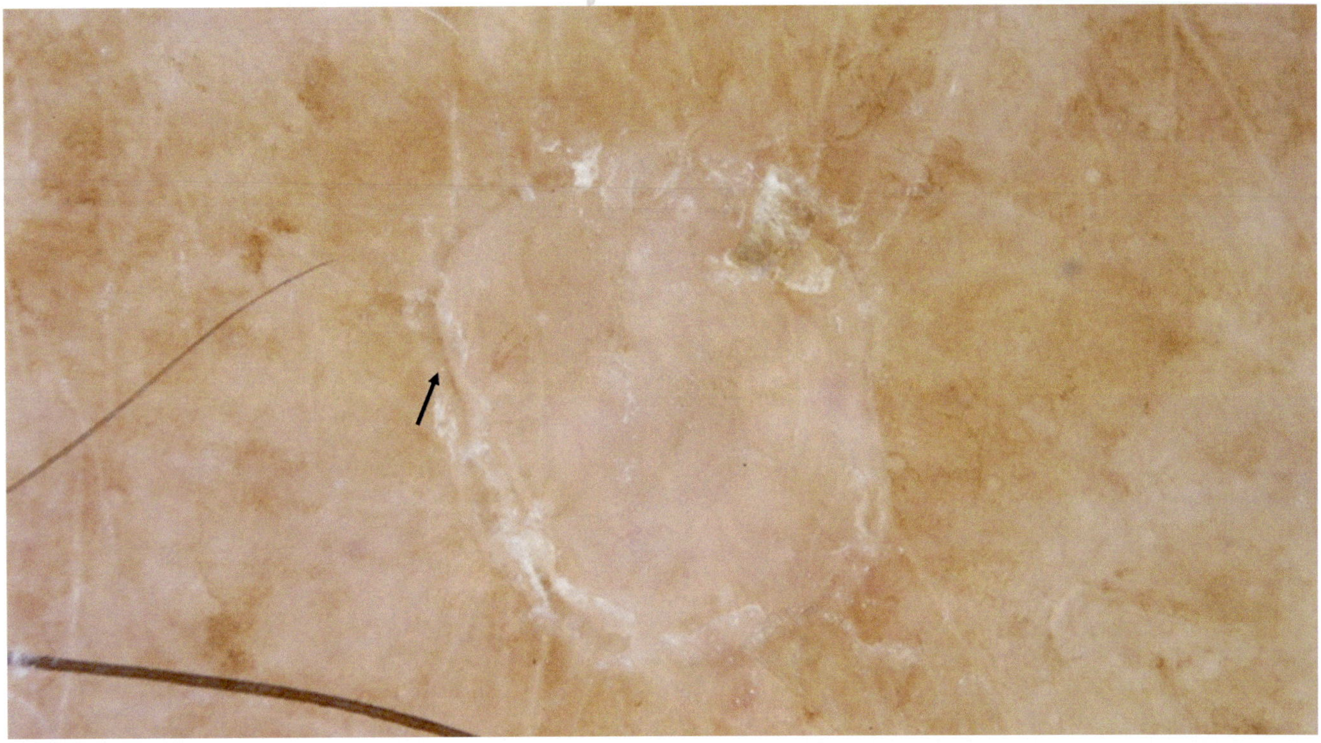

Fig. 11 White keratotic ring with double free edge: cornoid lamella of porokeratosis (arrow)

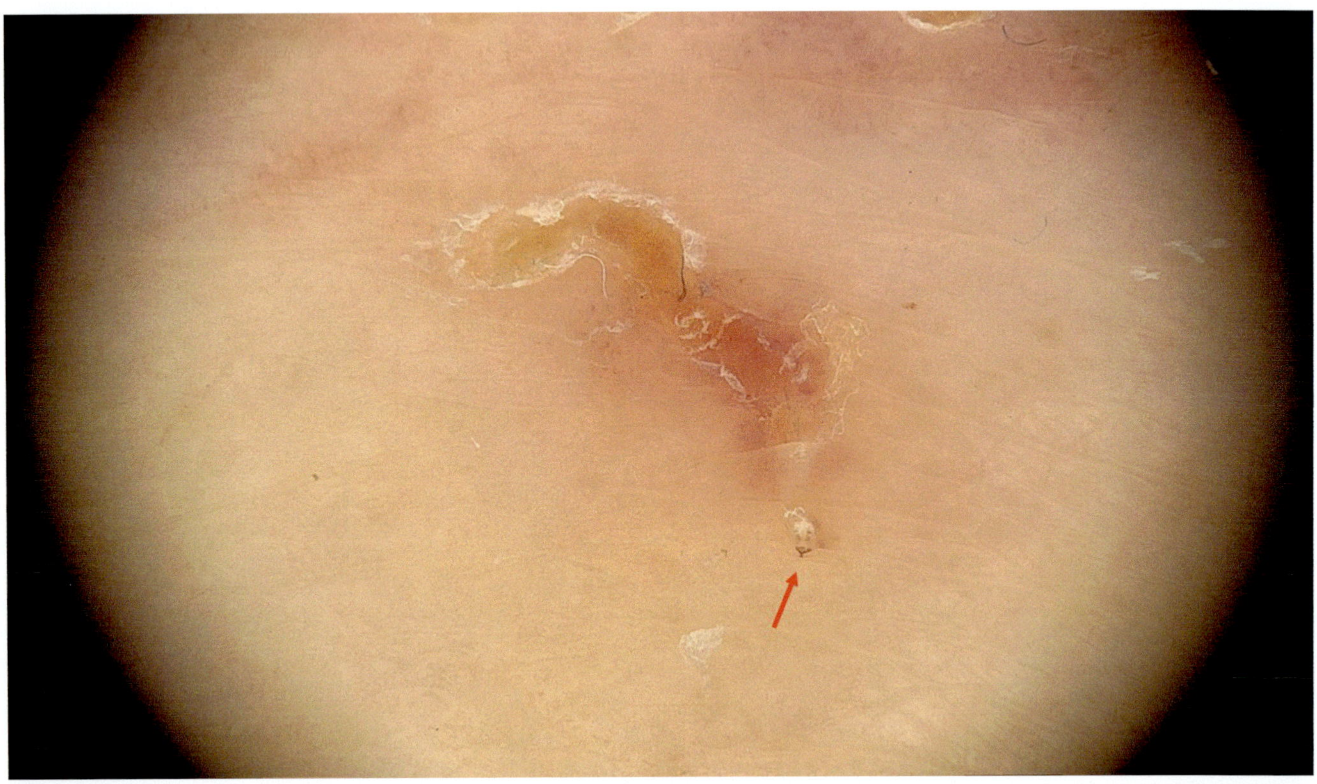

Fig. 12 Jet with contrail: in scabies–corresponding to the anterior part of the female mite in the gallery

Head and Neck Localization

Dominga Peirano Deck, Sebastián Vargas, Álvaro Abarzúa, Alejandra Villarroel, Cristián Navarrete-Dechent, Pablo Uribe, Francesco Lacarrubba, Anna Elisa Verzì, Giuseppe Broggi, Paula Anca, Gabriel Salerni, Polychronia Eftychidou, Renato Marchiori Bakos, Fernanda Staub, Papageorgiou Chryssoula, Ružica Jurakić Tončić, Theodosia Gkentsidi, Gisela D'Atri, and Horacio Cabo

Abstract

Different nonpigmented skin lesion in head and neck area such as Lymphoma, Pseudo lymphoma, Basal cell carcinoma, Basosquamous carcinoma, Squamous cell carcinoma, Keratoacanthoma, Seborrheic Keratosis, Clear cell acanthoma and Fibrosing alopecia are described. Histopathological clinical considerations are made and its dermaroscopic characteristics are also described.

Keywords

Lymphoma • Pseudo lymphoma • Basal cell carcinoma • Basosquamous carcinoma • Squamous cell carcinoma • Keratoacanthoma • Seborrheic Keratosis • Clear cell acanthoma • Fibrosing alopecia

D. P. Deck · S. Vargas · Á. Abarzúa · C. Navarrete-Dechent · P. Uribe
Department of Dermatology, Escuela de Medicina, Pontificia Universidad Católica de Chile, Diagonal Paraguay 362, 6th Floor, 8330077 Santiago, Chile
e-mail: dpeirano@miuandes.cl

S. Vargas
e-mail: sivargas@uc.cl

A. Villarroel
Department of Pathology, Escuela de Medicina, Pontificia Universidad Católica de Chile, 8330077 Santiago, Chile

F. Lacarrubba · A. E. Verzì
Dermatology Clinic, University of Catania, Catania, Italy

G. Broggi
Department "G.F. Ingrassia", Section of Anatomic Pathology, University of Catania, Catania, Italy

P. Anca
Department of Dermatology, "Iuliu Hațieganu" University of Medicine and Pharmacy, 37 Erich Bergel Street, apt 2, 400461 Cluj-Napoca, Romania

G. Salerni
Hospital Provincial del Centenario de Rosario, Universidad Nacional de Rosario, Urquiza 3101. C.P.: 2000, Rosario, Santa Fe, Argentina

P. Eftychidou
Resident of Dermatology-Venereology, 1st Department of Dermatology, Thessaloniki, Greece

R. M. Bakos
Department of Dermatology, Hospital de Clínicas de Porto Alegre, Universidade Federal do Rio Grande do Sul, Rua Ramiro Barcellos, 2350 CEP, Porto Alegre, 900035-903, Brazil
e-mail: rbakos@hcpa.edu.br

F. Staub
Medical Resident in Dermatology, Department of Dermatology, Hospital de Clínicas de Porto Alegre, Universidade Federal do Rio Grande do Sul, Rua Ramiro Barcellos, 2350 CEP, Porto Alegre, 900035-903, Brazil
e-mail: flstaub@hcpa.edu.br

P. Chryssoula
Second Dermatology Department, Medical School, Faculty of Health Sciences, Aristotle University of Thessaloniki, 76 Agiou Pavlou, Pavlos Melas, 564 29 Thessaloniki, Greece

R. J. Tončić
University Hospital Centre Zagreb and School of Medicine, University Department of Dermatovenereology, Kišpatićeva 12, 10000 Zagreb, Croatia

T. Gkentsidi
First Department of Dermatology, Aristotle University, Delfon 124 Str., Thessaloniki, Greece

G. D'Atri
6045 Nicaragua Street, Palermo, Buenos Aires, Argentina

H. Cabo (✉)
Clinical Dermatology, University of Buenos Aires, Arenales 1446 1 °C (1061) CABA, Buenos Aires, Argentina
e-mail: cabohoracio@gmail.com

H. Cabo and A. Lallas (eds.), *Dermatoscopic Atlas of Non-Pigmented Lesions*,
https://doi.org/10.1007/978-3-031-34310-0_3

Case 1

Authors: Dominga Peirano Deck, Sebastián Vargas, Álvaro Abarzúa, Alejandra Villarroel, Cristián Navarrete-Dechent, Pablo Uribe

Clinical record:

Sex: Male

Age: 35 years

Clinical description of the case or the lesion: A shiny, erythematous nodule of about 10 mm in diameter.

Body site: Right cheek

Surface: Nodular

Maximum diameter: 10 mm

Duration of the lesion: 6 weeks

History of morphologic changes: No, in particular it had no signs of recent bleeding or ulceration.

Personal history of skin cancer: No

Family history of skin cancer: Yes, nonmelanoma skin cancer (Father)

Skin Phototype: III

Clinical diagnosis: Skin tumor, suspicious of Cutaneous lymphoma

Dermoscopic findings: The presence of a homogeneous lesion with pink background, follicular plugs and some arborizing vessels, suggestive of cutaneous lymphoma as a differential diagnosis.

Other clinical findings: (-) (Figs. 1, 2 and 3)

Diagnosis: Primary cutaneous CD4 (+) small/medium sized T-cell lymphoproliferative disorder

Key message: This case corresponded to a primary cutaneous CD4 (+) small/medium sized T-cell lymphoproliferative disorder (CD4+ PCSM-LPD). It is a rare subtype of cutaneous T-cell lymphoma with indolent benign behavior.

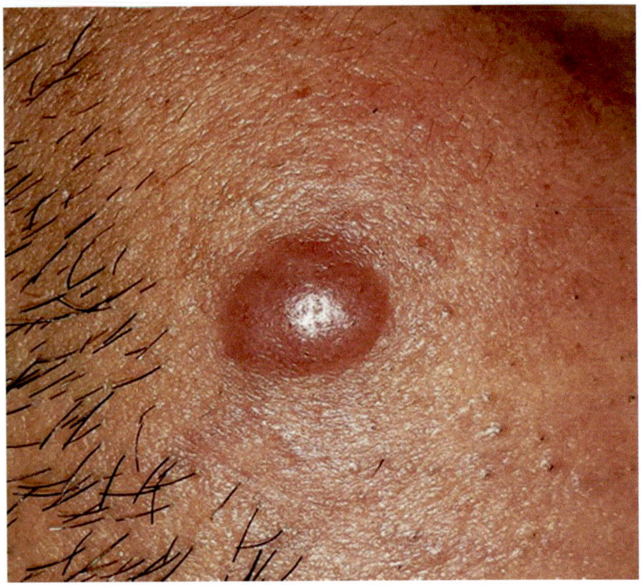

Fig. 1 A small, circumscribed, shiny-erythematous nodule of about 10 mm in diameter located in the right cheek

CD4+ PCSM-LPD classically presents as a solitary nodule on the face, neck or trunk. The dermoscopy of cutaneous T- and B-cell lymphomas and pseudolymphomas presenting as solitary nodules has been recently described. The diagnosis should be suspected in any lesion displaying the following dermoscopic features:

- Organized lesión
- Orange color or diffuse orange/salmon background
- Follicular plugs
- Vessels, commonly linear and arborizing vessels

The dermoscopic differential diagnosis includes cutaneous neoplasms such as basal cell carcinoma and also other diseases with dense cellular and/or granulomatous infiltrates such as sarcoidosis, granuloma faciale, and tuberculosis, among others.

Case 2

Authors: Dominga Peirano Deck, Sebastián Vargas, Alejandra Villarroel, Cristián Navarrete-Dechent, Pablo Uribe, Álvaro Abarzúa

Clinical record:

Sex: Male

Age: 70-year-old

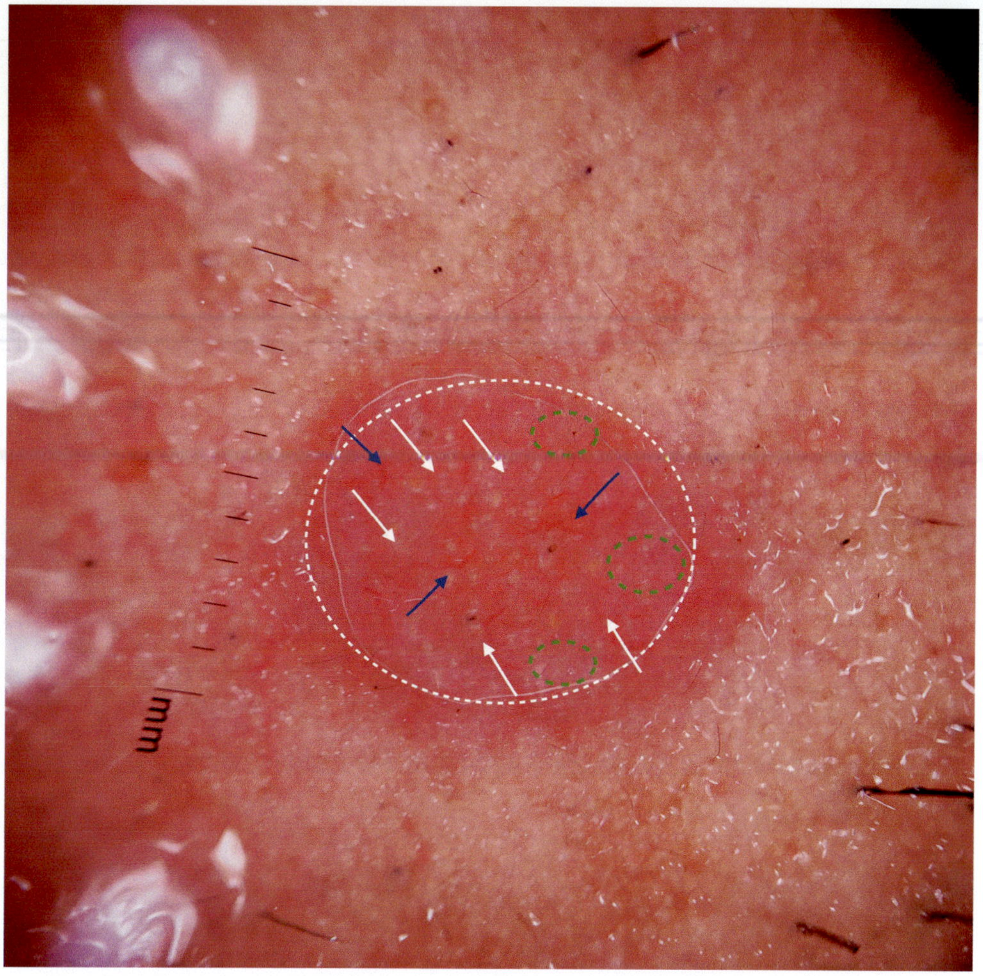

Fig. 2 Dermoscopy image (polarized light): an organized lesion with a pink background (white dotted circle), follicular plugs (white arrows), white structureless areas (green dotted circles) and linear, irregular and arborizing vessels (blue arrows), should make us suspect cutaneous lymphoma as a differential diagnosis

Clinical description of the case or the lesion: A well delimited, shiny erythematous nodule of about 1 cm in diameter in the right side of the glabella.

Body site: Forehead- Right side of glabella

Surface: Nodular

Maximum diameter: 1 cm

Duration of the lesion: 2 months

History of morphologic changes: It had no signs of recent bleeding or ulceration.

Personal history of skin cancer: No

Family history of skin cancer: No

Skin Phototype: II

Clinical diagnosis: Skin tumor

Dermoscopic findings: On dermoscopy, the lesion showed a reddish-orange background with in-focus vessels and follicular plugs, suggestive of cutaneous tumor.

Other clinical findings: None (Figs. 4, 5 and 6)

Diagnosis: Primary cutaneous CD4 (+) small/medium sized T-cell lymphoproliferative disorder (CD4 + PCSM-LPD)

Key message: This case corresponded to a **primary cutaneous CD4 (+) small/medium sized T-cell lymphoproliferative disorder (CD4+ PCSM-LPD)**. It's a rare subtype of cutaneous T-cell lymphoma with indolent benign behavior. CD4+ PCSM-LPD classically presents as a solitary nodule on the face, neck or trunk. The dermoscopy of cutaneous T- and B-cell lymphomas and pseudolymphomas presenting as solitary nodules has been recently described.

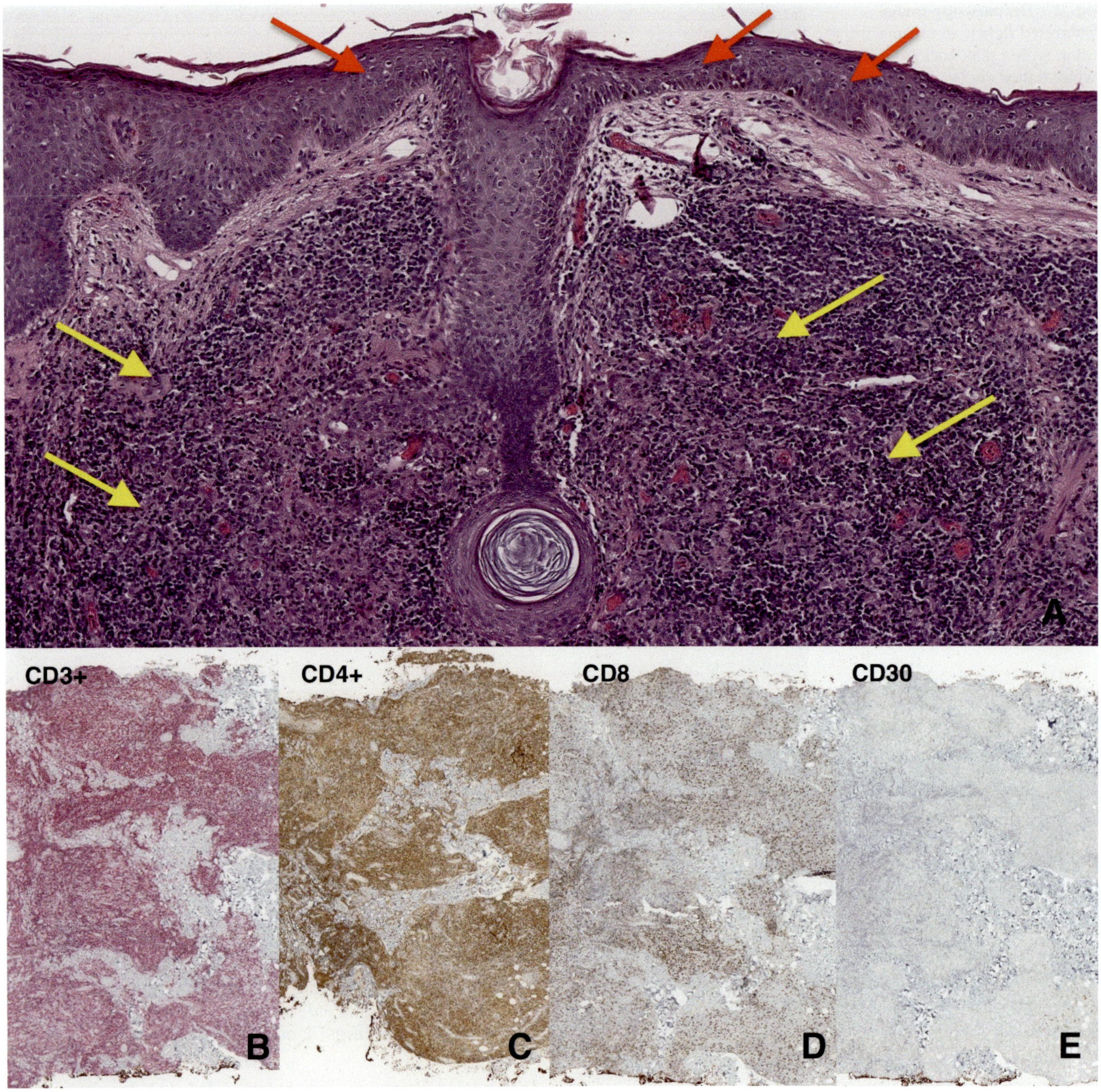

Fig. 3 Histopathology: A (H&E 20x) Photomicrograph showing skin with atrophic epidermis (red arrow) and an atypical dermal lymphoid infiltrate (yellow arrows). Immunohistochemistry showing positivity for CD3 (Image B), CD4 (Image C) and absence of CD8 (Image D) and CD30 (Image E) markers. Courtesy of Alejandra Villarroel, MD, Department of Pathology, Pontificia Universidad Católica de Chile

The diagnosis should be suspected in any lesion displaying the following dermoscopic features:

- Organized lesion
- Orange color or diffuse orange/salmon background
- Follicular plugs
- Vessels, commonly linear and arborizing vessels

The dermoscopic differential diagnosis includes cutaneous neoplasms such as basal cell carcinoma and also other

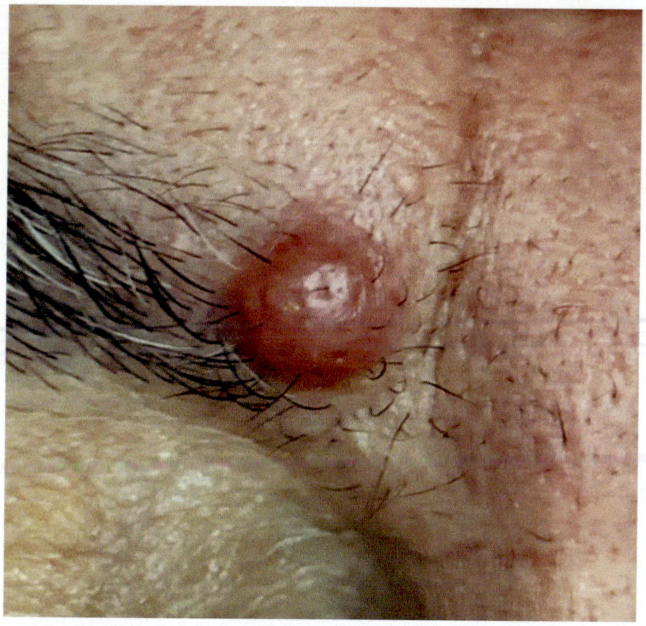

Fig. 4 A well delimited, shiny erythematous nodule of about 1 cm in diameter in the right side of the glabella

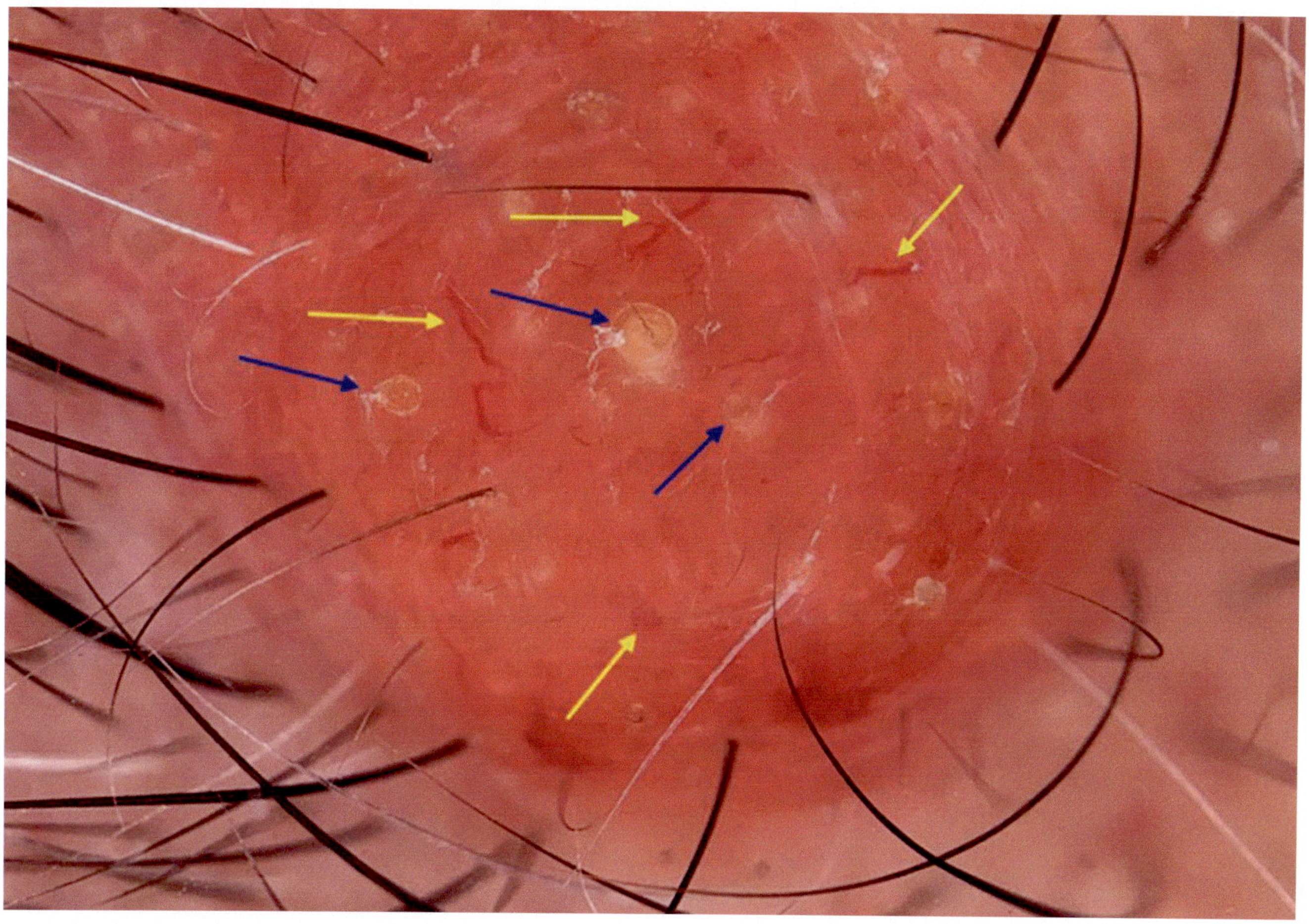

Fig. 5 **Dermoscopy (polarize light)** evidenced polymorphous in-focus vessels (yellow arrows) with follicular yellow plugs (blue arrows)

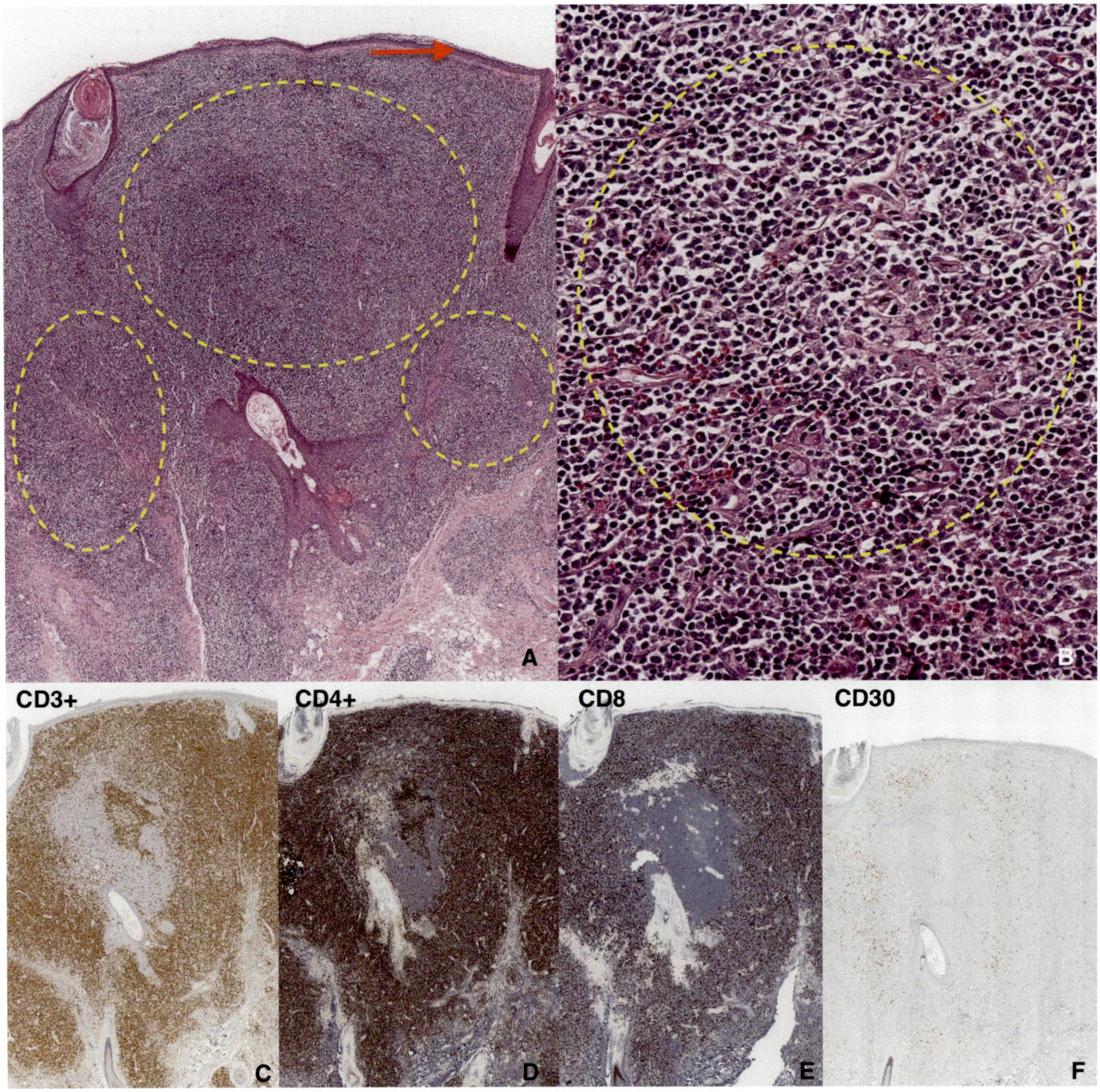

Fig. 6 Histopathology: Image A(H&E 2x) and B(20x). Photomicrograph showing skin with atrophic epidermis (red arrow) and an atypical dermal lymphoid infiltrate (yellow dotted circle). Immunohistochemistry showing positivity for CD3 (Image C), CD4 (Image D) and absence of CD8 (Image E) and CD30 (Image F) markers. Courtesy of Alejandra Villarroel, MD, Department of Pathology, Pontificia Universidad Católica de Chile

diseases with dense cellular and/or granulomatous infiltrates such as sarcoidosis, granuloma faciale, and tuberculosis, among others

Case 3

Authors: Francesco Lacarrubba, Anna Elisa Verzì, Giuseppe Broggi

Clinical record:

Sex: Female

Age: 55-years-old

Clinical description the case or the lesion: Solitary, asymptomatic, nodular lesion of the face showing a reddish color and smooth surface

Body site: Chin

Surface: Nodular

Maximum diameter: 8 mm

Duration of the lesion: 8 months

History of morphologic changes: Slow enlargement

Personal history of skin cancer: No

Family history of skin cancer: No

Skin Phototype: III

Clinical diagnosis: Nodular basal cell carcinoma

Dermoscopic findings: Orangish background, follicular plugs, and short unfocused linear vessels

Other clinical findings: N/A (Figs. 7, 8 and 9)

Diagnosis: Pseudolymphoma (cutaneous lymphoid hyperplasia)

Key message: The presence of orangish background, follicular plugs and linear vessels may help clinicians in the differential diagnosis of pseudolymphoma with other clinically similar lesions of the face that show a different dermoscopic pattern. Of note, the described dermoscopic features may be also observed in primary cutaneous B- and T-cell lymphomas.

Case 4

Author: Ilut Paula Anca

Clinical record:

Sex: Female

Age: 56-years-old

Clinical description the case or the lesion: nodular lesion located at the level of the right nasal wing, with a wide base, slow growth in the last 2 years and without clinical symptoms

Body site: Face (nose)

Surface: Nodular

Maximum diameter: 1.2 cm

Duration of the lesion: 2 years

History of morphologic changes: Slow growth

Personal history of skin cancer: None

Family history of skin cancer: None

Skin Phototype: II

Clinical diagnosis: Nodular-cystic Basal Cell Carcinoma

Dermoscopic findings:

- pink translucent background
- linear arborizing vessels, typically seen in focus
- small ulceration in the superior part
- lack of pigment

Other clinical findings: None (Figs. 10 and 11)

Diagnosis: Basal cell carcinoma

Key message: In focus branching linear vessel are typical for basal cell carcinoma and for the nodular-cystic subtype, they are usually seen on a translucent background with or without

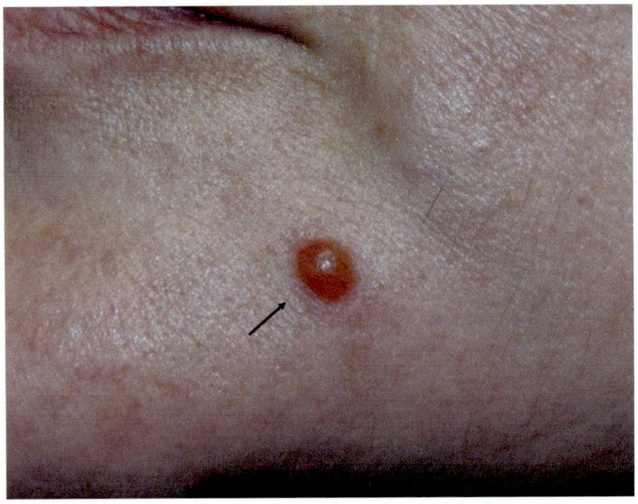

Fig. 7 Clinical view: reddish, nodular lesion of the face showing a smooth surface (black arrow)

ulceration. Sometimes the vessels are so prominent that can be visible even without a dermatoscope like in this case

Case 5

Author: Ilut Paula Anca

Clinical record:

Sex: Female

Age: 81-years-old

Clinical description the case or the lesion: Nodular lesion with significant ulceration and bleeding, which started as a small nodule and grew gradually over several years

Body site: Face – preauricular region

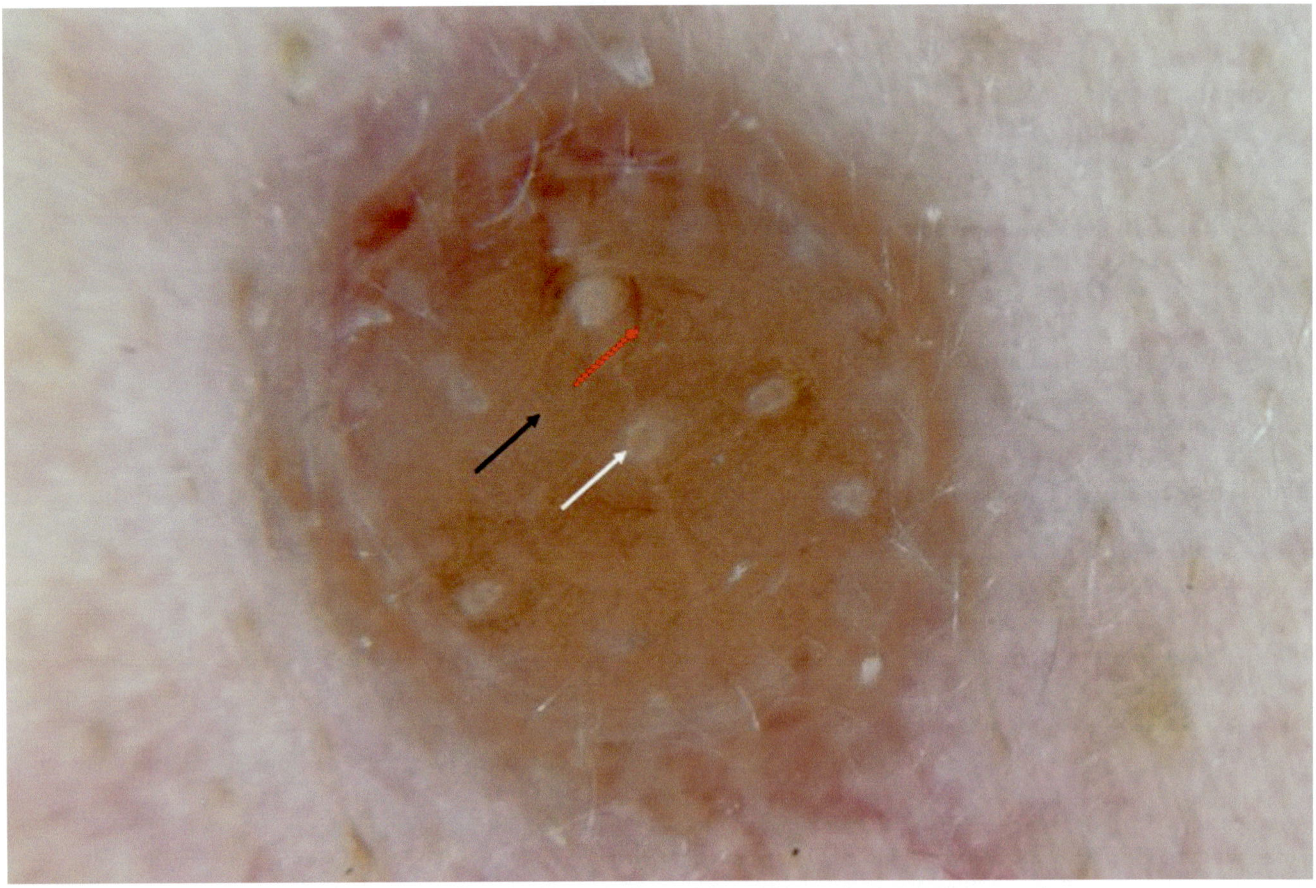

Fig. 8 Polarized dermoscopy showing an oranges background (black arrow); follicular plugs (white arrow) and short unfocused linear vessels (red arrow) (original magnification x10)

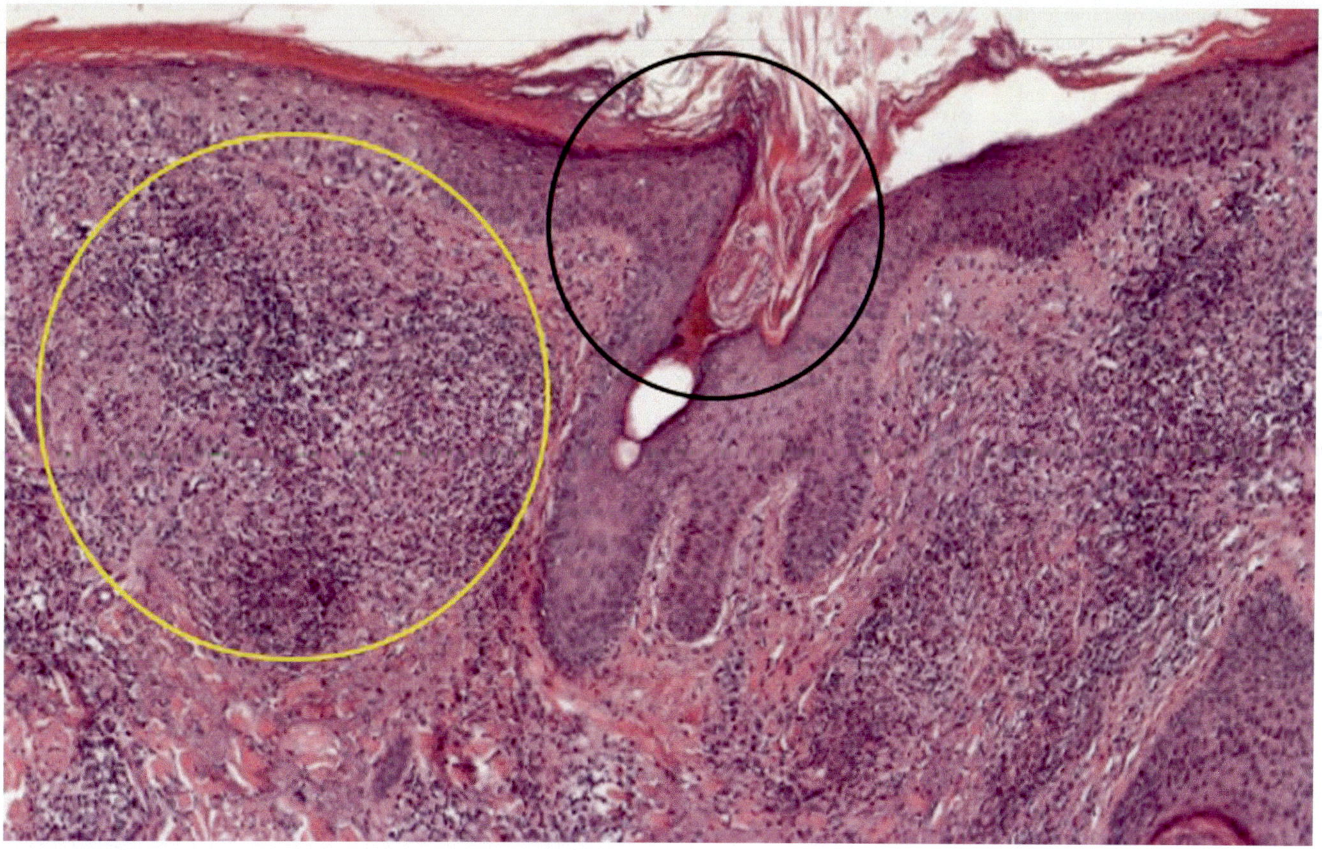

Fig. 9 Histopathology showing dermal lymphocytic and histiocytic inflammatory infiltrate with plasma cells and scattered granulocytes (yellow circle); the overlying epidermis, which exhibits hyperkeratosis with follicular plugs, is spared (black circle) (H&E staining; original magnification 200x)

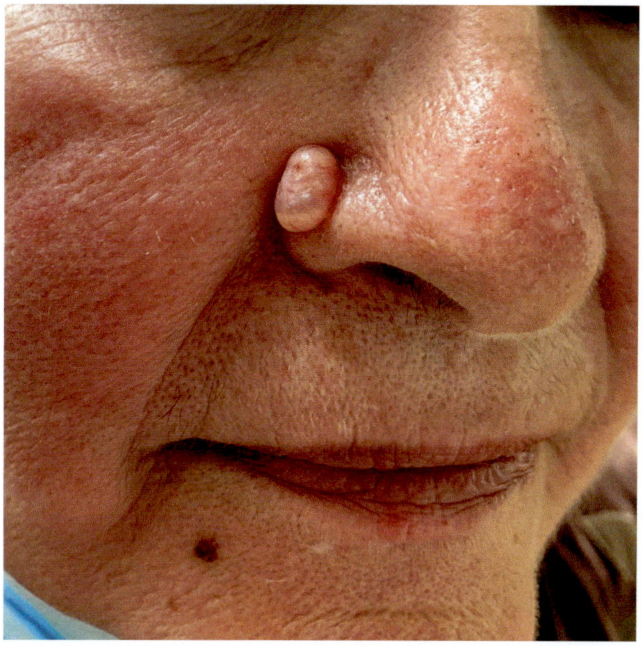

Fig. 10 Clinical image of a nodular-cystic Basal Cell Carcinoma with a translucent appearance. The linear vessels can be visible with the naked eye

Surface: Nodular

Maximum diameter: 2 cm

Duration of the lesion: 4 years

History of morphologic changes: Slow growth

Personal history of skin cancer: None

Family history of skin cancer: None

Skin Phototype: II

Clinical diagnosis: Nodular Basal Cell Carcinoma

Dermoscopic findings:

- ulceration that covers most of the lesion
- linear thick and thin arborizing vessels
- shiny white blotches
- few pigmented dots

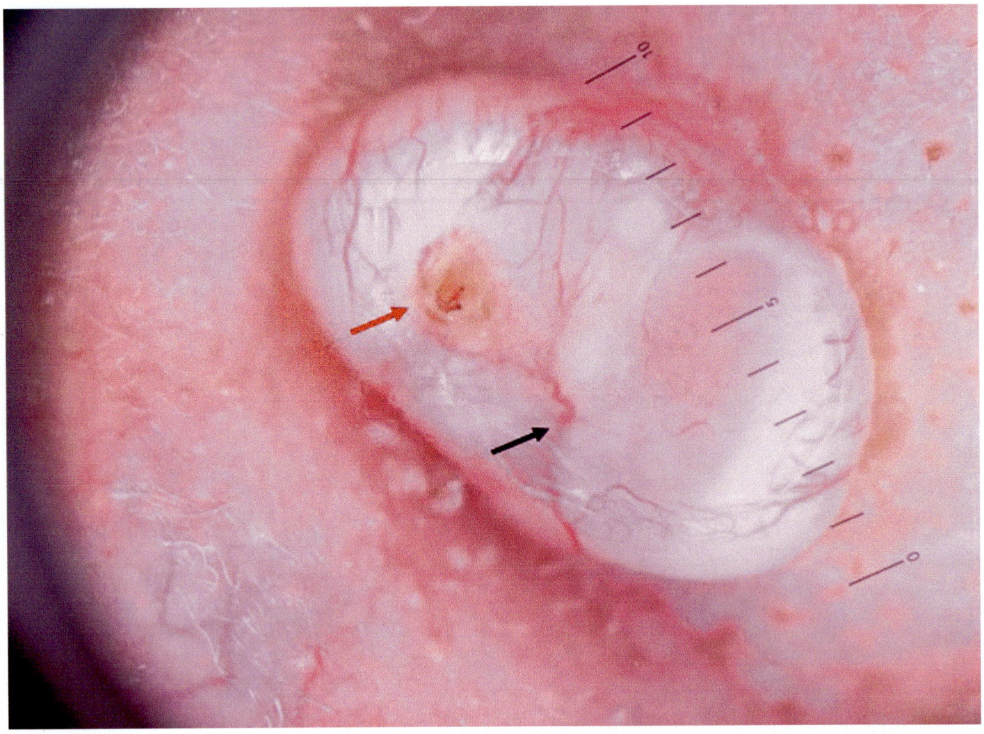

Fig. 11 Dermatoscopic image of a nodular basal cell carcinoma characterized by linear in focus arborizing vessels in a translucent background (black arrow) and a small ulceration (red arrow)

Other clinical findings: None (Figs. 12, 13 and 14)

Diagnosis: Nodular basal cell carcinoma

Key message: Nodular basal cell carcinomas that display large ulcerations are often difficult to diagnose considering that at the level of an ulceration, a polymorphous vascular pattern is frequently observed which does not provide specific citerias for identifying the type of the lesion. In such cases, it is very important to carefully analyze the entire lesion and try to find non-ulcerated areas (in this case at the periphery) that can reveal important clues and thus facilitate the diagnosis.

Case 6

Author: Gabriel Salerni

Clinical record:

Sex: Female

Age: 58-years-old

Clinical description the case or the lesion

Body site: Left lateral side of the neck

Surface: Nodular

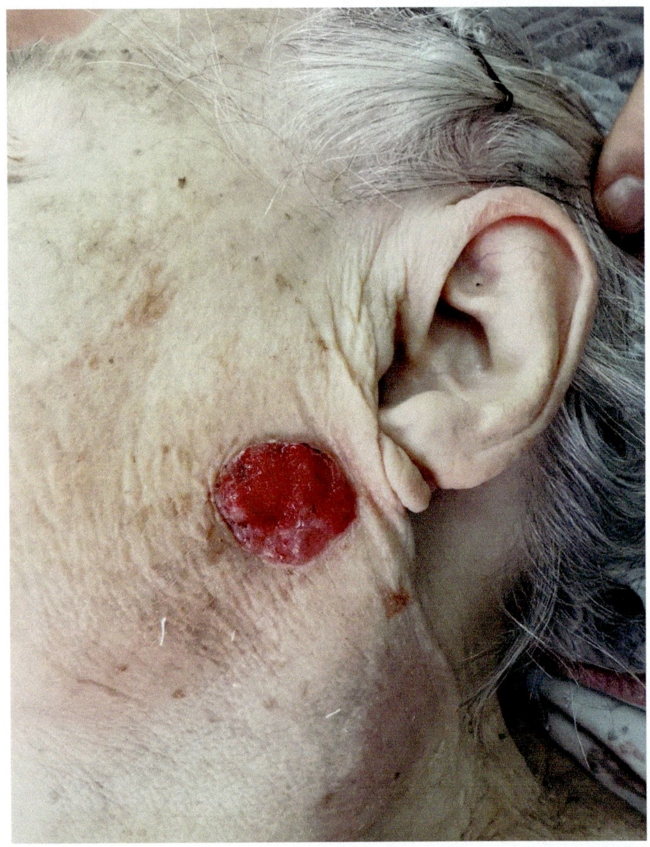

Fig. 12 Clinical image of a nodular BCC that could be easily misdiagnosed as a SCC, Amelanotic Melanoma or Merkel Cell Carcinoma

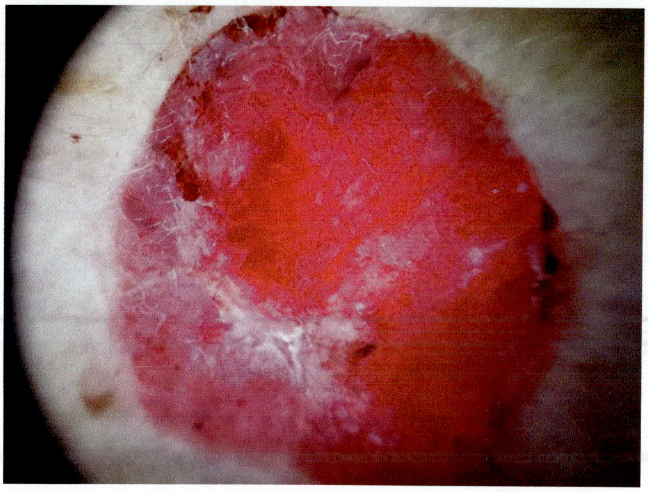

Fig. 13 Dermatoscopy of a nodular basal cell carcinoma with ulceration, arborizing vessels, shiny white blotches or strands and some signs of pigment (structureless areas and dots)

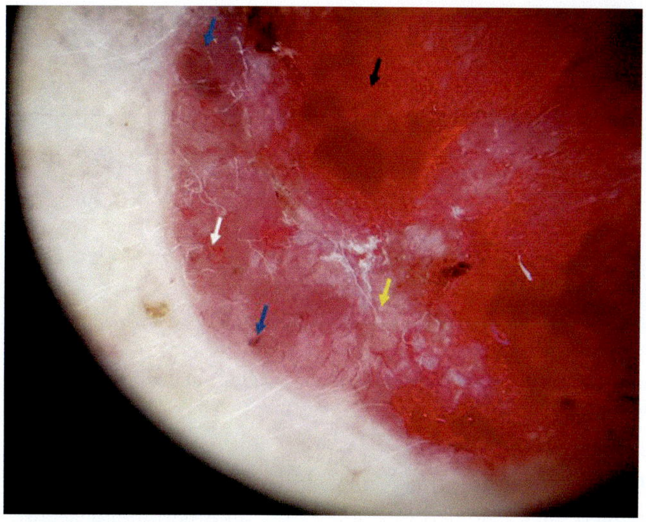

Fig. 14 Dermatoscopic image of the periphery of a nodular basal cell carcinoma with a significant ulceration (black arrow) that covers almost the entire lesion. The lesion is characterized by arborizing vessels (white arrow); shiny white blotches (yellow arrow) and pigmented dots (blue arrows)

Maximum diameter: 4 mm

Duration of the lesion: 6 months

History of morphologic changes: Occurrence 6 months ago and progressive increasing in size

Personal history of skin cancer: None

Family history of skin cancer: None

Skin Phototype: II

Clinical diagnosis: Amelanotic melanoma, CEC, CBC, eccrine poroma

Dermoscopic findings: Dermoscopy showed arborizing vessels, linear serpentine vessels, and multiple linear looped vessels with a diverse morphology: single-stranded, double-stranded, bending and forming multiple loops appearing uncoiled and overlapping. Histopathology revealed a nodular adenoid BCC (Figs. 15, 16 and 17).

Other clinical findings:

Diagnosis: Nodular adenoid basal cell carcinoma

Key message: Polymorphous hairpin vessels, although rarely, can be observed in BCCs

Case 7

Author: Polychronia Eftychidou

Clinical record:

Sex: Male

Age: 78-years-old

Clinical description the case or the lesion: Flat lesion located on the nose, which was clinically suspicious for basal cell carcinoma (BCC) as it exhibited macroscopically visible erosions and peripheral arborizing vessels.

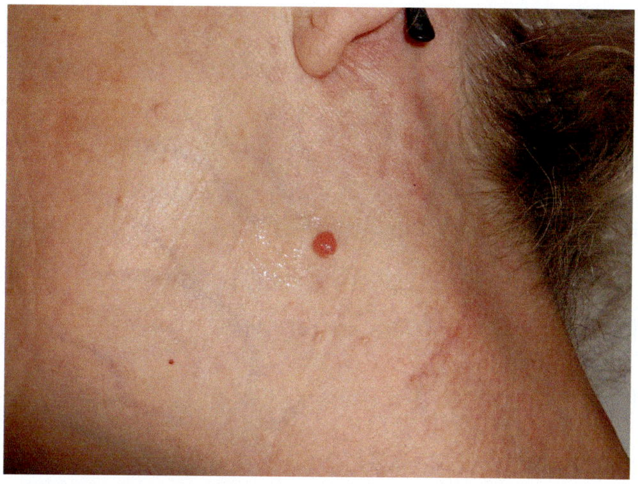

Fig. 15 Pink papule in the left lateral side of the neck

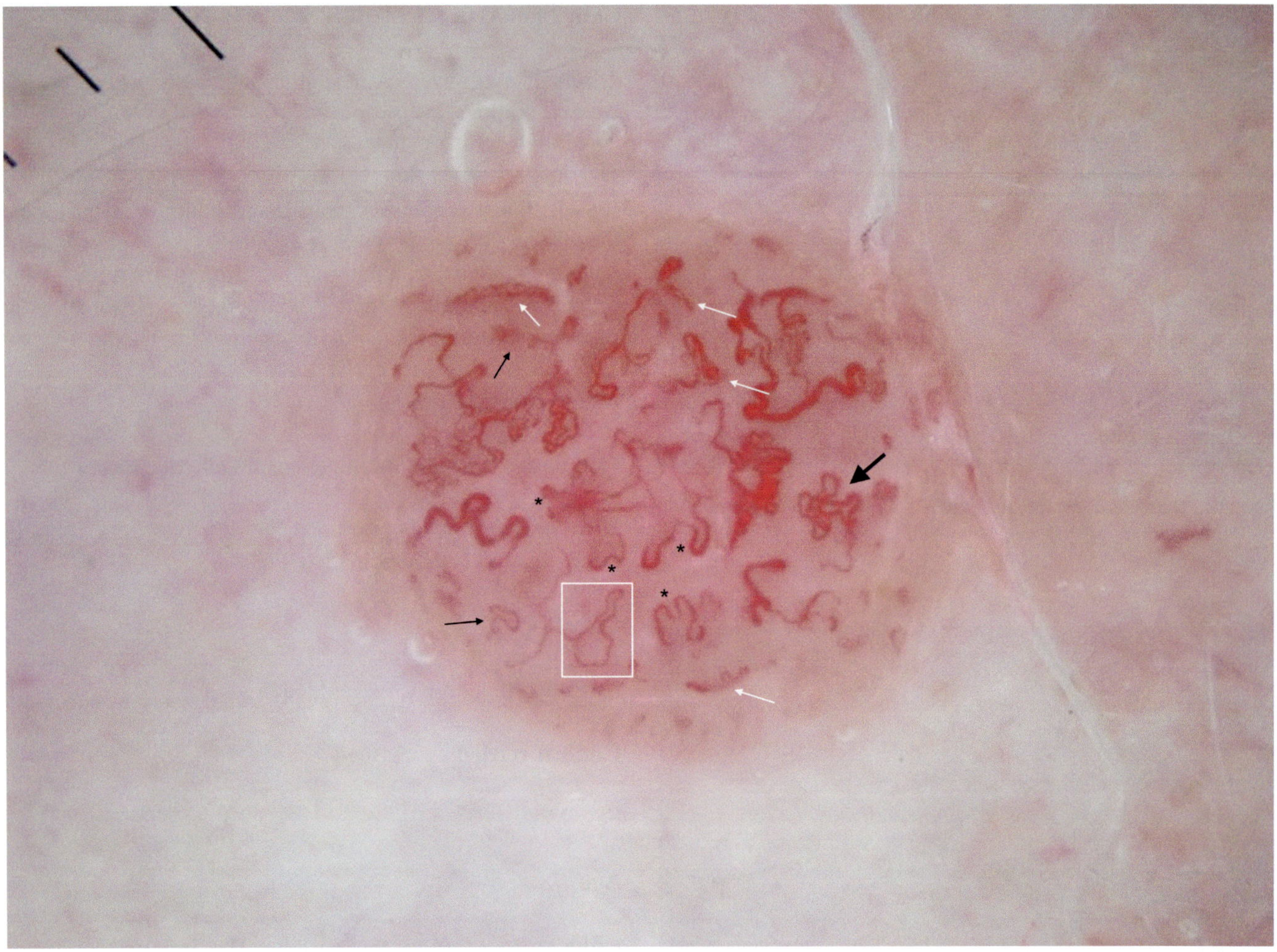

Fig. 16 Arborizing vessels, serpentine vessels (white arrow) and multiple hairpin vessels morphology: single-stranded (black arrow), double-stranded (asterisk), bending (square) and uncoiled overlapping (thick arrow)

Body site: Nose

Surface: Flat

Maximum diameter: 1.5 cm

Duration of the lesion: 1 year

History of morphologic changes: Gradual enlargement of the lesion and appearance of erosions

Personal history of skin cancer: None

Family history of skin cancer: None.

Skin Phototype: Type III

Clinical diagnosis: Basal cell carcinoma (BCC)

Dermoscopic findings: On dermoscopy, the lesion displayed BCC- related characteristics, like peripheral arborizing vessels and erosions, but also exhibited squamous cell carcinoma - related features, namely white circles (targetoid hair follicles), rosettes and blood spots in keratin masses.

Other clinical findings: Photodamaged skin (Figs. 18 and 19)

Diagnosis: Basosquamous carcinoma

Key message: The presence of white structures – white circles in a lesion otherwise considered BCC- like should raise suspicion of Basosquamous carcinoma, which is considered a relatively rare BCC variant. Basosquamous carcinoma, also known as metatypical BCC, is considered as an aggressive subtype, with a higher potential for lymph node and distant metastasis and recurrence as compared to nodular BCC.

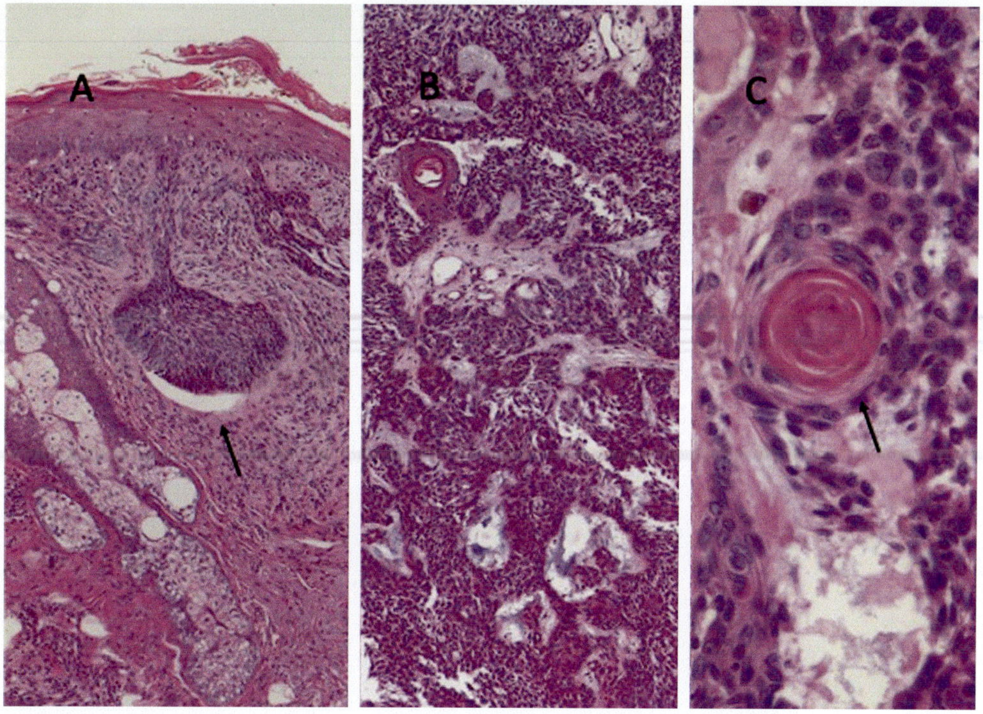

Fig. 17 A- Tumor Island with clefting (black arrow); B- panoramic view of basaloid cells; C-Prominent vessels (black arrow). Histopathology revealed a nodular adenoid basal cell carcinoma with prominent vessels

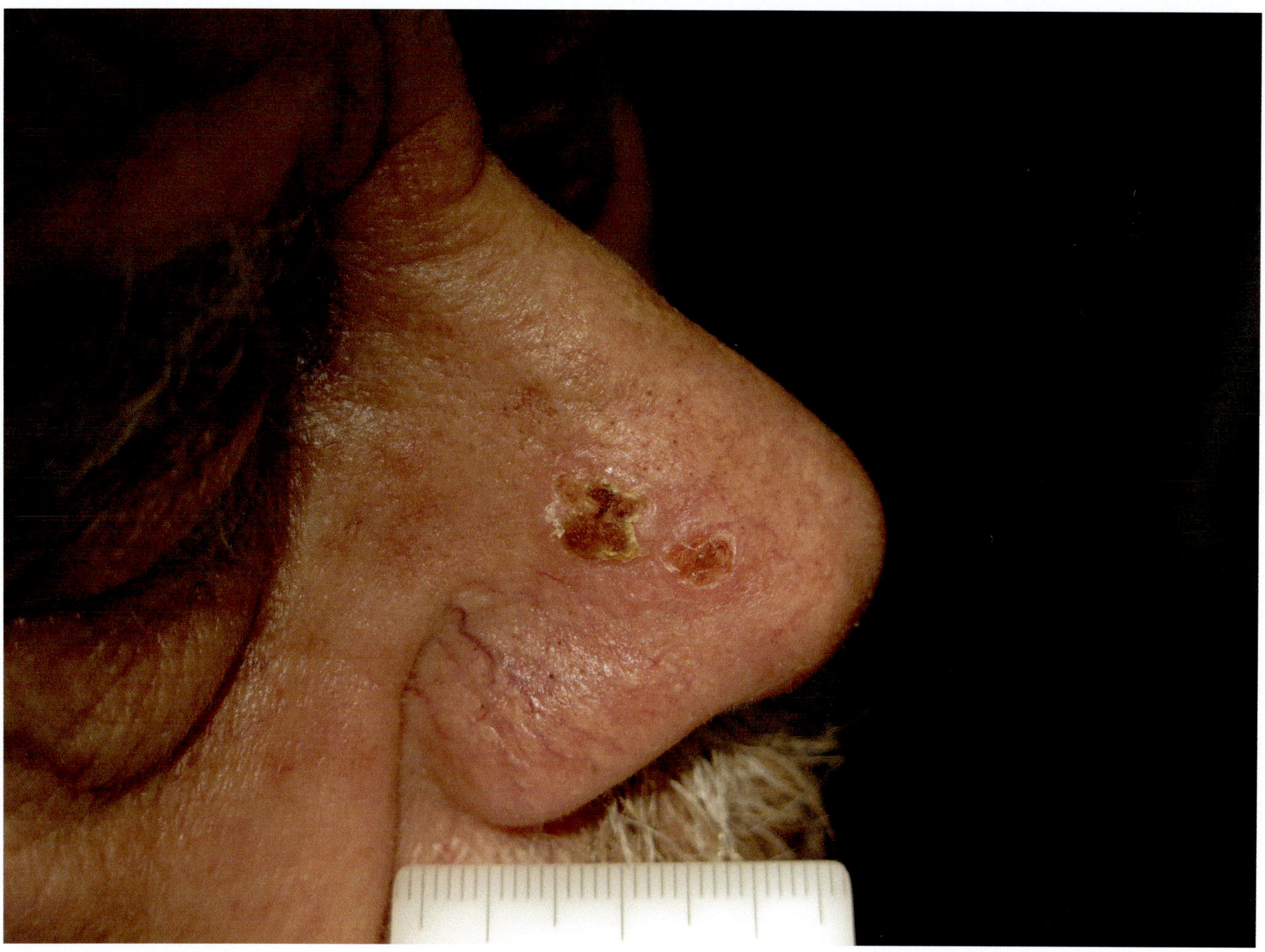

Fig. 18 Clinical image

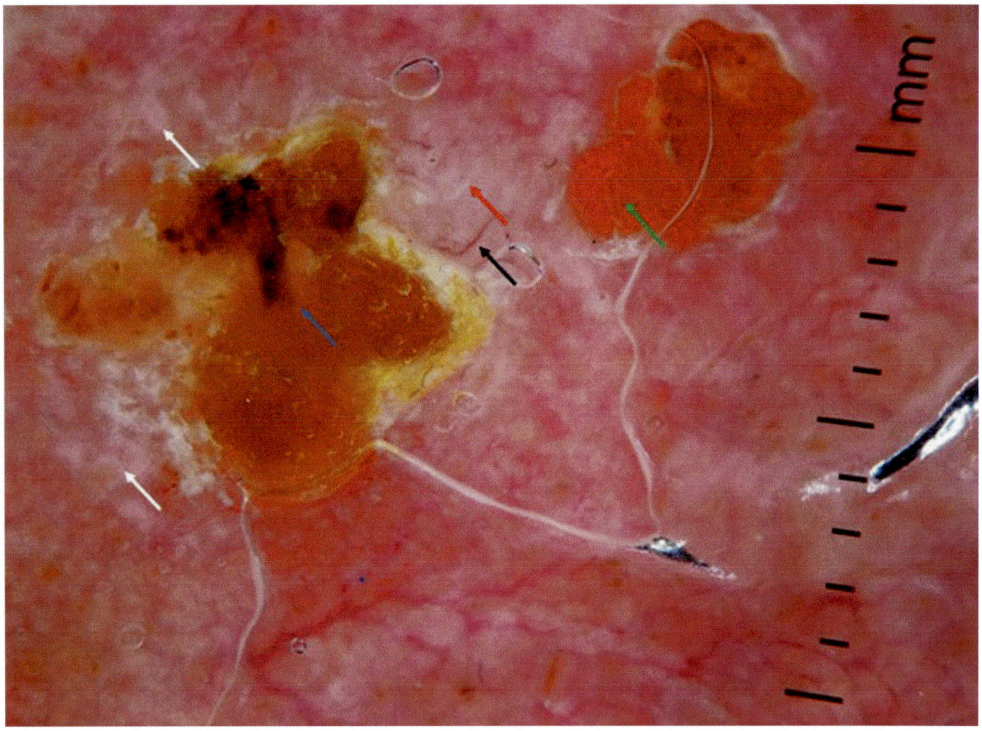

Fig. 19 Dermatoscopic image: arborizing vessels (black arrow); erosions (green arrow); white shiny streaks (red arrow); white circles (white arrows) and blood spots in keratin masses (blue arrow)

Dermoscopy facilitates early diagnosis, accurate management and better prognosis of this tumor.

Case 8

Authors: Renato Marchiori Bakos, Fernanda Staub

Clinical record:

Sex: Male

Age: 59-years-old

Clinical description the case or the lesion: Ulcerated atrophic plaque

Body site: Left temporal region

Surface: Infiltrated borders, central ulceration

Maximum diameter: 2.5 cm

Duration of the lesion: Around 1 year

History of morphologic changes: Increase in size

Personal history of skin cancer: No

Family history of skin cancer: Mother – non-melanoma skin cancer

Skin Phototype: III

Clinical diagnosis: Infiltrative basal cell carcinoma

Dermoscopic findings: Ulceration and arborizing telangiectasias on the ulcer

Other clinical findings: Perilesional hypoesthesia (Figs. 20 and 21)

Diagnosis: Infiltrative basal cell carcinoma

Key message: Aggressive BCC variants may also show usual BCC dermoscopic features.

Case 9

Author: Ilut Paula Anca

Clinical record:

Sex: Male

Age: 33-years-old

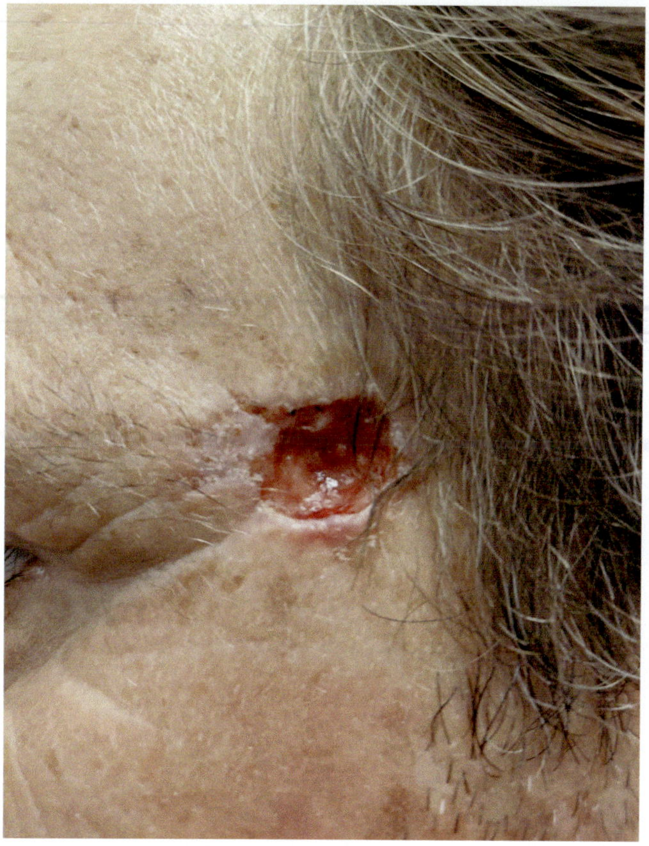

Fig. 20 Clinical image of the ulcerated lesion

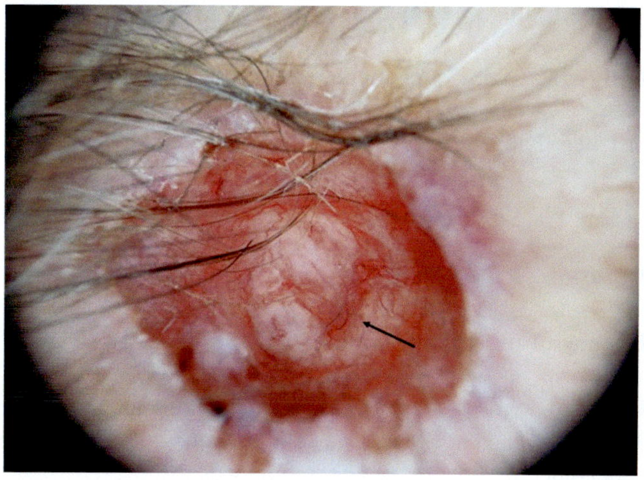

Fig. 21 Dermoscopic image of the ulcer showing erythema on the borders and arborizing telangiectasias on the bottom (black arrow)

Clinical description the case or the lesion: A very small nodular lesion with a thin crust in the center

Body site: Face

Surface: Nodular

Maximum diameter: 3 mm

Duration of the lesion: Half a year

History of morphologic changes: Rapid growth

Personal history of skin cancer: None

Family history of skin cancer: Father with a Basal Cell Carcinoma

Skin Phototype: III

Clinical diagnosis: Keratoacanthoma

Dermoscopic findings:

- central yellow keratin mass
- hairpin vessels at the periphery arranged concentrically

Other clinical findings: None (Figs. 22 and 23)

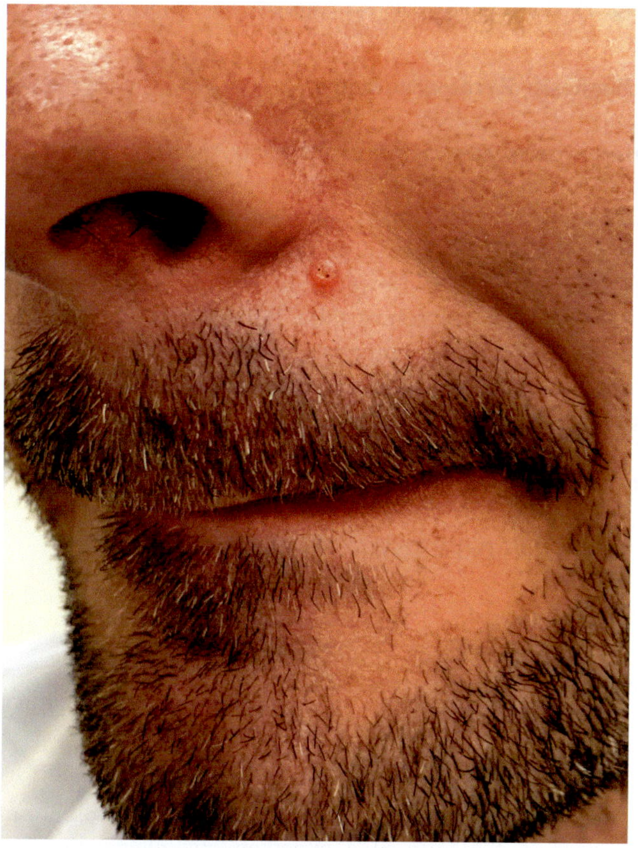

Fig. 22 Small keratoacanthoma developing near the nasolabial crease

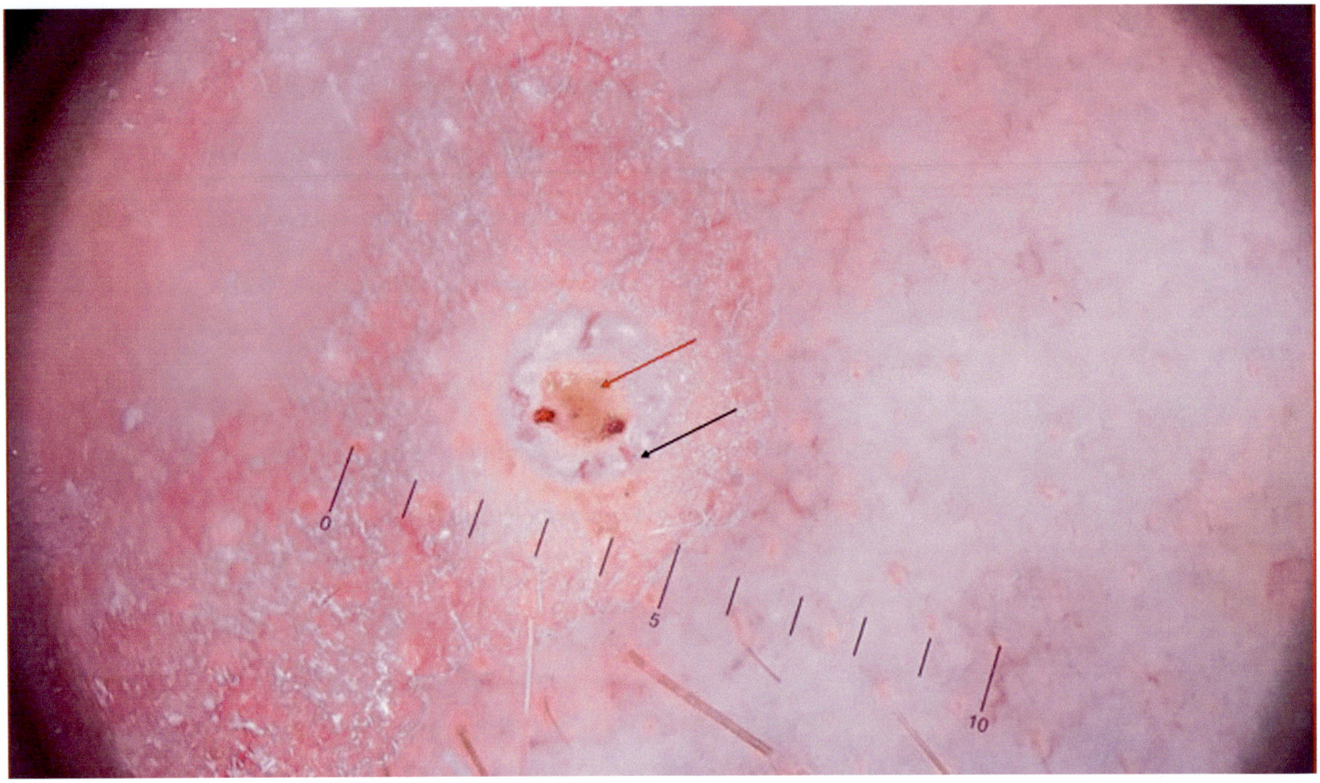

Fig. 23 Small keratoacanthoma displaying few hairpin vessels at the periphery (black arrow) and a central keratin mass (red arrow)

Diagnosis: Keratoacanthoma

Key message: Keratoacanthoma is considered a well-differentiated variant of Squamous cell carcinoma with the possibility of spontaneous involution. It typically presents a central keratin mass surrounded by linear vessels (hairpin or irregular. However, taking into account the fact that a small proportion of these lesions could turn into an invasive carcinoma, appropriate therapy with the removal of the lesion should be considered, of course adapted to each individual case

Case 10

Author: Ilut Paula Anca

Clinical record:

Sex: Male

Age: 65-years-old

Clinical description the case or the lesion: The presence of a lesion in the form of a hyperkeratotic plaque that has persisted for more than 5 years is observed; the patient describes the fact that every time he tries to remove the crust from the surface, the lesion bleeds intensely, after which the crust is restored again.

Body site: Face – preauricular area

Surface: Palpable

Maximum diameter: 1.7 cm

Duration of the lesion: More than 5 years

History of morphologic changes: Slow growth

Personal history of skin cancer: Concomitant, a nodular lesion on the neck with a clinical and dermatoscopic appearance of Basal Cell Carcinoma was discovered

Family history of skin cancer: None

Skin Phototype: II

Clinical diagnosis: Well-differentiated squamous cell carcinoma

Dermoscopic findings:

- white-yellow amorphous keratin mass (yellow arrow)
- white-yellow scales (red arrow)
- white circles surrounding follicles (targetoid follicular openings) (black arrows)
- telangiectasia on sun damaged surrounding skin (green arrow)

Other clinical findings: None (Figs. 24 and 25)

Diagnosis: Well-differentiated squamous cell carcinoma

Key message: Well-differentiated squamous cell carcinoma displays most often criteria associated to keratinization such as keratin masses, scales, white circles surrounding both follicles and vessels are typically characterized by white color. In contrast to this, the poorly differentiated SCCs are characterized by the red color, they have more of a vascular pattern and the criteria associated with keratinization are often missing.

Case 11

Author: Papageorgiou Chryssoula

Clinical record:

Sex: 61

Age: Male

Clinical description the case or the lesion: Non-pigmented palpable lesion on the forehead surrounded by multiple solar lentigos.

Body site: Forehead

Surface: Palpable

Maximum diameter: 5 mm

Duration of the lesion: 2 months on the forehead (black circle)

History of morphologic changes: None

Personal history of skin cancer: None

Family history of skin cancer: None

Skin Phototype: II

Clinical diagnosis: Actinic keratosis

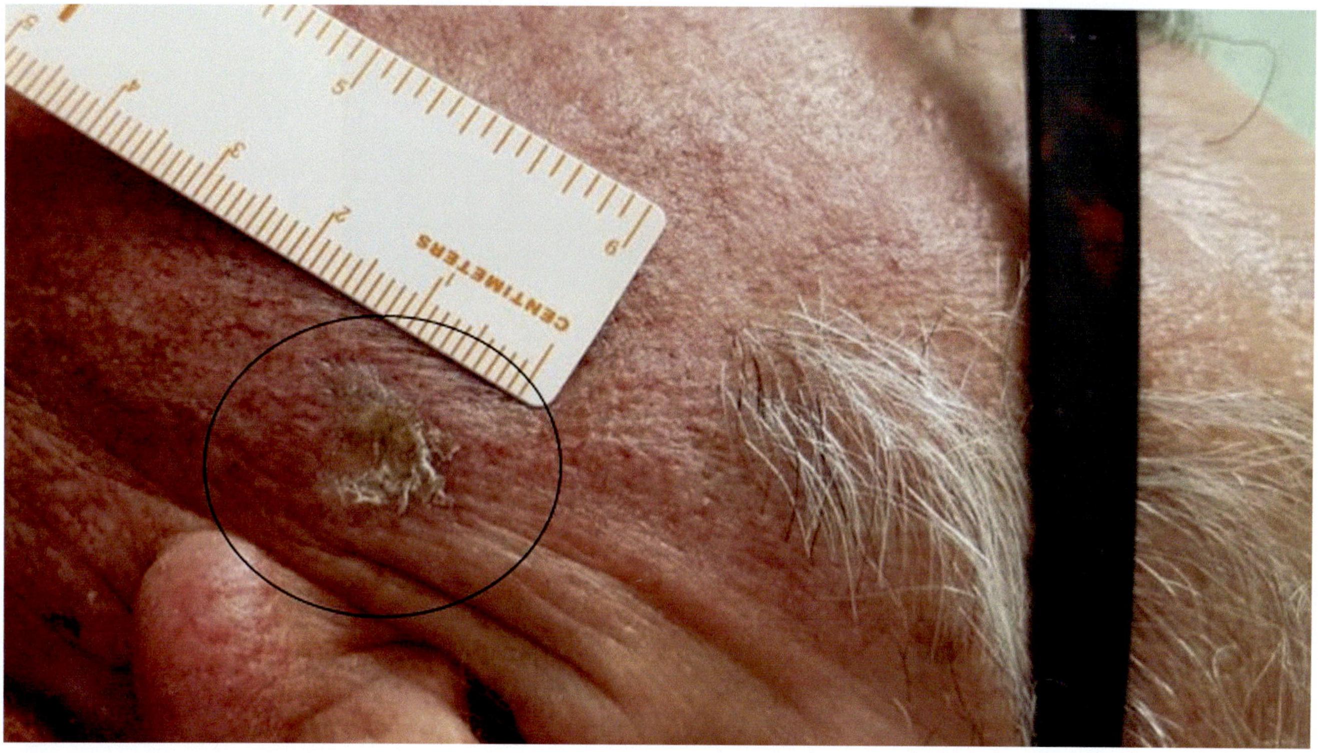

Fig. 24 Clinical image of a squamous cell carcinoma with an adherent crust on the surface

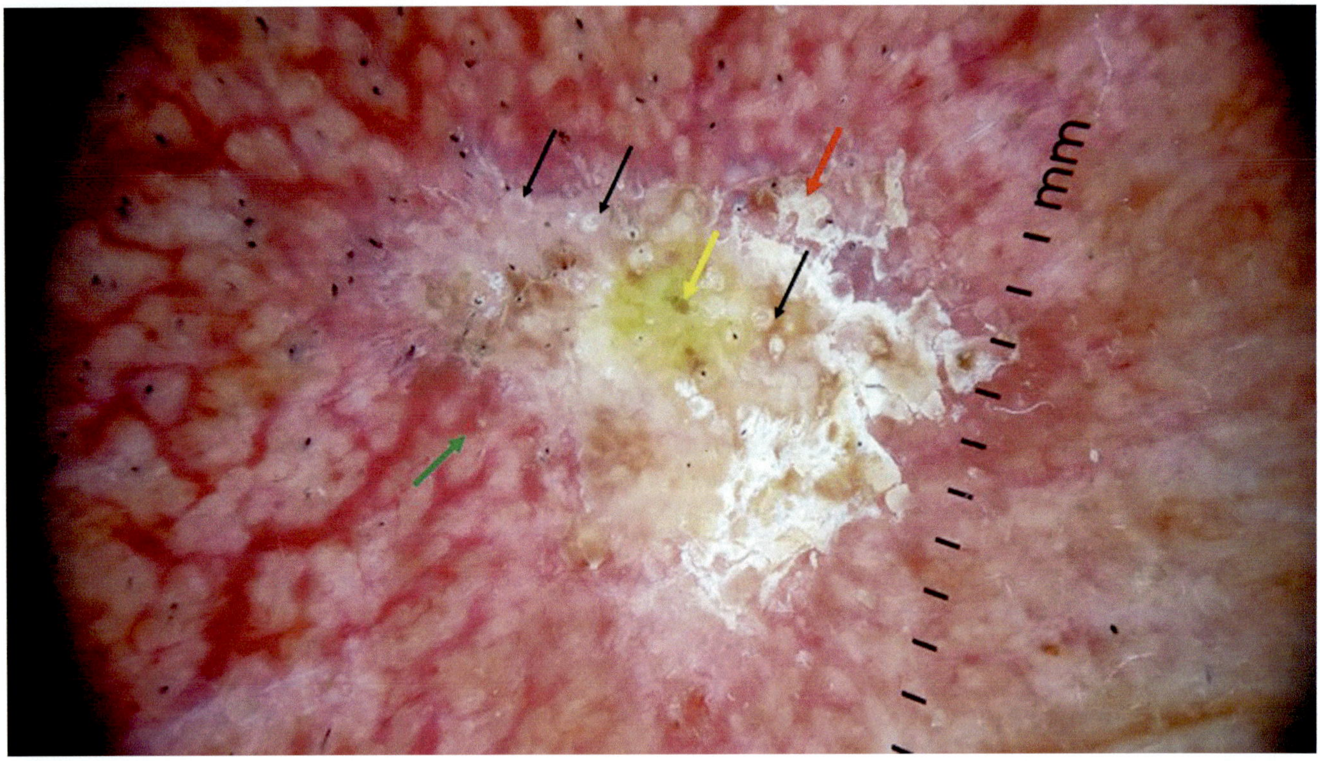

Fig. 25 Dermatoscopic image of a well-differentiated squamous cell carcinoma displaying white circles surrounding follicles (dark arrows); white-yellow scales (yellow arrow); white-yellow amorphous keratin mass (red arrow) and telangiectasia on sun damaged surrounding skin (green arrow)

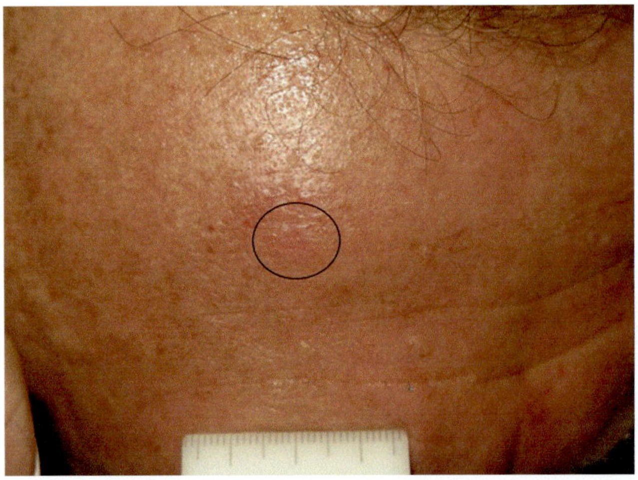

Fig. 26 On clinical examination, there is a symmetric, non-pigmented, erythematous plaque Sun damage with multiple solar lentigos on the surrounding skin is also observed

Dermoscopic findings: Multiple white circles surrounding follicles, shiny white streaks/ Squamous cell carcinoma arising on an actinic keratosis

Other clinical findings: None (Figs. 26 and 27)

Diagnosis: Squamous cell carcinoma arising on an actinic keratosis

Key message: White color in dermoscopy represents a sign of keratinization. In this case, white structures such as

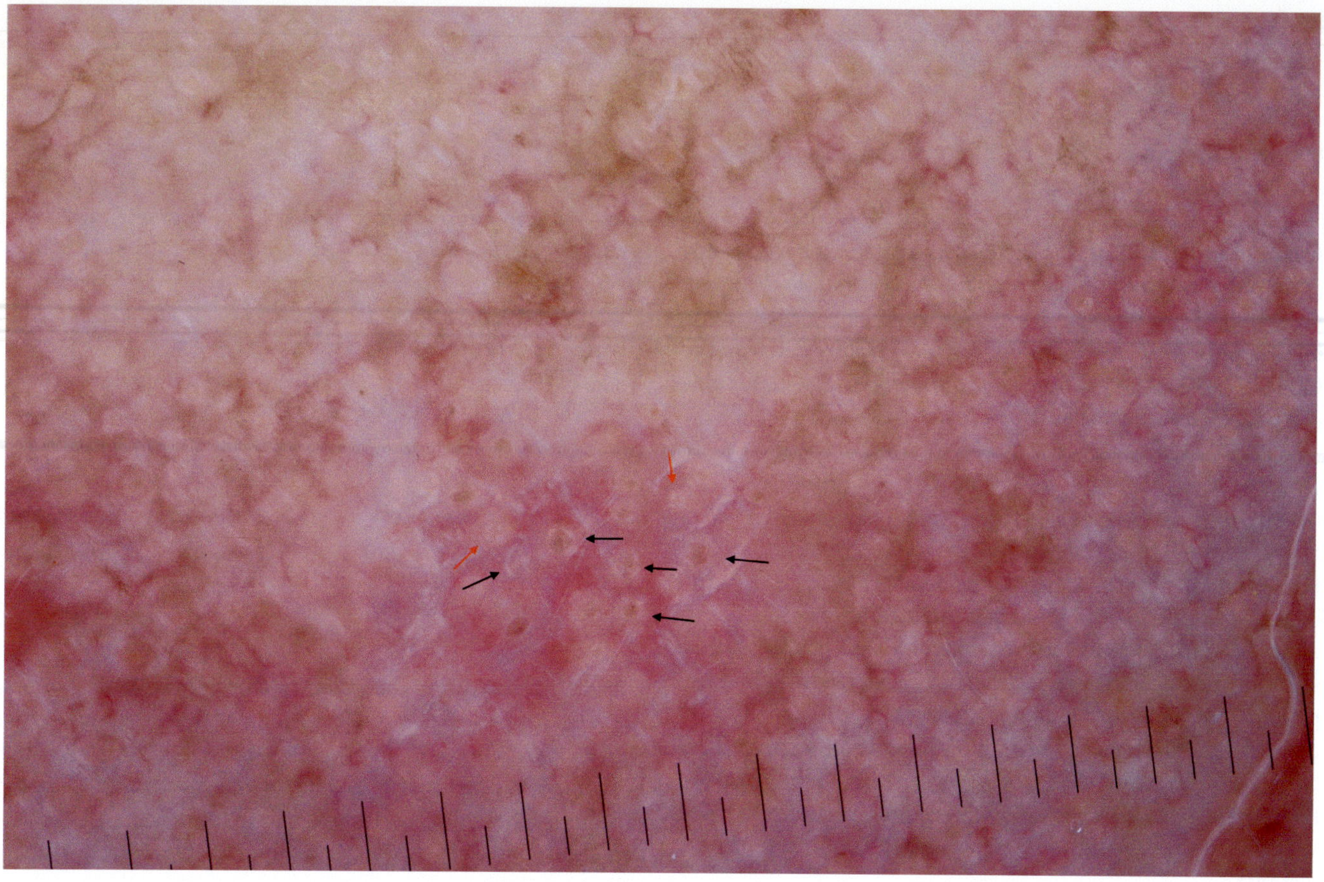

Fig. 27 Dermoscopy reveals few rosettes (red arrows) and multiple white circles surrounding follicles (black arrows). Multiple shiny white streaks are also observed

rosettes, white circles and shiny white streaks are present suggesting, thus, a keratinocytic tumor. Although rosettes are indicative of actinic keratosis, the concomitant presence of white circles around the follicles is highly suggestive of squamous cell carcinoma. The lesion proved to be a squamous cell carcinoma arising on an actinic keratosis after the histopathological examination highlighting, thus, that the presence of white circles is a strong predictor of squamous cell carcinoma.

Case 12

Author: Ružica Jurakić Tončić

Clinical record:

Sex: Female

Age: 30-years-old

Clinical description the case or the lesion: The patient has a dystrophic epidermolysis bullosa on the scalp and he is not sure when the lesion on the occipital area appeared

Body site: Scalp

Surface: flat and ulcerated

Maximum diameter: N/A

Duration of the lesion: Not known, but longstanding lesion, patient not sure about having since the ulcerations are part of the chronic course of the dystrophic epidermolysis bullosa

History of morphologic changes: Multiple non-healing ulcerations

Personal history of skin cancer: None

Family history of skin cancer: None

Skin Phototype: III

Clinical diagnosis: Poorly differentiated squamous cell carcinoma in dystrophic epidermolysis bullosa

Dermoscopic findings: Dermoscopically very worrisome picture due to the atypical presentation of multiple, irregular vessels. The background is reddish, some parts of the lesion expose pink or whitish regions, but no keratin scales due to the fact this is poorly differentiated squamous cell carcinoma (Figs. 28, 29, 30, 31 and 32)

Diagnosis: Poorly differentiated squamous cell carcinoma

Key message: Dermoscopy can be used as extremely useful diagnostic tool in differentiation of ulcerations and suspicious lesions in dystrophic epidemolysis patients since squamous cell carcinoma is the main cause of death in these patients. Dermoscopy should be regarded as useful tool in choosing the right place to make biopsy since ulcerations are commonly found as a part of clinical presentation. Making the diagnosis as early as possible is the major message and we cannot stress the importance of early diagnosis in these patients.

Case 13

Author: Theodosia Gkentsidi

Sex: Male

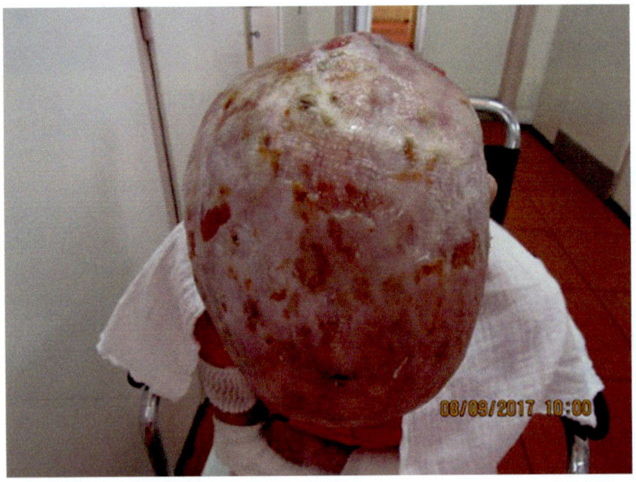

Fig. 28 Clinical aspect of the scalp shows multiple ulcerations covering the entire ski. Clinical diagnosis: dystrophic epidemolysis bullosa

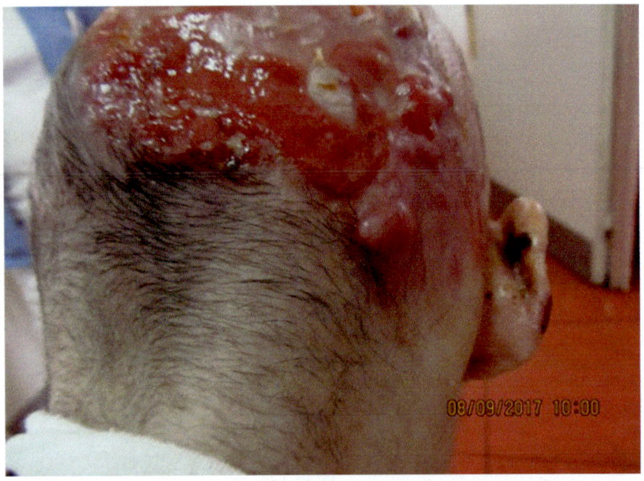

Fig. 29 Clinical view of the occipital area with a large and elevated red lesion

Age: 61

Clinical description the case or the lesion: Male patient, 61 years old, presents with a nodular lesion at his right cheek, which he first observed a year ago. The lesion has grown over the year and during the last month started bleeding. Clinically the lesion presents with central erosion and dotted vessels. Scales and pigmentation are not clinically observed.

Body site: Face

Surface: Nodular

Maximum diameter: 5 mm

Duration of the lesion: One year

History of morphologic changes: Lesion has grown over the last year, bleeding during the last month

Personal history of skin cancer: None

Family history of skin cancer: None

Skin Phototype: III

Clinical diagnosis: Seborrheic keratosis (sk), squamous cell carcinoma (scc)

Dermoscopic findings: Irritated seborrheic keratosis (isk) Dermatoscopy of the lesion revealed a diffuse regular vessel arrangement and white halos surrounding vessels covering the whole surface of the lesion. The type of the

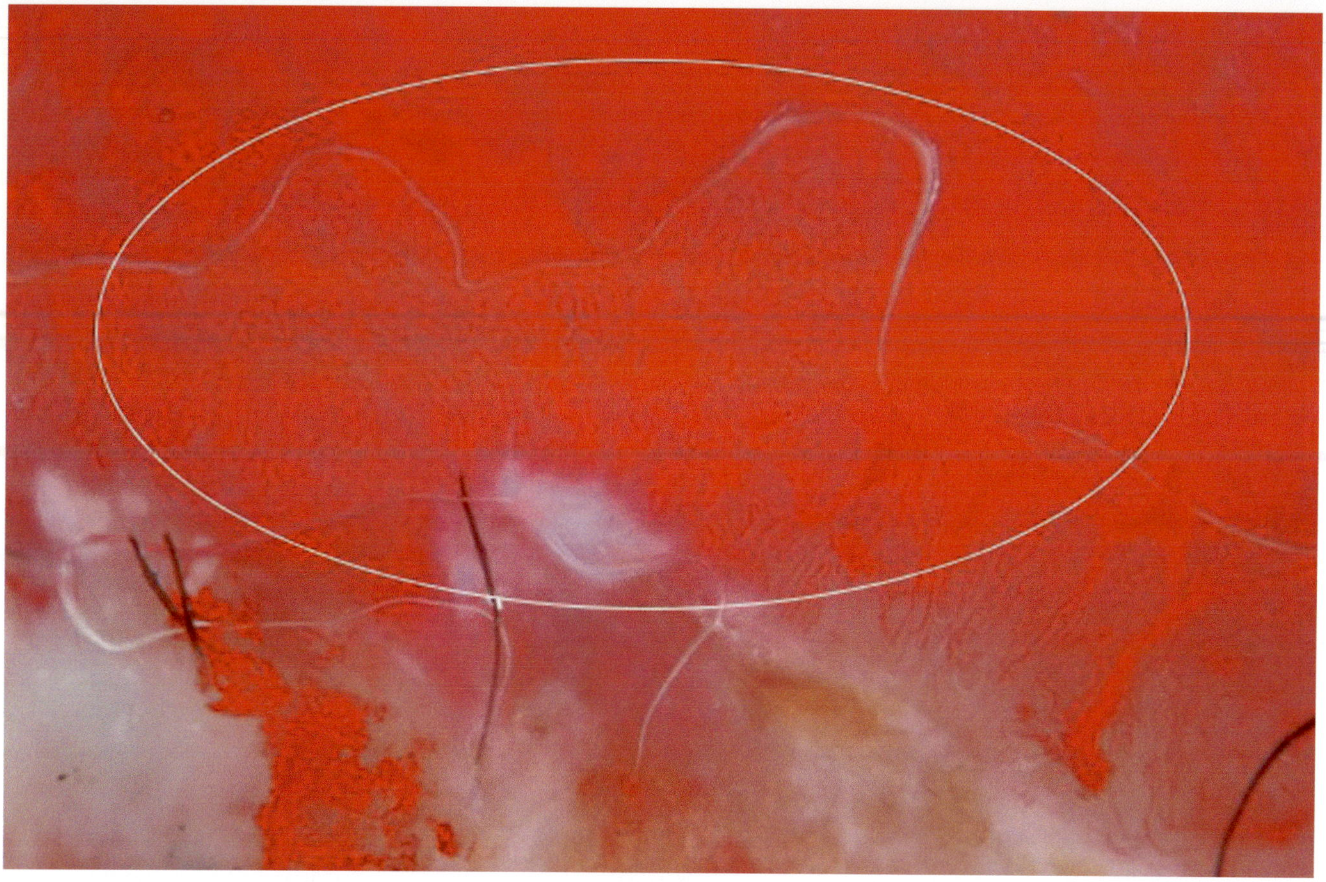

Fig. 30 Dermoscopic presentations showing atypical and morphologically abnormal vessels, red, pinkish and whitish background (white oval)

vessels is hairpin, dotted and glomerular. Central erosion is also observed. No scales, no rosettes, no white circles around the follicles and no white structureless areas were observed.

Other clinical findings: A few seborrheic keratosis on the face and back and three actinic keratosis on the scalp (Figs. 33 and 34)

Diagnosis: Seborrheic keratosis

Key message: A significant morphologic overlap between seborrheic keratosis and well differentiated scc does exist since both tumors display signs of keratinization and similar vessel types (hairpin and glomerular). A high number and a regular distribution of the vascular structures favor the diagnosis of seborrheic keratosis.

Case 14

Author: Gisela D'Atri

Clinical record:

Sex: Female

Age: 58-year-old

Clinical description: Hair thinning of the central scalp area, intermittent mild pruritus

Disease duration: 3 years

Pull test: Negative

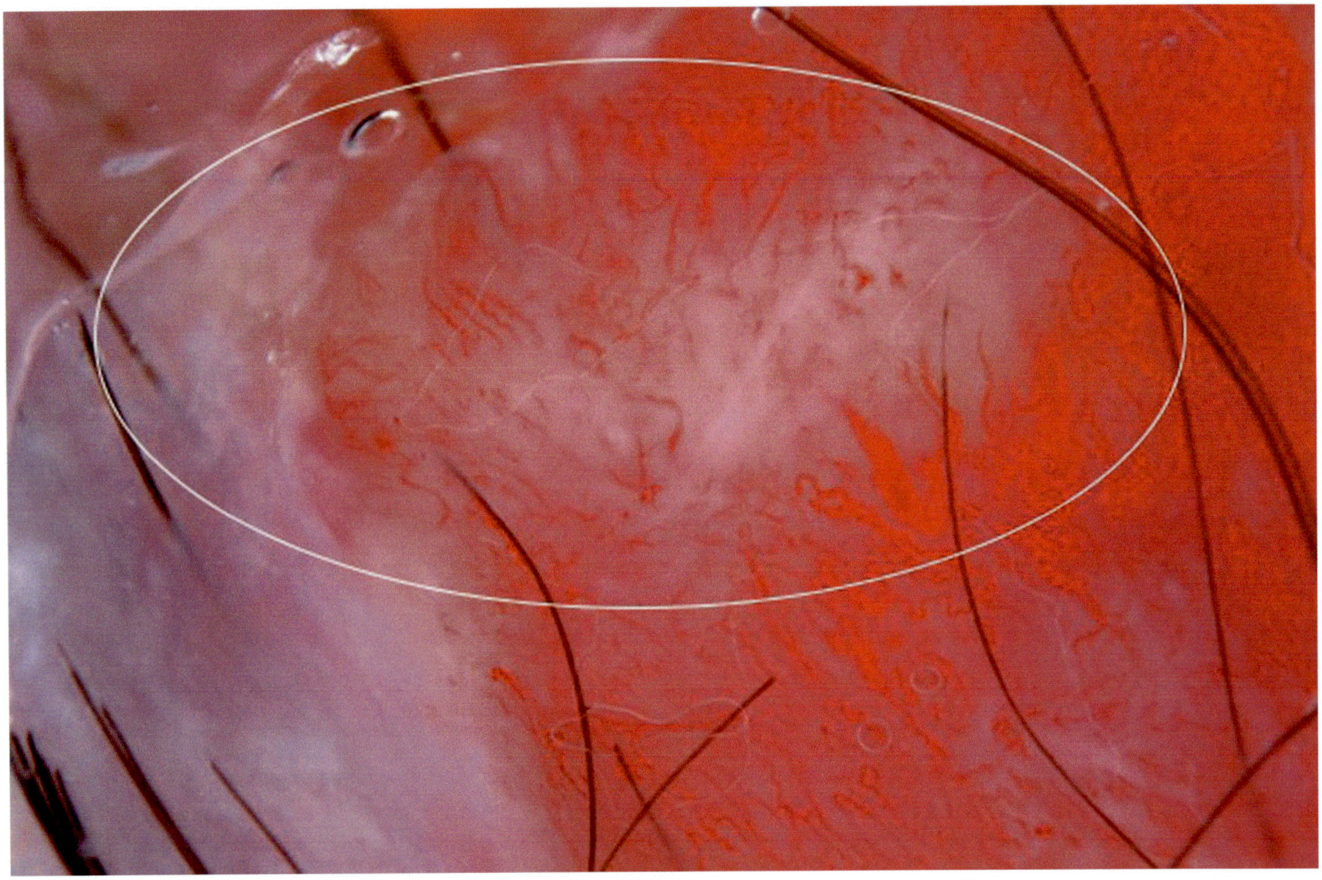

Fig. 31 Dermoscopic presentations showing atypical and morphologically abnormal vessels, red, pinkish and whitish background (white oval)

Personal history of alopecia (if yes please specify): No

Family history of alopecia (if yes please specify): Mother with female pattern hair loss

Clinical diagnosis: Female pattern hair loss

Other clinical findings: No

Dermoscopic findings: Fibrosing alopecia in a pattern distribution (Figs. 35, 36 and 37).

Diagnosis: Fibrosing alopecia in a pattern distribution

Key message: FADP is considered a peculiar variant of lichen planopilaris (LPP) that is hidden in the form of a pure androgenetic alopecia (AGA). It overlaps characteristics of both LPP and AGA. Lichen lesions are confined to androgen-dependent areas only, are subtle, and do not produce the typical alopecic patches of the classic form of LPP. In the predermoscopic era, this entity was not diagnosed and is not uncommon. That is why we recommend a dermoscopic examination in all AGA cases, since early diagnosis and timely treatment helps to reduce permanent hair loss.

Case 15

Author: Ilut Paula Anca

Clinical record:

Sex: Male

Age: 41-years-old

Clinical description the case or the lesion: Indurated lesion at the level of the vertex, on an area of androgenic alopecia, which shows a slight hyperpigmented edge and a more hypopigmented center

Body site: Scalp

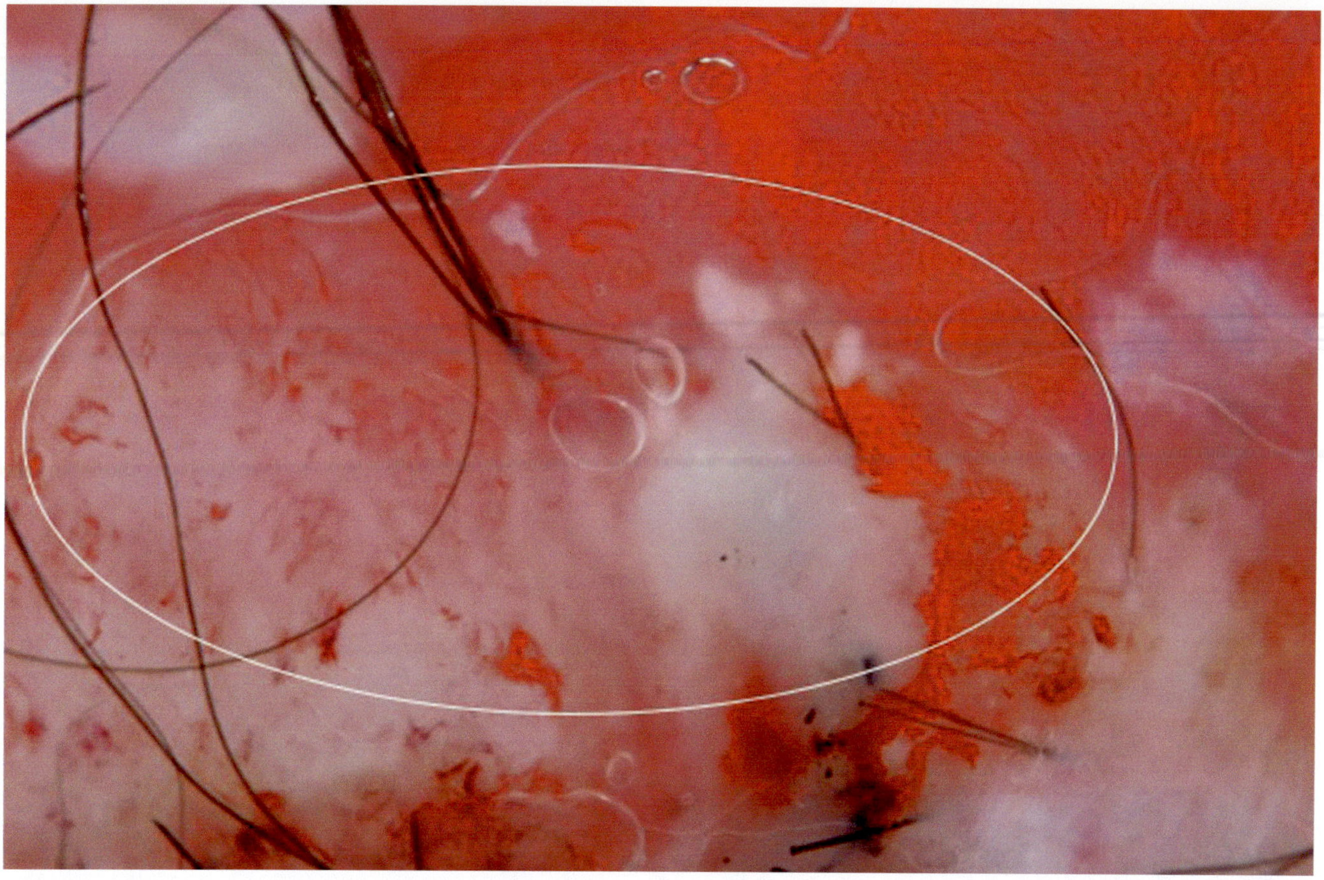

Fig. 32 Dermoscopic presentations showing atypical and morphologically abnormal vessels, red, pinkish and whitish background (white oval)

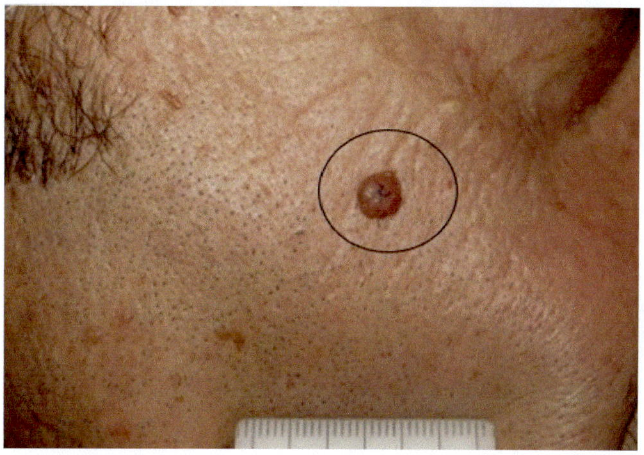

Fig. 33 Clinical image

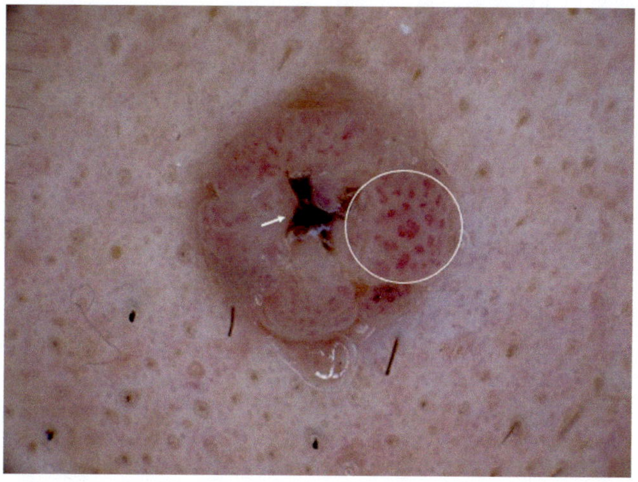

Fig. 34 **Dermatoscopic image:** diffuse regular vessel arrangement and white halos surrounding vessels covering the whole surface of the lesion

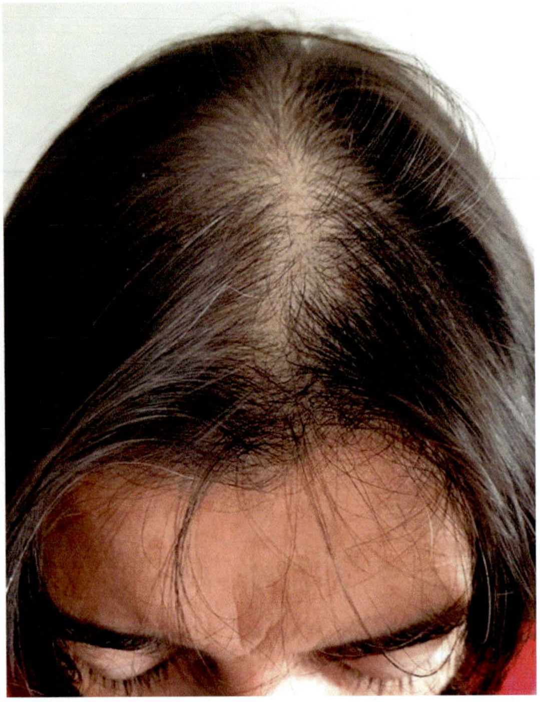

Fig. 35 Clinical image

Surface: Palpable

Maximum diameter: 0.8

Duration of the lesion: Unknown

History of morphologic changes: Unknown

Personal history of skin cancer: None

Family history of skin cancer: None

Skin Phototype: III

Clinical diagnosis: Clear Cell Acanthoma, Dermatofibroma, Adnexal tumor, Actinic Keratosios

Dermoscopic findings:

- dotted vessels arranged in a "string of pearls" surrounding follicular openings
- thin scales and a small erosion
- hyperpigmentation at the periphery

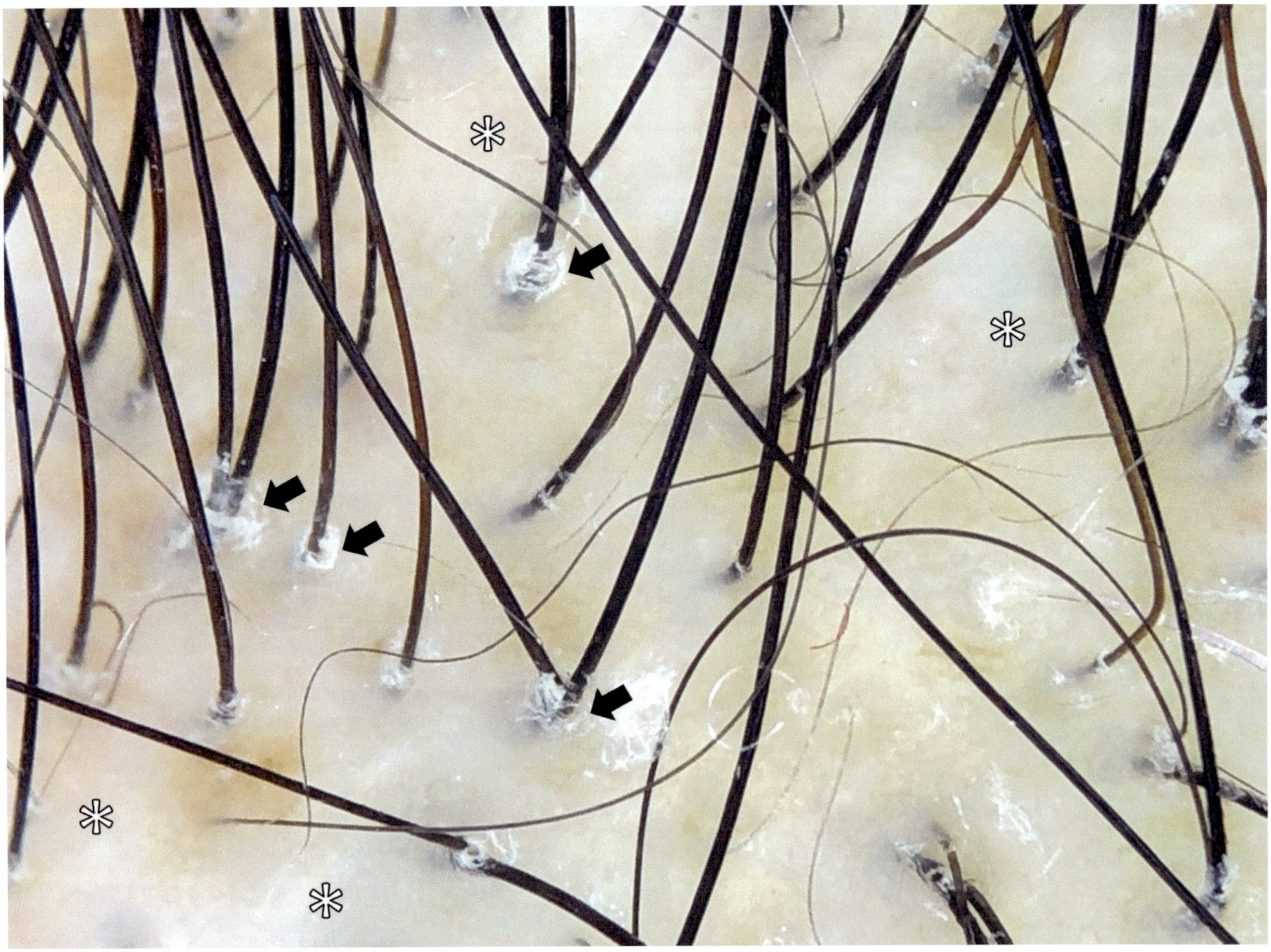

Fig. 36 Dermoscopy showing hair diameter diversity (anisotrichosis), multiple peripilar casts presenting as concentrically arranged layers of scales surrounding the hair shaft emergence with formation of tubular structures (arrows) and white areas with loss of follicular openings (asterisks)

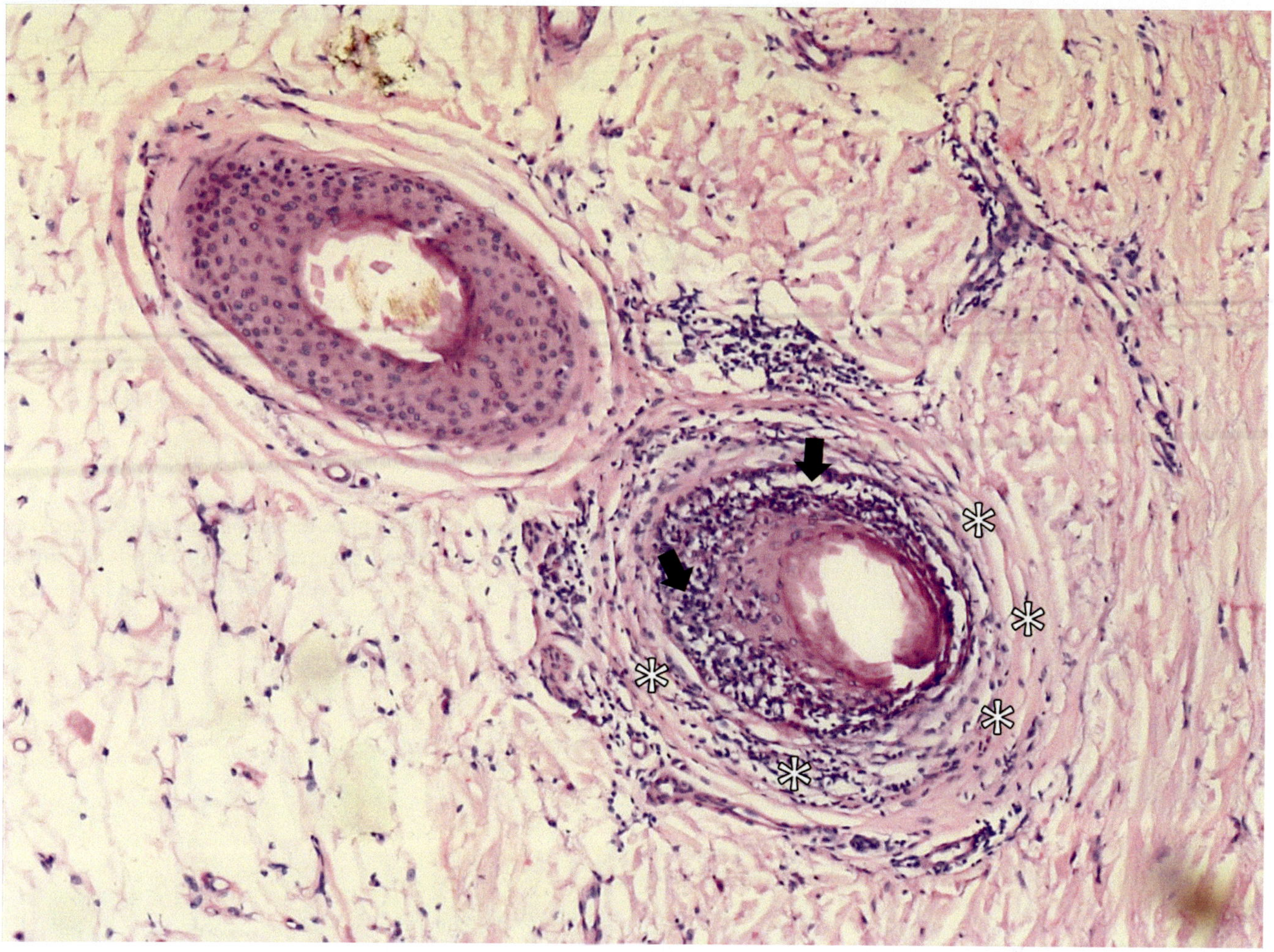

Fig. 37 Histopathologic examination showing hair follicle miniaturization and a lichenoid inflammatory infiltrate targeting the upper follicle region of the hair follicles (arrows) with perifollicular lamellar fibrosis (asterisks) supporting the diagnosis of fibrosing alopecia in a pattern distribution (FAPD)

Other clinical findings: None (Figs. 38 and 39)

Diagnosis: Clear cell acanthoma

Key message: Clear Cell Acanthoma is a benign tumor rarely seen on the scalp. The presence of dotted vessels arranged in a "string of pearls" is pathognomonic for this lesion.

Case 16

Author: Horacio Cabo

Sex: Male

Age: 65-years-old patient

Clinical description the case or the lesion: Asymptomatic nodular pink lesion on the forehead

Body site: Forehead

Surface: Nodular

Maximum diameter: 8 mm

Duration of the lesion: More than 8 months

History of morphologic changes: Growing

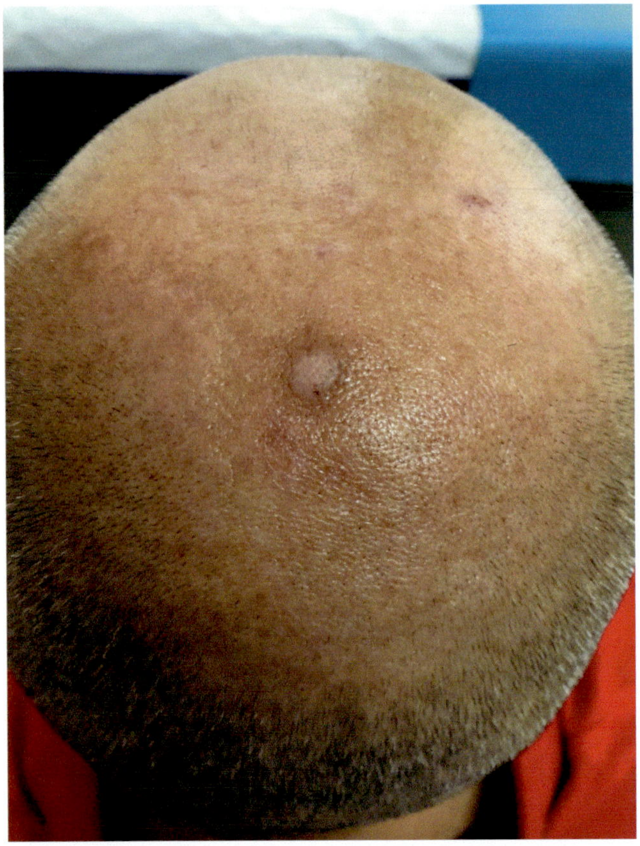

Fig. 38 Clinical image of a Clear Cell Acanthoma localized on the scalp that could be easily misdiagnosed as a dermatofibroma or a trichilemmoma

Personal history of skin cancer: Melanoma

Family history of skin cancer: No

Skin Phototype: III

Clinical diagnosis: Squamous cell Carcinoma, Basal cell carcinoma, Merkel Carcinoma

Dermoscopic findings: Central erosion, white areas, peripheral vessels

Other clinical findings: None (Figs. 40 and 41)

Diagnosis: Invasive Squamous Cell Carcinoma

Key message: Nodular pink lesion on the head & neck are difficult because many different lesions could be similar clinically. Dermatoscopy is very useful to arrive to the right diagnosis

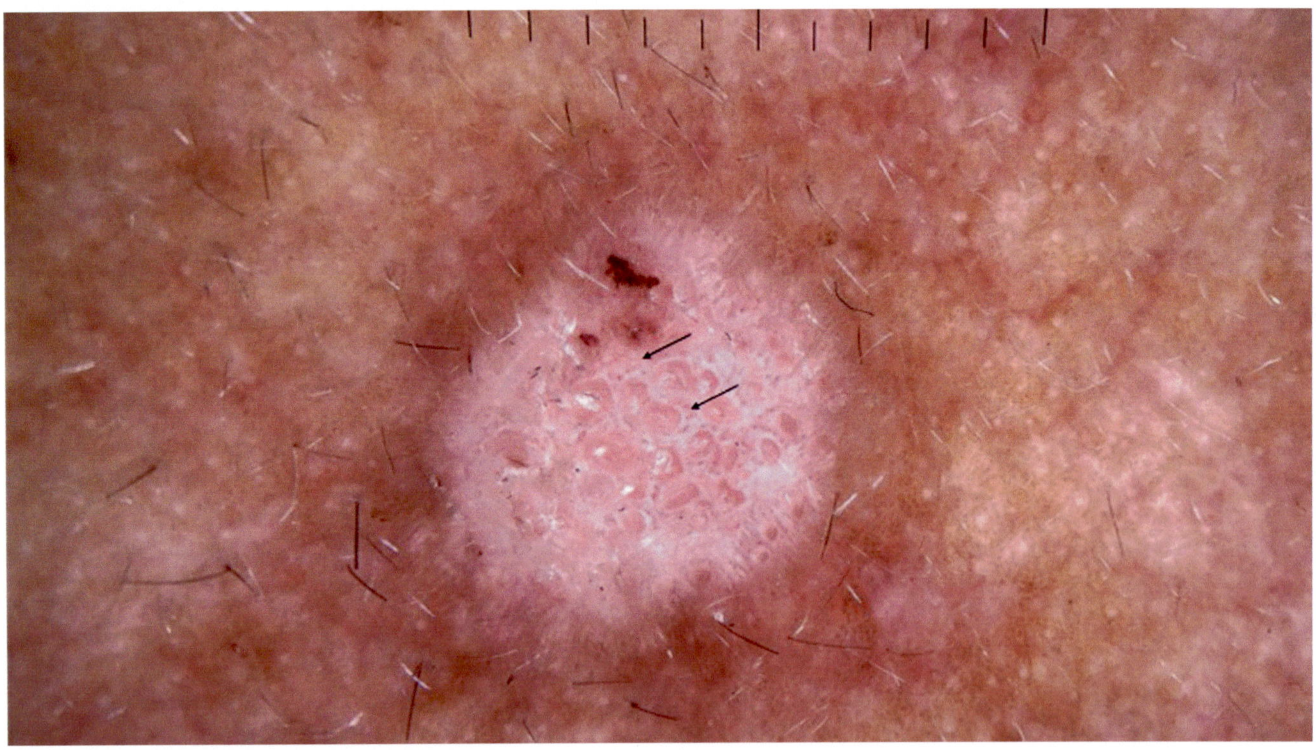

Fig. 39 Dermatoscopic image of a Clear Cell Acanthoma displaying dotted vessels that outline a linearly "string of pearls" arrangement that appear to surround follicular openings (Black arrows)

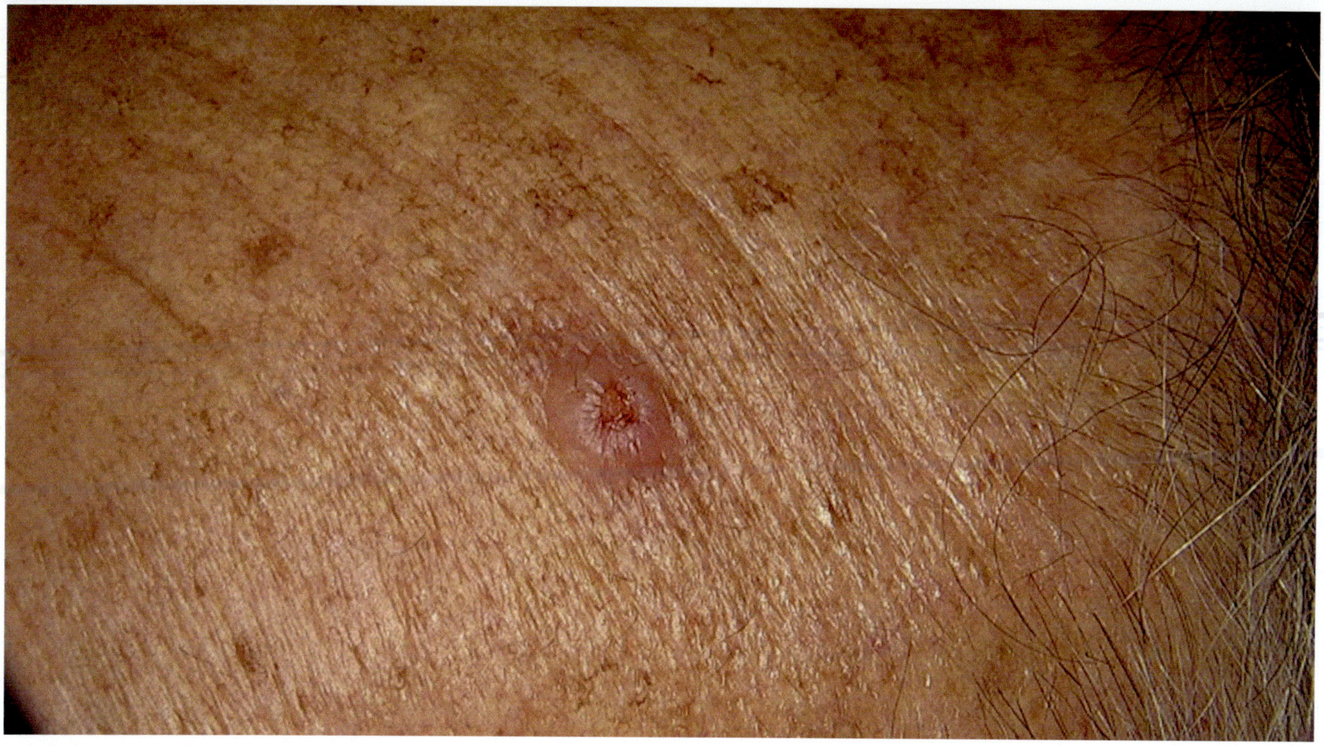

Fig. 40 Clinical view

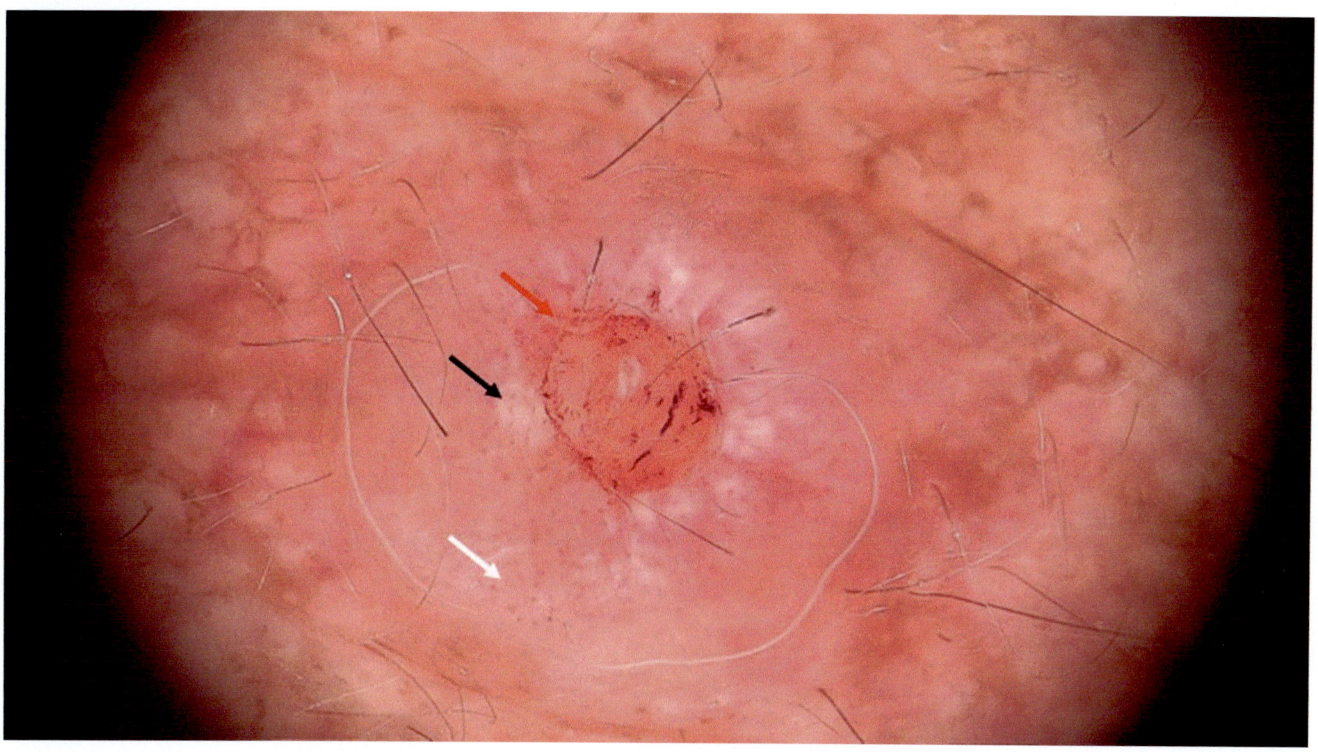

Fig. 41 Dermoscopic view: Central erosion (red arrow) white areas (black arrow) and peripheral vessels (white arrow)

Trunk Lesions

Ahmed Sadek, Emilia Noemi Cohen Sabban, Horacio Cabo, Enzo Errichetti, Dominga Peirano, Sebastian Vargas, Alvaro Abarzua, Cristian Navarrete Dechent, Pablo Uribe, Verche Todorovska, Pedro Zaballos, John Paoli, Elvira Moscarella, Juan Sebastian Andreani Figueroa, Jelena Stojkovic Filipovic, Dusan Skiljevic, Guiseppe Micali, Ana Elisa Verzi, Livia Liguori, Roger Gonzalez Ramirez, Maria Sofia Nicoletti Russi, Ricardo Quiñones Venegas, and Deyamira Gabriela Quiñones Hernandez

Abstract

Different nonpigmented skin lesion in trunk area such as Extra Genital Lichen Sclerosis et Atrophicus, Lichen planus, Basal cell carcinoma, MAY globules, Invasive Squamous Cell Carcinoma, Fibroephitelioma of Pinkus, Hypomelanotic melanoma, Collision lesions, Bowen disease, Molluscum contagiosum, Lynmphangioma, Clear Cell Acanthoma, Paget's disease are described. The main dermoscopic characteristics of these pink lesions are mentioned.

Keywords

Extra Genital Lichen Sclerosis et Atrophicus • Lichen planus • Basal cell carcinoma • MAY globules • Invasive Squamous Cell Carcinoma • Fibroephitelioma of Pinkus • Hypomelanotic melanoma • Collision lesions • Bowen disease • Molluscum contagiosum • Lynmphangioma • Clear Cell Acanthoma • Paget's disease

A. Sadek
Dr. Sadek Clinics: 5 Lateef Pasha Selim, Off Al-Nozha St., Heliopolis, Cairo, 11341, Egypt

E. N. Cohen Sabban
Chief of Dermatology Division of the "Instituto de Investigaciones Médicas A. Lanari", University of Buenos Aires, Arenales 1446 1 °C, Buenos Aires, Argentina

H. Cabo (✉)
Clinical Dermatology, University of Buenos Aires, Arenales 1446 1 °C (1061) CABA, Buenos Aires, Arenales, Argentina
e-mail: cabohoracio@gmail.com

E. Errichetti
Institue of Dermatology, "S. Maria della Misericordia", University Hospital, Udine, Italy

D. Peirano · S. Vargas · A. Abarzua · C. Navarrete Dechent · P. Uribe
Department of Dermatology, Escuela de Medicina, Escuela de Medicina, Pontificia Universidad Católica de Chile, Diagonal Paraguay 362, 6th floor, Santiago, Chile
e-mail: dpeirano@miuandes.cl

S. Vargas
e-mail: sivargas@uc.cl

V. Todorovska
Private Practice, Skopje, Macedonia

P. Zaballos
Dermatology Department, Hospital Sany Pau i Santa Tecla, Tarragona, Spain
e-mail: PZaballos@aedv.es

J. Paoli
Department of Dermatology and Venereology, Institute of Clinical Sciences, Sahlgrenska Academy, University of Gothenburg, Gothenburg, Sweden
e-mail: john.paoli@vgregion.se

E. Moscarella
Dermatologo Ricercatore RTD A, Dip. L.240/2010
SALUTE MENTALE E FISICA E MEDICINA PREVENTIVA, Università degli studi della Campania Luigi Vanvitelli, Naples, Italy

J. S. A. Figueroa
Dermatology Department, Facultad de Medicina Clínica Alemana, Universidad del Desarrollo, Santiago, Region Metropolitana, Chile

J. Stojkovic Filipovic · D. Skiljevic
Clinic of Dermatovenereology, University Clinical Center of Serbia, Medical Faculty, University of Belgrade, Pasterova 2, Belgrade, Serbia

G. Micali · A. E. Verzi · L. Liguori
Dermatology Clinic, University of Catania, Via Santa Sofia, 78, 95123 Catania, Italy

H. Cabo and A. Lallas (eds.), *Dermatoscopic Atlas of Non-Pigmented Lesions*,
https://doi.org/10.1007/978-3-031-34310-0_4

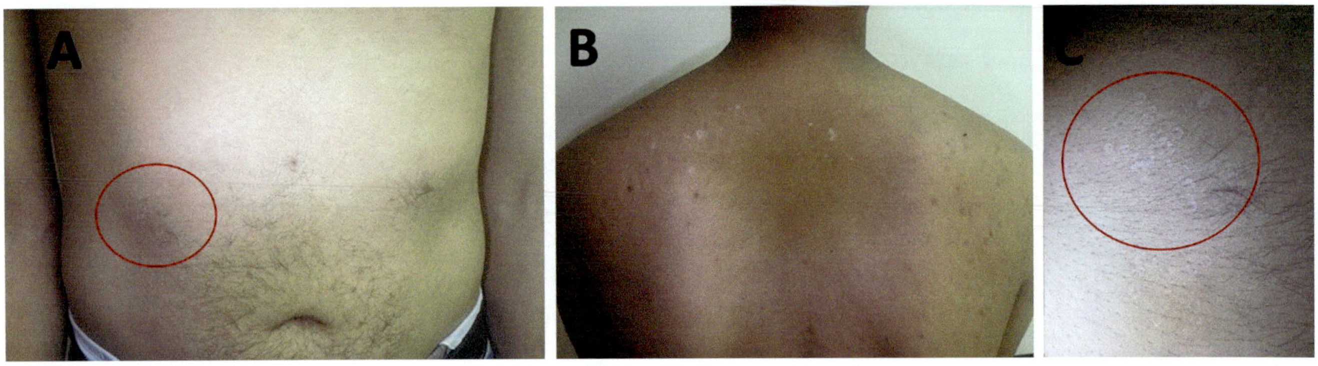

Fig. 1 A) Clinical Image of The Abdomen, B) Clinical Image of the Shoulders, C) Macro Clinical Image of the Abdomen

Case 1

Author: Ahmed Sadek

Clinical record:

Sex: Male

Age: 26

Clinical description the case or the lesion: Hypopigmented macules of the abdomen, shoulders and back

Body site: Trunk

Surface: Flat, Slightly Atrophic

Maximum diameter: 4 mm

Duration of the lesion: 1 year

History of morphologic changes: Hypopigmented Slowly Progressive Macules of the Abdomen, Shoulders & Back

Personal history of skin cancer: None

Family history of skin cancer: None

Skin Phototype: IV

Clinical diagnosis: Pityriasis Versicolor or Vitiligo

Dermoscopic findings: Extra Genital Lichen Sclerosis et Atrophicus. Diffuse Hypopigmentation, Loss of reticular pigment network, Faint follicular Plugs

Other clinical findings: None (Figs. 1, 2, 3 and 4)

Diagnosis: Extra Genital Lichen Sclerosis et Atrophicus

Key message: Assess all hypopigmented lesions thoroughly

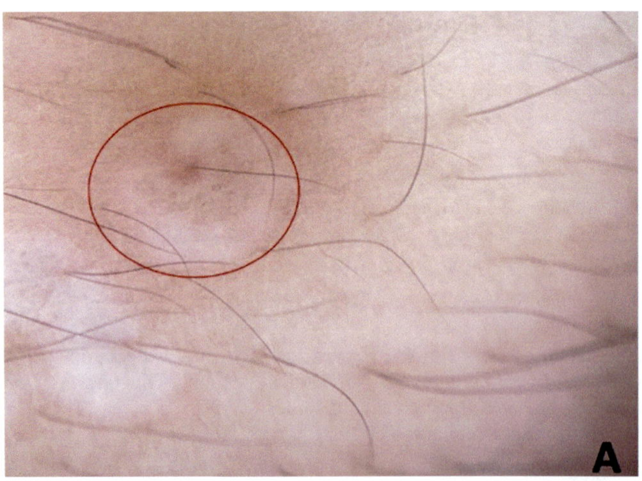

Fig. 2 Polarized Contact Dermoscopic Image of the Abdomen, A) 10x Diffuse Hypopigmentation, Loss of reticular pigment network, Faint follicular Plugs (red circle)

R. G. Ramirez
Departamento de Introducción a la Clínica, Facultad de Medicina, Universidad Autónoma de Nuevo León, San Nicolás de los Garza, México

M. S. N. Russi
Departamento de Dermatologia Hospital Britanico, Montevideo, Uruguay

R. Q. Venegas · D. G. Q. Hernandez
Instituto Dermatológico de Jalisco "Dr. José Barba Rubio", Avenida Federalismo Norte 3102, Atemajac del Valle, CP, Zapopan, Jalisco, México

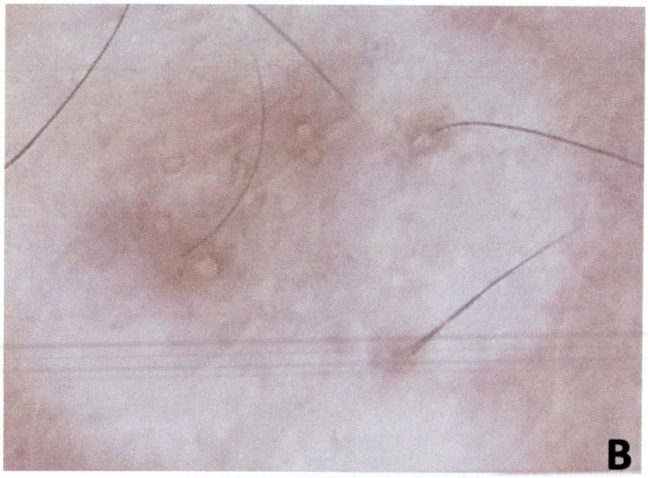

Fig. 3 Polarized Contact Dermoscopic Image of the Abdomen, B) 30x Diffuse Hypopigmentation, Loss of reticular pigment network, Faint follicular Plugs

Case 2

Authors: Emilia Noemi Cohen Sabban; Horacio Cabo

Clinical record:

Sex: Female

Age: 68-years-old

Clinical description the case or the lesion: Multiple whitish papules and plaques, with rough surface. Asymptomatic

Body site: Trunk

Surface: Palpable

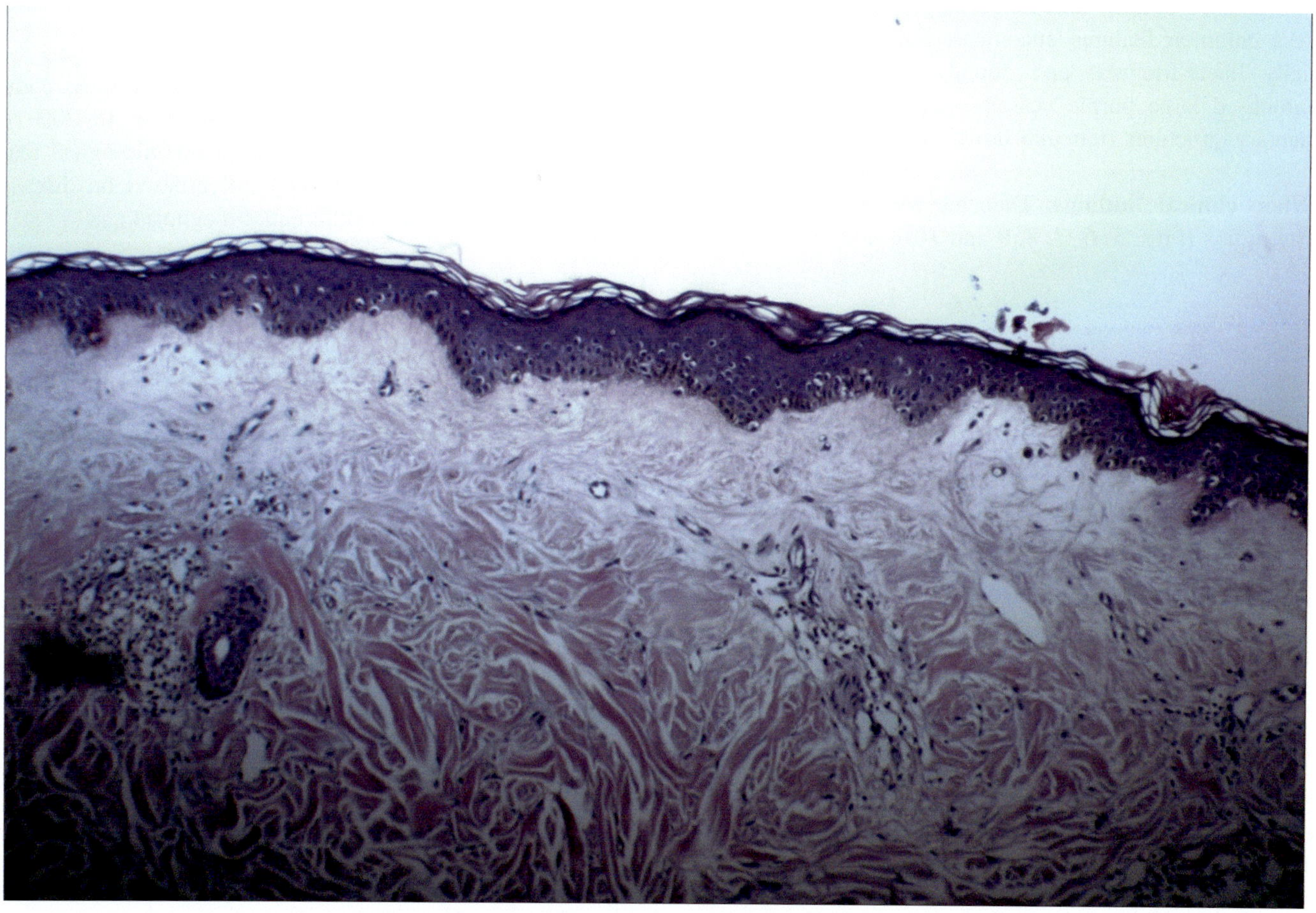

Fig. 4 Histopathological Image of H&E section (10x) taken by Dermoscopy Guided Punch Biopsy from the Abdominal Lesions showing epidermal loss of rete ridges with focal vacuolar alteration of basal cell layer, oedema and homogenization of the collagen, little perivascular lymphocytic Infiltrate with blood vessels set at lower than usual level

Maximum diameter: Lesion size is about 2 to 3 cm each

Duration of the lesion: 5 years

History of morphologic changes: Yes

Personal history of skin cancer: BCC on the dorsum of the noise

Family history of skin cancer: None

Skin Phototype: II-III

Clinical diagnosis: Extragenital Lichen sclerosus

Dermoscopic findings: The hallmark of dermoscopic findings of lichen sclerosus are well-defined, bright white patches, resulting from superficial fibrosis, and keratotic follicular plugs, corresponding to follicular hyperkeratosis. Additionally scaling and hemorrhagic spots can be seen. Less common features encompass focused vessels (especially linear-irregular and dotted), crystalline structures, unfocused large purple vessels, yellowish areas, and pigmentary structures (reticular brown areas and brown dots).

Other clinical findings: Diabetes Mellitus, Hashimoto's Thyroiditis (Figs. 5, 6, 7, 8, 9 and 10)

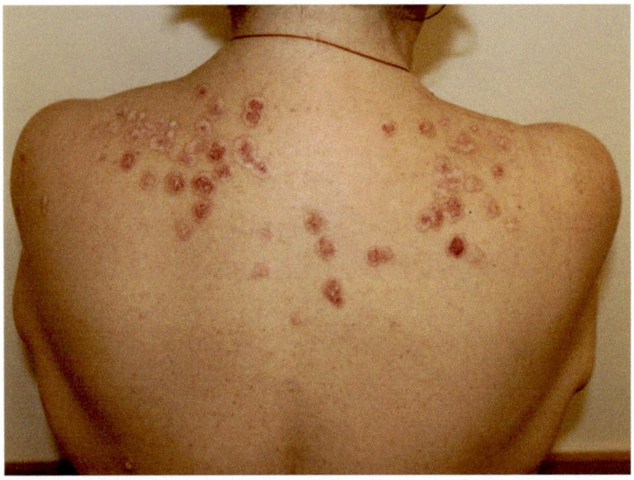

Fig. 5 Clinical view: Multiple patches of lichen sclerosus on the dorsum

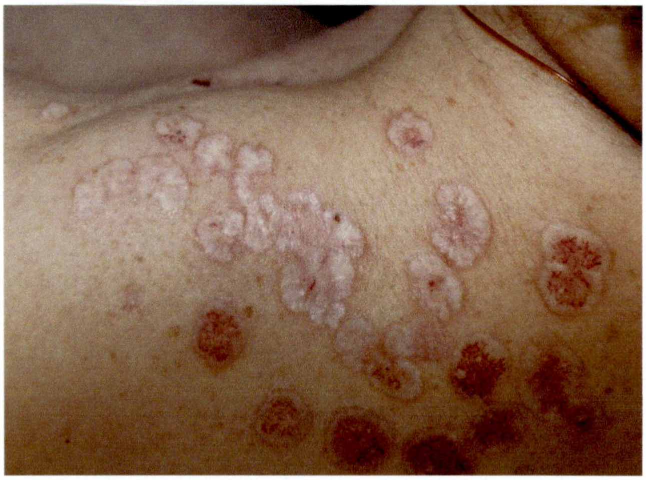

Fig. 6 A close up of the clinical view: Plaques with erythematous border and atrophic center. Some of them show hemorrhagic crusts and scales on their surface

Diagnosis: Extragenital Lichen sclerosus

Key message: Extragenital Lichen sclerosus is a less common variant of Lichen sclerosus, accounting for 15–20% of the cases. Clinical, dermoscopic and histopathological features are well described, but they differ based on disease stage. Morphea is it main differential diagnosis.

Case 3

Author: Enzo Errichetti

Clinical record:

Sex: Male

Age: 67

Clinical description the case or the lesion: Two asymptomatic purple patches

Body site: Back

Surface: Slightly palpable

Maximum diameter: 18 mm (large lesions)

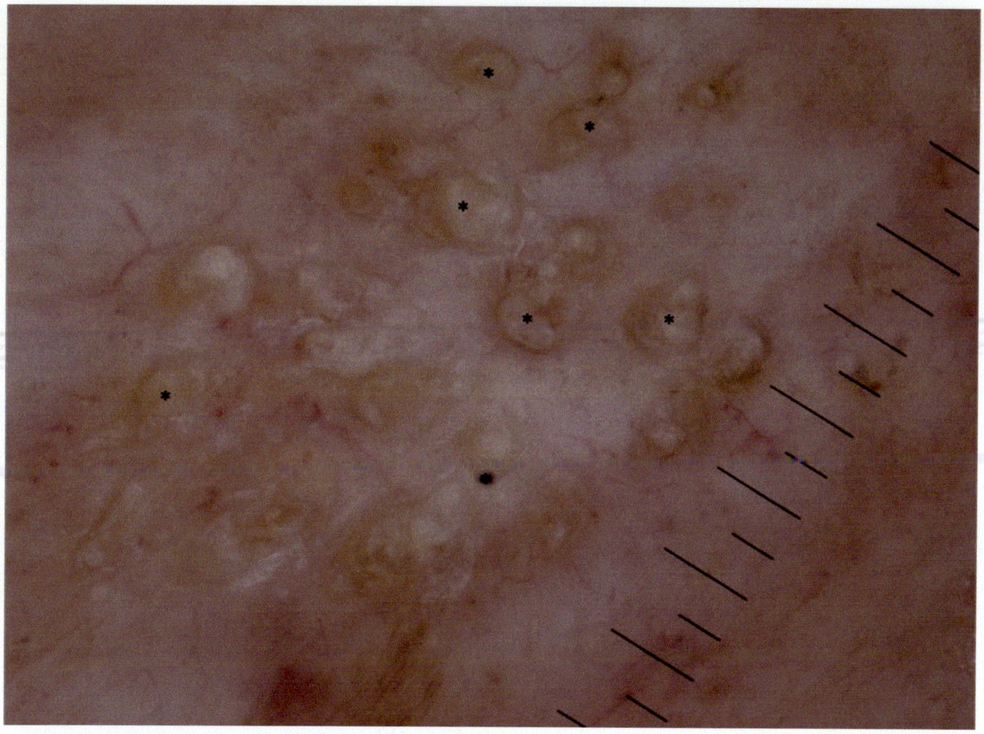

Fig. 7 Non-polarized light *Keratotic follicular plugs

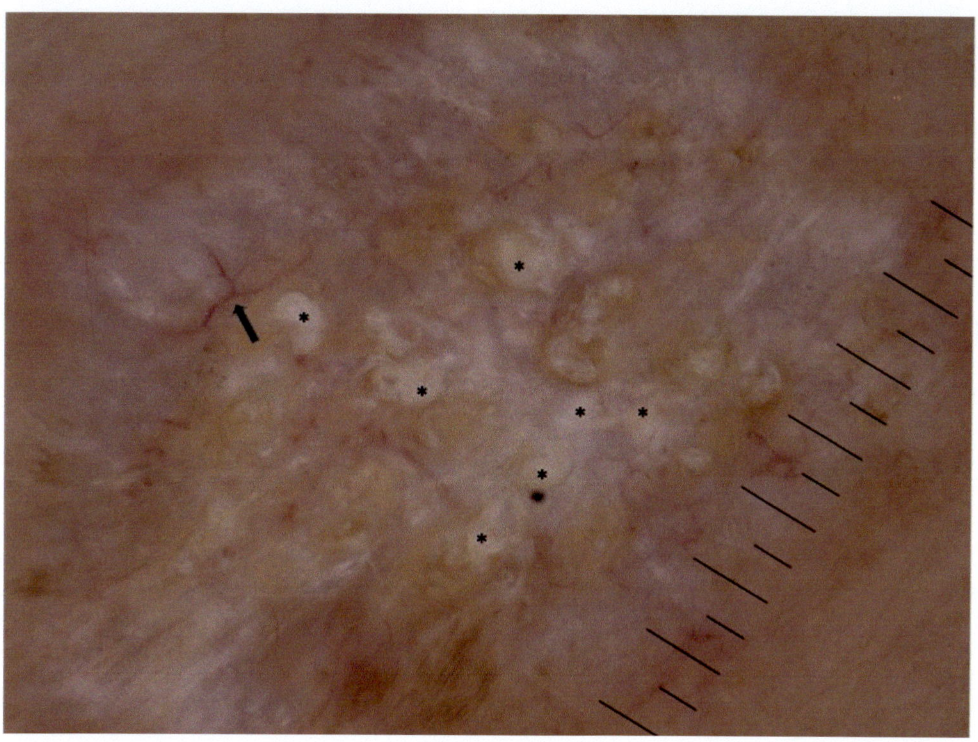

Fig. 8 Polarized light * Well-defined, bright white patches. Linear vessels (black arrow)

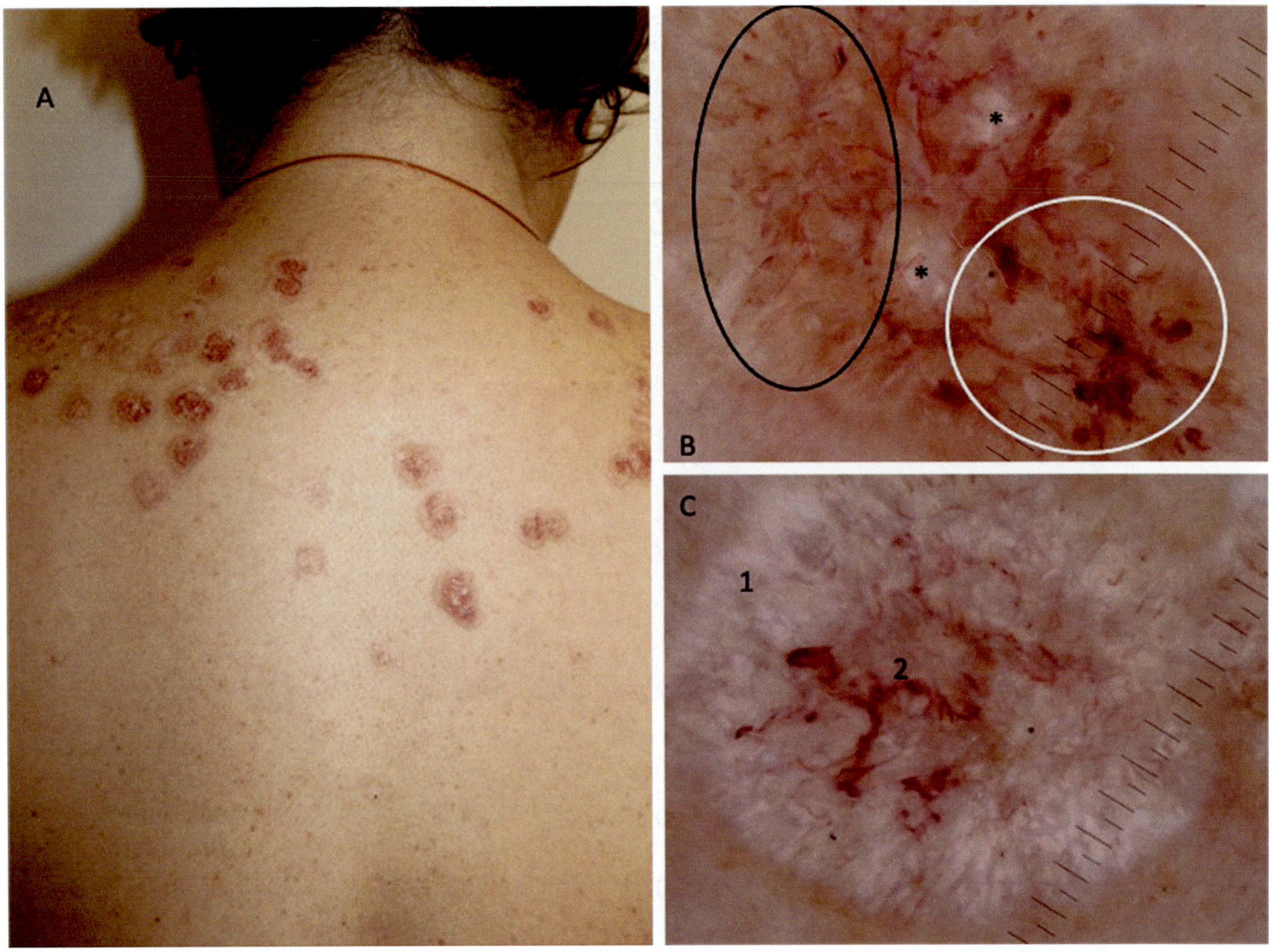

Fig. 9 **A** Clinical view: Multiple plaques, some are bright and atrophic; and others show hemorrhagic spots. **B** Polarized light. White bright structures (*), linear irregular vessels (black oval) and hemorrhagic spots (white circle). **C** Non-polarized light. White bright structures at the periphery(1); multiple vessels, hemorrhagic spots and pigmented structureless areas at the center (2)

Duration of the lesion: 3 months

History of morphologic changes: Stable

Personal history of skin cancer: No

Family history of skin cancer: No

Skin Phototype: III

Clinical diagnosis: Kaposi sarcoma

Dermoscopic findings: Lichen planus; crossing white lines (Wickham striae) and patchy dotted vessels over a brown background

Other clinical findings: None (Figs. 11 and 12)

Diagnosis: Lichen planus

Key message: Lichen planus may manifest with unspecific clinical presentation, yet dermoscopy features the characteristic white crossing lines (Wickham striae) histologically corresponding to a peculiar finding, that is hypergranulosis.

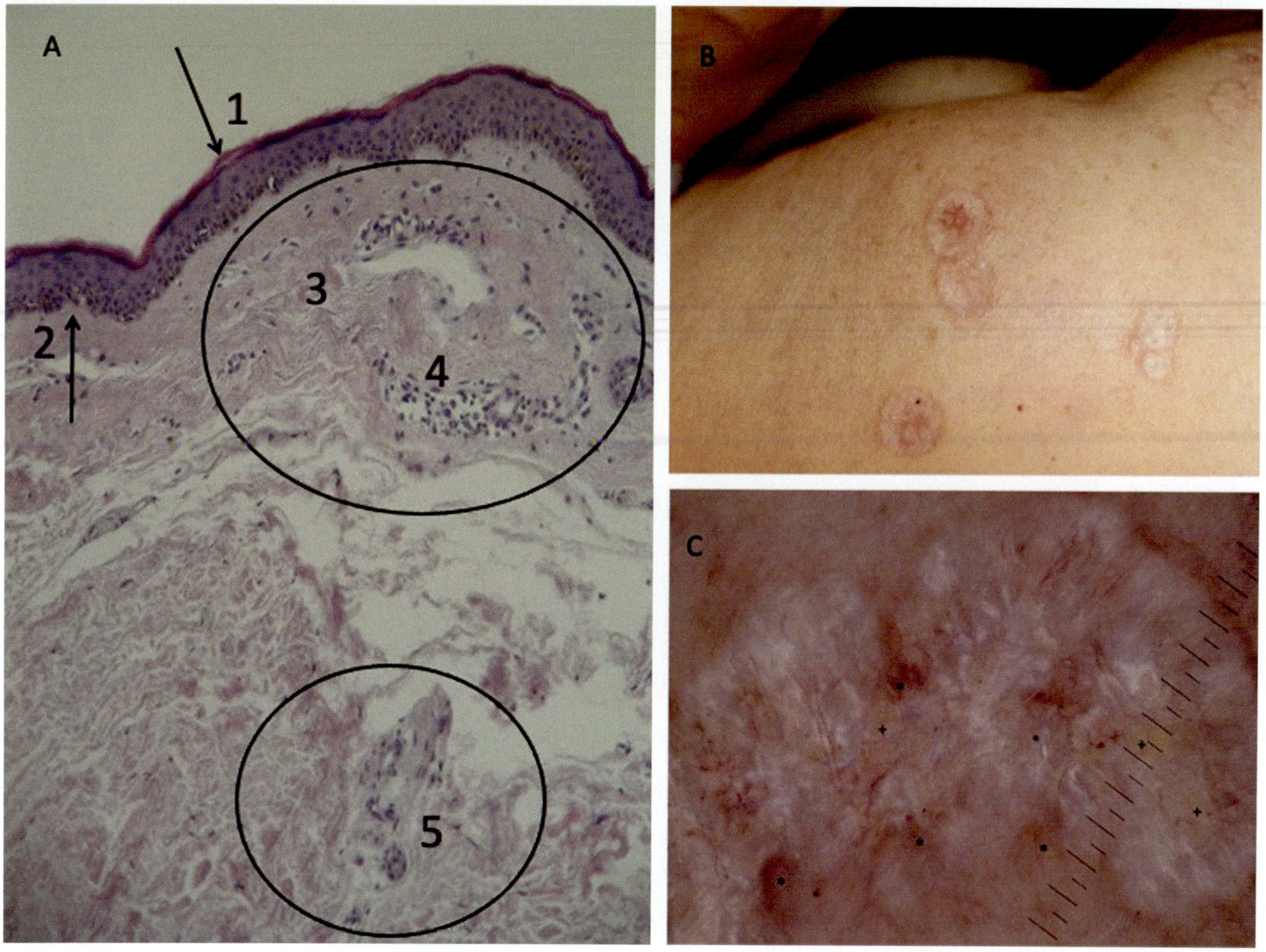

Fig. 10 A Histopathology: 1 Hyperkeratosis. 2 Rete ridges flattening 3 hyalinization and homogenization of collagen fibers (sclerosis) 4 lymphocytic infiltrate in the upper dermis in a perivascular distribution 5 Skin appendages are not involved. **B** Clinical View; **C** Polarized light. Bright white structures. Linear and irregular vessels. Pigmented areas (*); Yellowish areas (+)

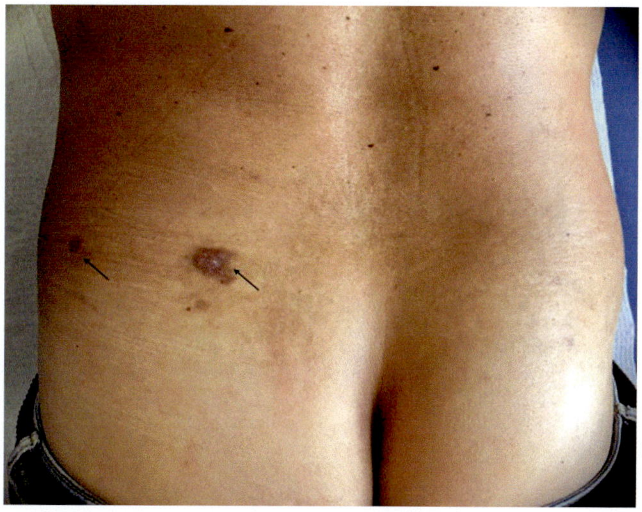

Fig. 11 Clinical examination shows two purple patches of the back (black arrow)

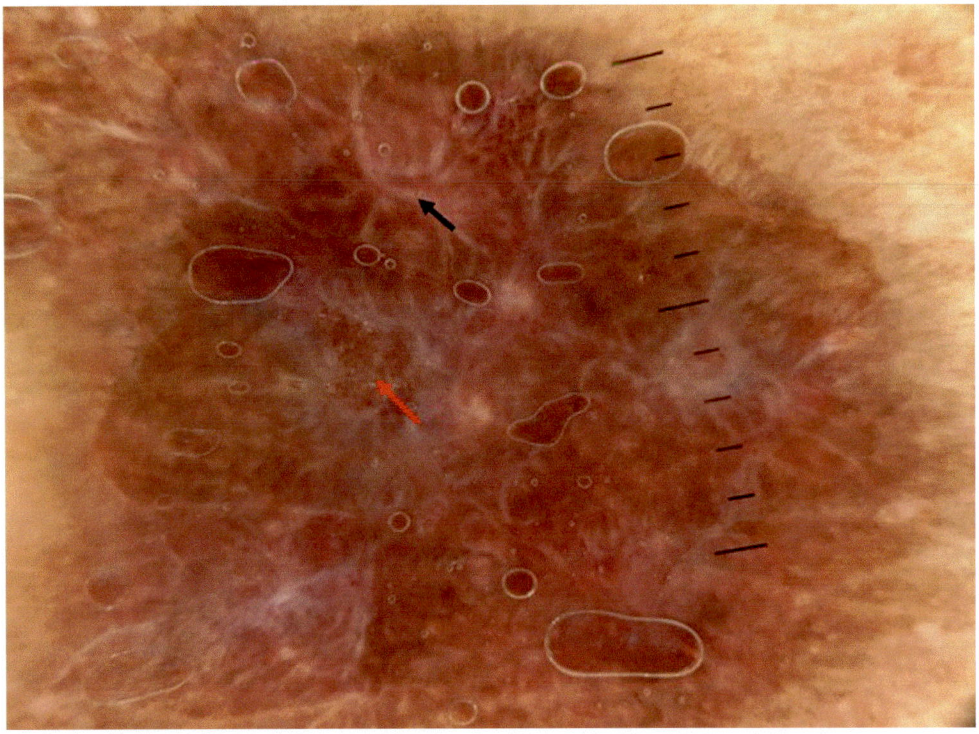

Fig. 12 Dermoscopic examination (10x magnification) displays crossing white lines (Wickham striae) (black arrow) and patchy dotted vessels over a brown background (red arrow)

Case 4

Authors: Dominga Peirano, Sebastián Vargas, Álvaro Abarzúa, Cristián Navarrete Dechent, Pablo Uribe

Clinical record:

Sex: Male

Age: 71 years-old

Clinical description of the case or the lesion: Asymptomatic small pink papule on the abdomen, without history of bleeding or ulceration.

Body site: Right upper quadrant of abdomen

Surface: Palpable

Maximum diameter: 1 cm

Duration of the lesion: Unknown

History of morphologic changes: No history of changes, bleeding or ulceration

Personal history of skin cancer: Yes, Basal cell carcinoma

Family History of Skin Cancer

Skin Phototype: II

Clinical diagnosis: Basal Cell Carcinoma

Dermoscopic findings: Multiple arborizing vessels and in-focus vessels, with shiny white structures on polarized dermoscopy, and the presence of Multiple Aggregated Yellow-white (MAY) globules, highly suggestive of basal cell carcinoma.

Other clinical findings: None (Figs. 13, 14, 15 and 16)

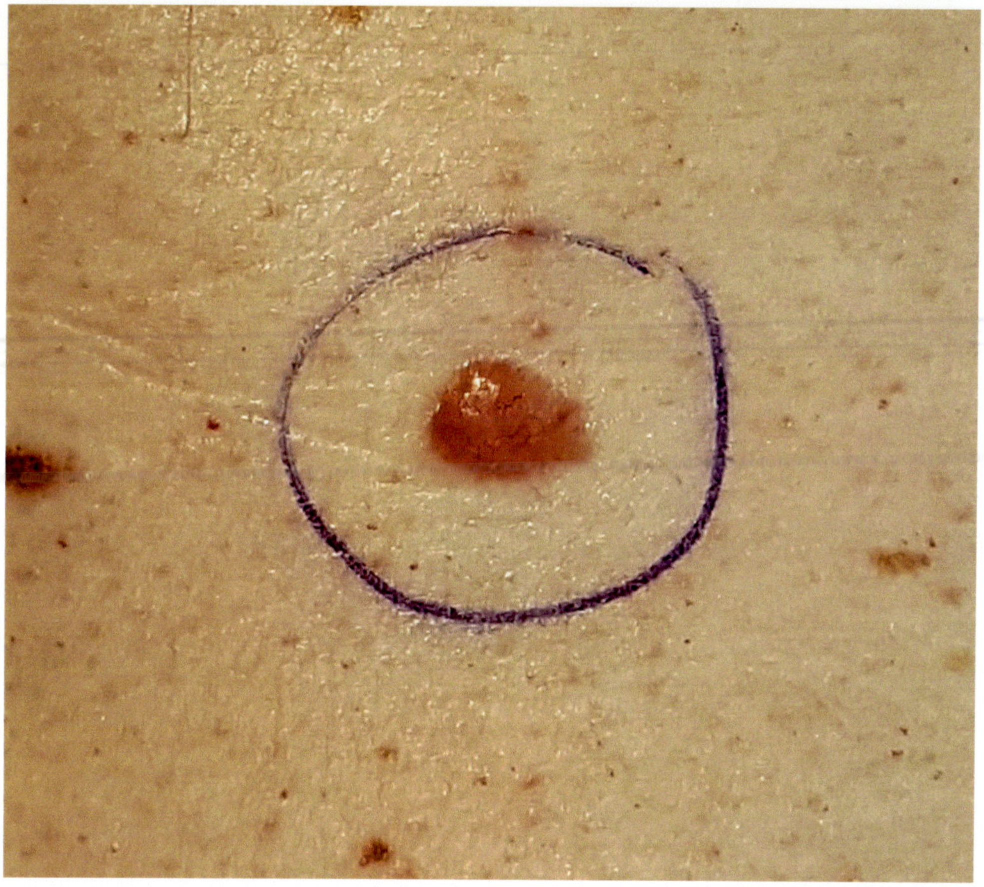

Fig. 13 **Clinical image**. A shiny erythematous papular lesion of about 1 cm in diameter was observed in the right upper quadrant of abdomen. (blue circle)

Diagnosis: Basal cell carcinoma (MAY globules)

Key message: Dermoscopy is a non-invasive tool useful for improving the diagnostic accuracy for Basal Cell Carcinoma (BCC) diagnosis. It provides visualization of structures and clues not visible to the naked eye. Some BCCs display multiple aggregated yellow-white (MAY) globules, a recently described BCC feature, characterized by multiple, aggregated, white-to-yellowish globules (circles) arranged in clusters, correlating with calcification sites on histopathology. Unlike milia-like cysts, MAY globules can be seen both in polarized and nonpolarized light. It has been described that MAY globules are seen in 21% of nonpigmented BCCs, with a similar frequency to other BCC-specific criteria, and they also have been associated with high-risk histologic subtypes. Thus, the presence of MAY globules may be an important clue toward the diagnosis of BCC by narrowing the differential diagnosis toward other skin neoplasms.

Case 5

Author: Verche Todorovska

Clinical record:

Sex: Male

Age: 70-years-old

Clinical description the case or the lesion: Solitary, pink, ulcerated nodule, on a heavily sun-damaged skin.

Body site: Back

Surface: Nodular

Maximum diameter: 20 mm

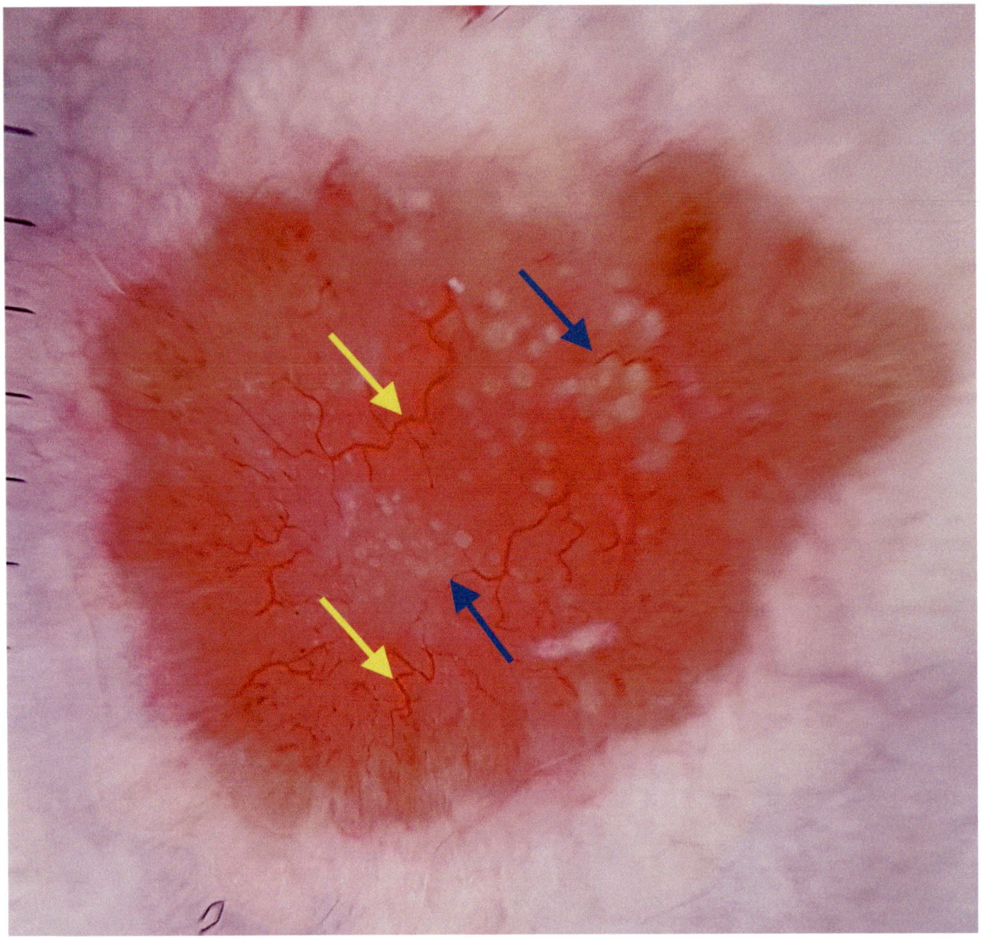

Fig. 14 **Dermoscopy image (polarized light):** Multiple arborizing vessels and in-focus vessels (yellow arrows) and Multiple Aggregated Yellow-white (MAY) globules (blue arrows)

Duration of the lesion: 2 years

History of morphologic changes: Slowly growing

Personal history of skin cancer: No

Family history of skin cancer: No

Skin Phototype: II

Clinical diagnosis: Fibroma, nodular BCC

Dermoscopic findings: Large caliber arborizing and linear irregular in focus vessels on a translucent background. Red structureless area of ulceration (bleeding), intense white shiny lines and strands visible only with polarized light.

Other clinical findings: Solitary, stand out, sessile, pink ulcerated nodule covered with a crust, medium firm on palpation (Figs. 17, 18, 19 and 20).

Diagnosis: Nodular Basal Cell Carcinoma

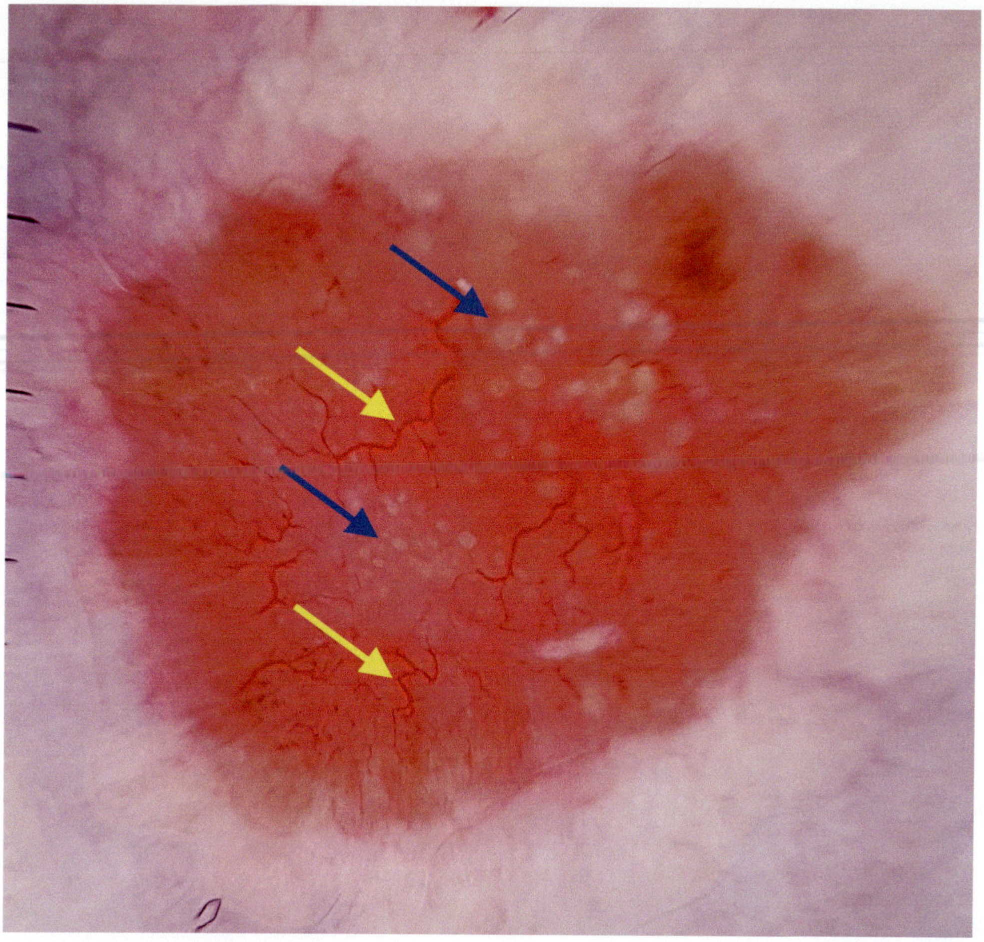

Fig. 15 **Dermoscopy image (non-polarized light)**. The presence of arborizing vessels (yellow arrows) and multiple aggregated yellow-white (MAY) globules (blue arrows) gives the dermoscopy evaluation of this lesion a high specificity for Basal Cell Carcinoma

Key message: Polarizing specific white lines and vessels morphology are crucial in distinguishing benign lesion from a malignant tumor in non-pigmented lesions, as demonstrated in this case of a nodular Basal Cell Carcinoma

Case 6

Author: Pedro Zaballos

Clinical record:

Sex: Female

Age: 60-years-old

Clinical description the case or the lesion: Solitary asymptomatic erythematous tumor located on the lower back

Body site: Lower Back

Surface: Palpable

Maximum diameter: 1 cm

Duration of the lesion: 4 months

History of morphologic changes: None

Personal history of skin cancer: None

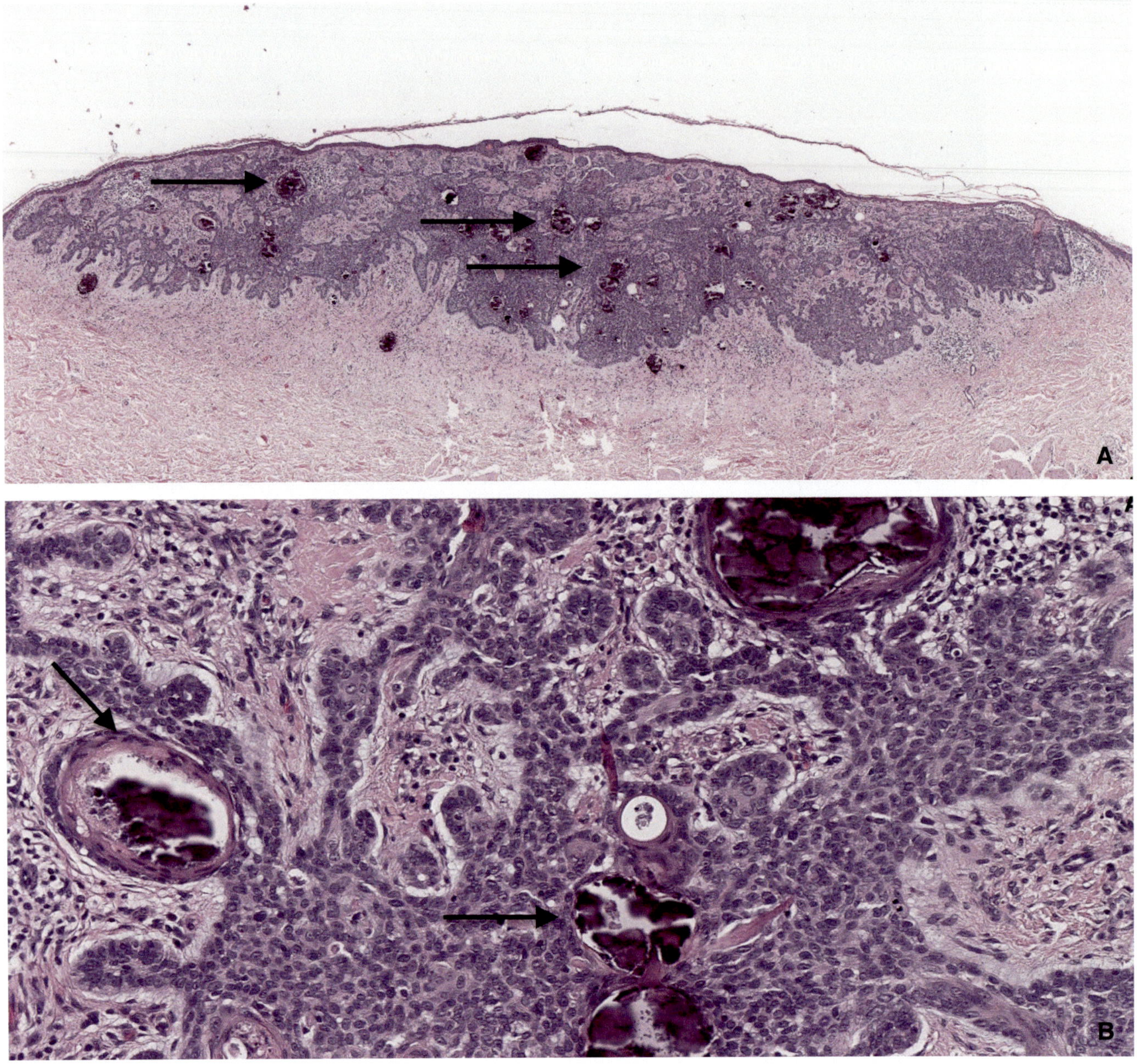

Fig. 16 H&E, original magnification 2x (Image A) and 10x (Image B) Histopathology showing a basaloid cell proliferation with intratumoral calcium deposits (black arrows)

Family history of skin cancer: None

Skin Phototype: III

Clinical diagnosis: Basal cell carcinoma

Dermoscopic findings: Polarized dermoscopy demonstrates fine focused arborizing vessels; some dotted vessels; shiny white streaks and a micro-ulceration

Other clinical findings: None (Figs. 21, 22 and 23)

Diagnosis: Fibroepithelioma of Pinkus

Key message: The dermoscopic pattern composed of fine arborizing vessels and shiny white streaks is very characteristic of Fibroepithelioma of Pinkus, which is an uncommon variant of basal cell carcinoma.

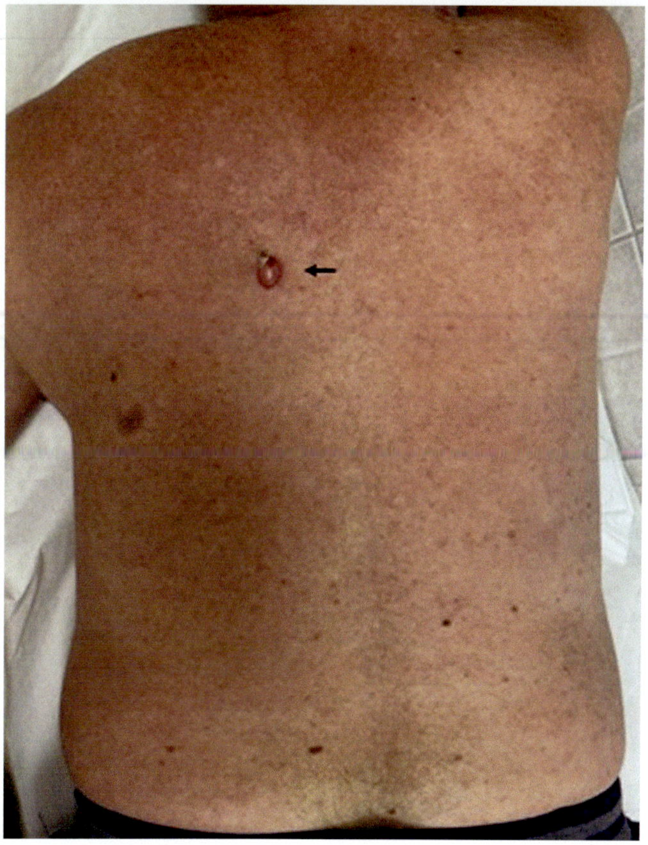

Fig. 17 Clinically: standout, solitary, pink, ulcerated nodule, on a heavily sun-damaged skin (arrow)

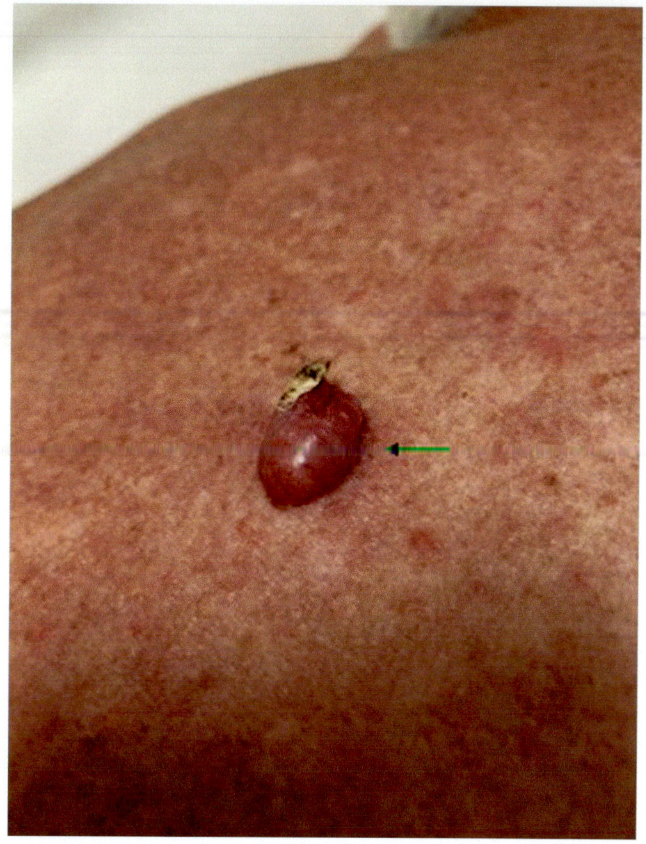

Fig. 18 Close-up of the clinical view: standout, solitary, pink, ulcerated nodule, on a heavily sun-damaged skin (arrow)

Case 7

Author: John Paoli

Clinical record:

Sex: Male

Age: 54-year-old

Clinical description the case or the lesion: Nhite macule on the upper back

Body site: Upper back

Surface: Flat

Maximum diameter: 8 mm

Duration of the lesion: Unknown

History of morphologic changes: Unknown

Personal history of skin cancer: None

Family history of skin cancer: None

Skin Phototype: III

Clinical diagnosis: Melanoma, Basal cell carcinoma

Dermoscopic findings: Polarized dermoscopy revealed a pink and shiny white structureless background with a few,

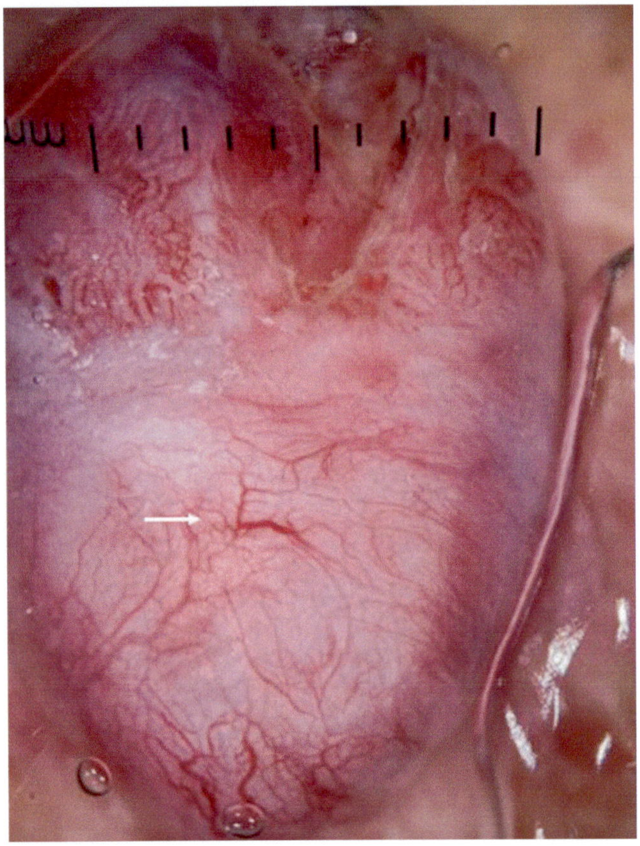

Fig. 19 Dermoscopy, non-polarized image: in focus arborizing vessels on a white–pink background (white arrows)

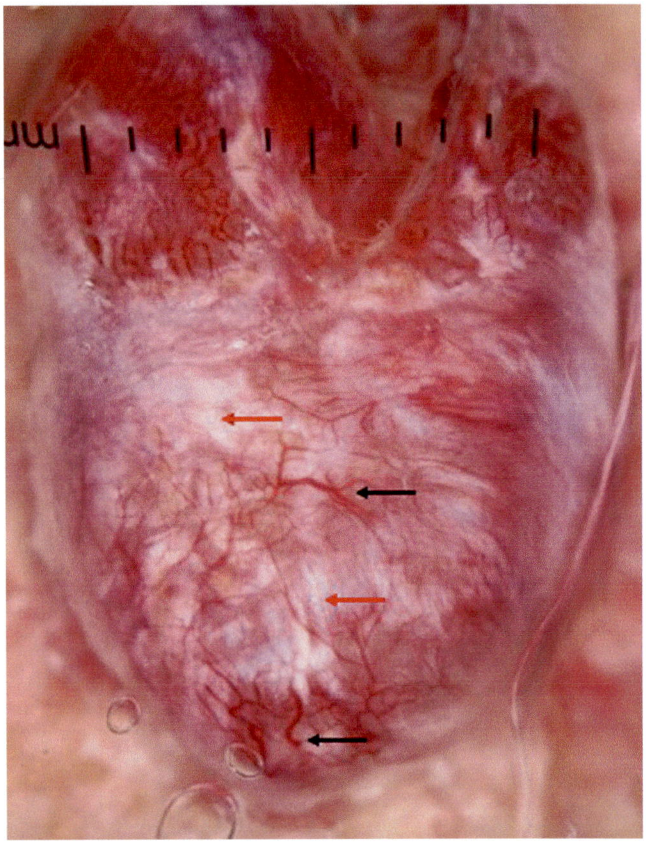

Fig. 20 Dermoscopy, polarized image: shiny white lines and strands (red arrows); bright red in focus vessels on a translucent stroma (black arrows)

irregularly distributed dotted and linear vessels and a peripheral negative network.

Other clinical findings: None (Figs. 24 and 25)

Diagnosis: Hypomelanotic melanoma

Key message: In the presence of a pink lesion on the skin damaged by the sun, we must take into account different diagnoses. Dermoscopy is useful in distinguishing between different lesions, such as basal cell carcinoma, squamous cell carcinoma, and hypomelanotic melanoma.

Case 8

Author: Elvira Moscarella

Clinical record:

Sex: Male

Age: 70-years-old

Clinical description the case or the lesion: A 70-year-old man with previous history of non-melanoma skin cancer underwent regular annual skin check. A pink amelanotic papule was noted on his lower back. At close-up examination the lesion presented two components, a flat light brown area and an amelanotic papule. Clinical differential diagnosis included melanoma and a collision tumor of nevus and basal cell carcinoma. The latter hypothesis was favored by the history of the patient who had excised several basal cell carcinomas in the past.

Body site: Lower back

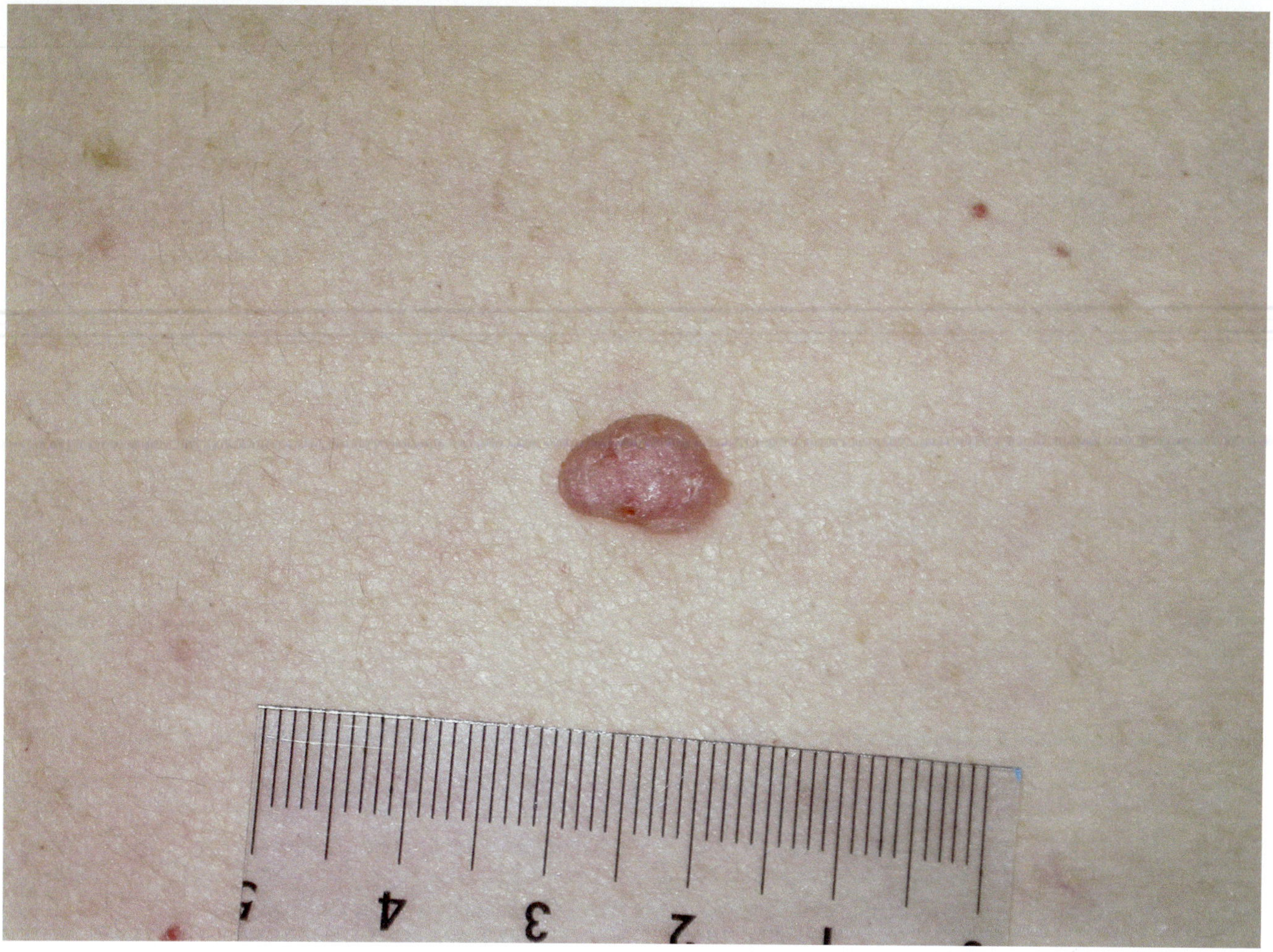

Fig. 21 Solitary asymptomatic erythematous tumor located on the lower back of a 60-year-old woman

Surface: Palpable

Maximum diameter: 6 mm

Duration of the lesion: Unknown

History of morphologic changes: Unknown

Personal history of skin cancer: Basal cell carcinomas

Family history of skin cancer: None

Skin Phototype: II

Clinical diagnosis: Differential diagnosis included melanoma versus collision tumor (nevus + BCC)

Dermoscopic findings: asymmetric lesion, composed by a flat pigmented area with brown structureless area and atypical network. On the other side, an amelanotic pink area was seen, characterized by the presence of dotted and linear irregular vessels.

Other clinical findings: Sun damaged skin (Figs. 26, 27 and 28)

Diagnosis: Amelanotic melanoma 0.6 mm Breslow thickness

Key message: Vascular pattern is crucial in the evaluation of amelanotic tumors. Dotted and linear irregular vessels can be seen in amelanotic melanoma. Their detection should prompt toward excision and histopathologic examination.

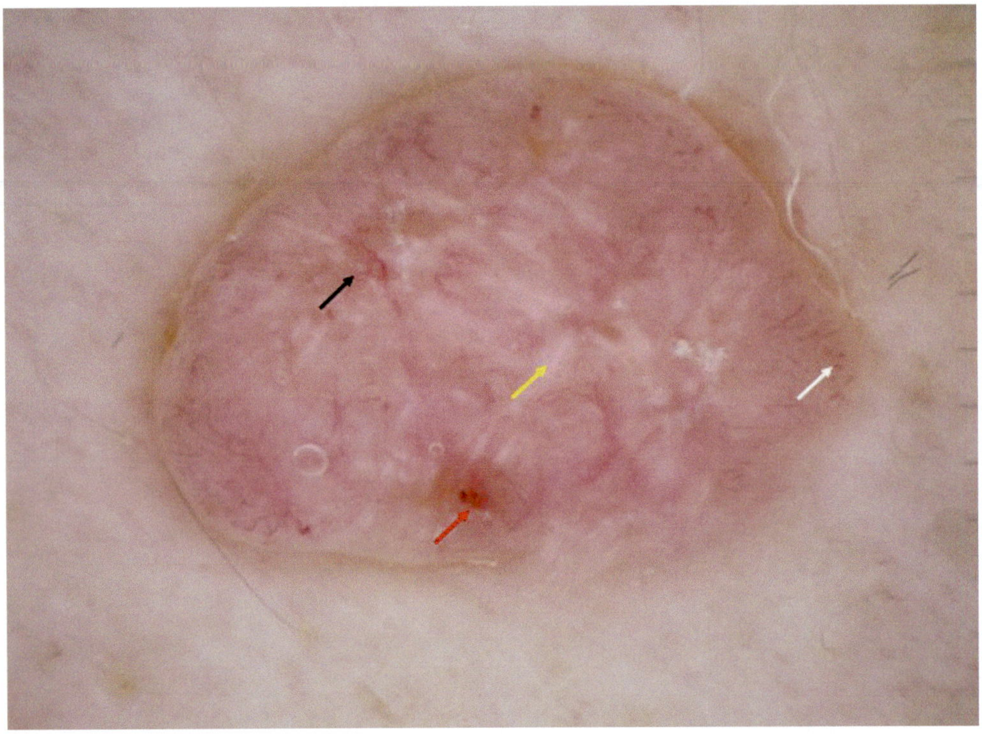

Fig. 22 Polarized dermoscopy demonstrates fine focused arborizing vessels (black arrow); some dotted vessels (white arrow); shiny white streaks (yellow arrow) and a micro-ulceration (red arrow)

Case 9

Author: Juan Sebastián Andreani Figueroa

Clinical record:

Sex: Male

Age: 43 years

Clinical description of the case: A mole in the back (Fig. 1)

Body site: Lumbar

Surface: Flat

Maximum diameter: Pigmented zone 8 × 4 mm, non-pigmented zone 11 × 5 mm

Duration of the lesion: Unknown

History of morphologic changes: No

Personal history of skin cancer: No

Family history of skin cancer: No

Skin Phototype: III

Clinical diagnosis: Melanoma with extensive regression vs Melanoma collision with irritated seborrheic keratosis

Dermoscopic findings: Pigmented lesion of 8 × 4 mm with atypical reticular structure in the periphery with brown areas without structure and in the central area black dots in focus that converge in a black blotch, in contact with a non-pigmented lesion with punctiform and curved linear vessels, some surrounded by a whitish halo distributed in an orderly manner with isolated scales on the surface.

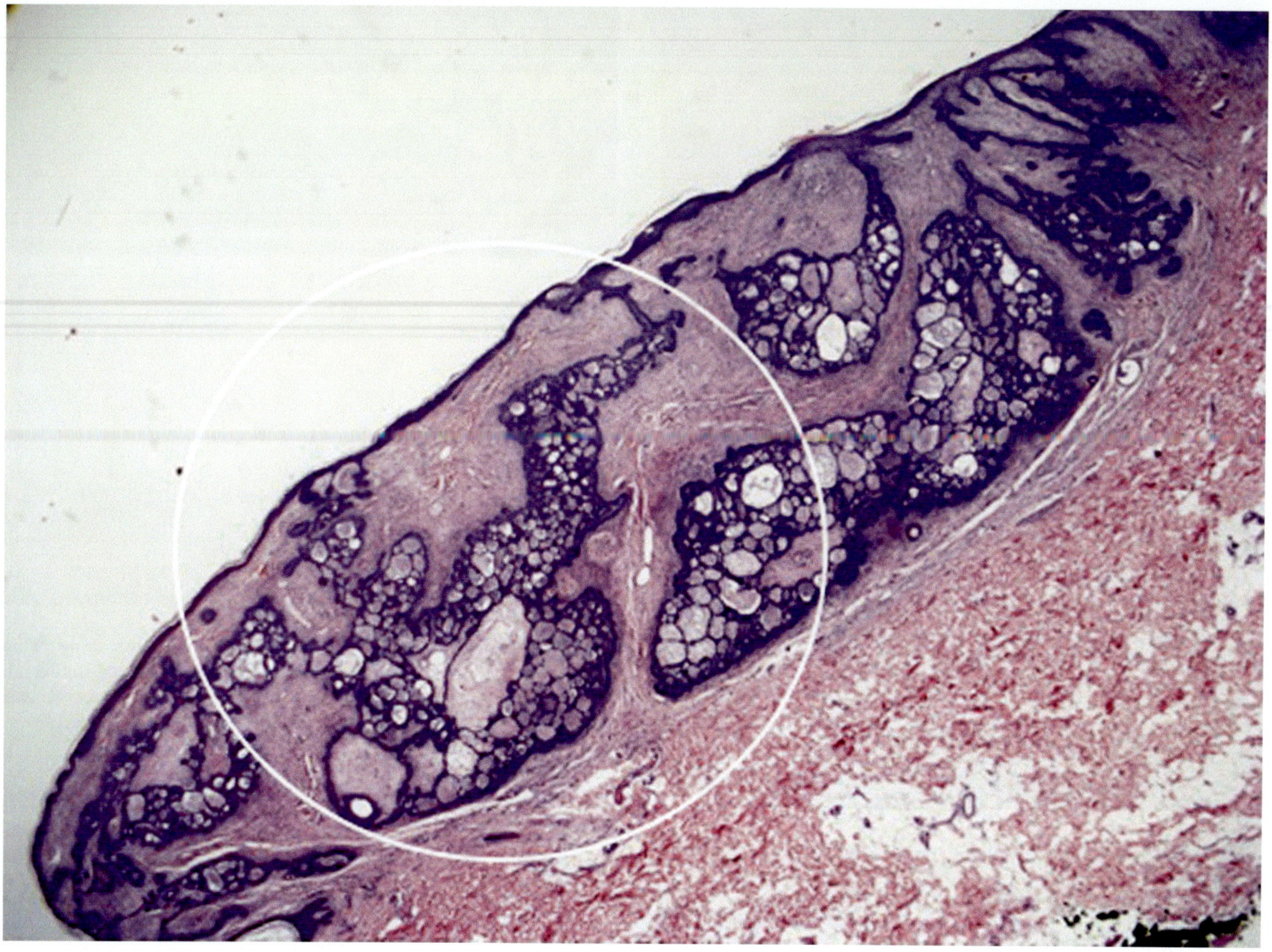

Fig. 23 The tumor shows a fenestrated pattern of anastomosing epithelial strands embedded in a fibrous stroma (white circle)

In dermatoscopy with UV light, it is observed the presence of bright circular lesions that are compatible with a seborrheic keratosis stands out in the non-pigmented area.

Other clinical findings: Reflectance confocal microscopy was performed and shows in the epidermis of the pigmented area, large bright cells with prominent dark nuclei and multiple dendritic cells, in addition to epidermal disarray and loss of ring pattern in the dermal–epidermal junction, which guides the diagnosis of melanoma. In the non-pigmented area, multiple dendritic cells associated with hyperkeratosis and rope-like structures were observed in the epidermis, which support the diagnosis of an irritated seborrheic keratosis.

The histological report confirms an in-situ melanoma in collision with an irritated seborrheic keratosis (Figs. 29, 30, 31 and 32).

Diagnosis: In-situ melanoma in collision with an irritated seborrheic keratosis

Key message: The presence of seborrheic keratoses in collision to melanoma has been published as more than a coincidence.[1] Many times this collision, as in the case presented, can clinically simulate being part of the malignant tumor, simulating a regression area, which can even lead to take an excisional biopsy including the area of

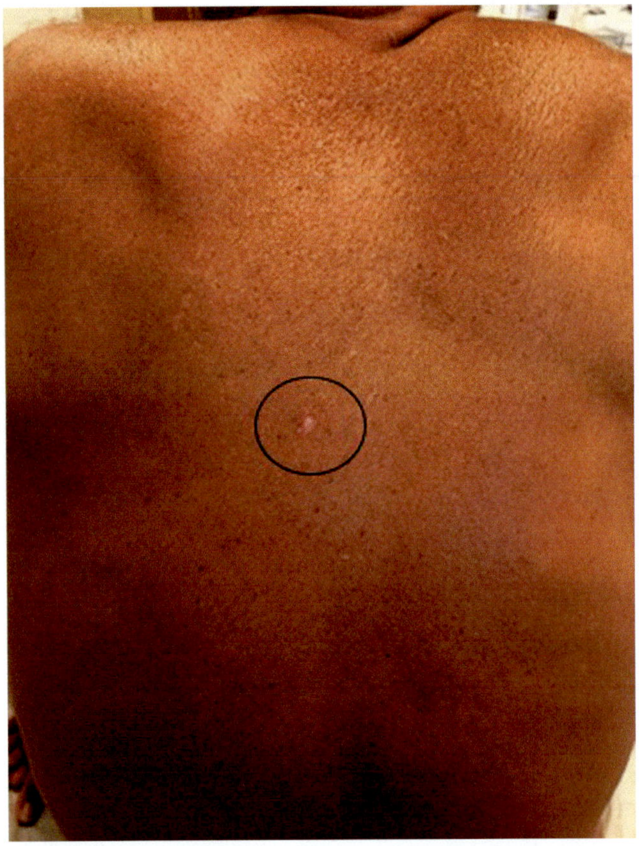

Fig. 24 Hypopigmented and slightly scaly macule on the upper back (black circle)

seborrheic keratosis, generating an unnecessary initial surgical defect.

In this case, dermatoscopy becomes relevant, remembering that we must first use the dermatoscope without cleaning the surface with alcohol, since the presence of scaling helps us to think of a diagnosis of a non-melanocytic lesion. In addition, when using the dermatoscope with polarized light, with alcohol, we see structures of irritated seborrheic keratosis, as is described in the literature.[2]

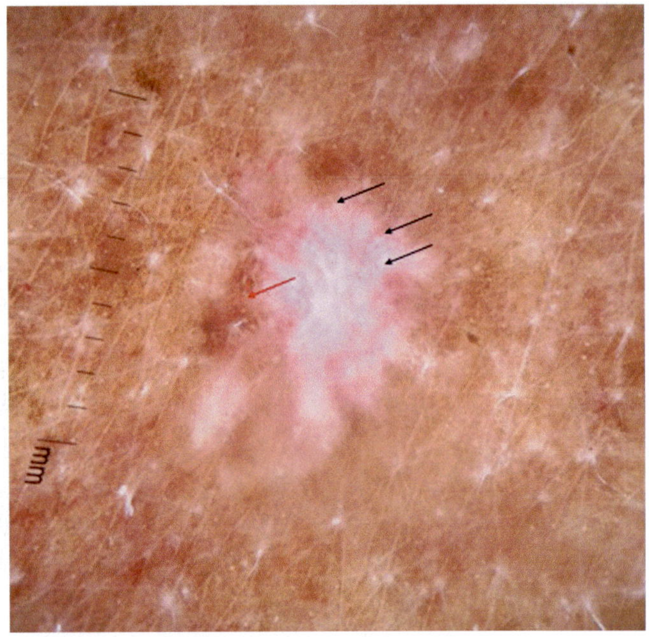

Fig. 25 Polarized dermoscopy revealed a pink and shiny white structureless background with a few, irregularly distributed dotted and linear vessels (black arrows). A peripheral negative network was observed (red arrow)

UV spectral range light in dermatoscopy can also provide a new contrast for diagnosing skin diseases, and these bright shiny round structures could be taken into account as a key to diagnosing seborrheic keratosis.

Case 10

Authors: Jelena Stojkovic-Filipovic, Dusan Skiljevic

Clinical record:

Sex: Male

Age: 76-years-old

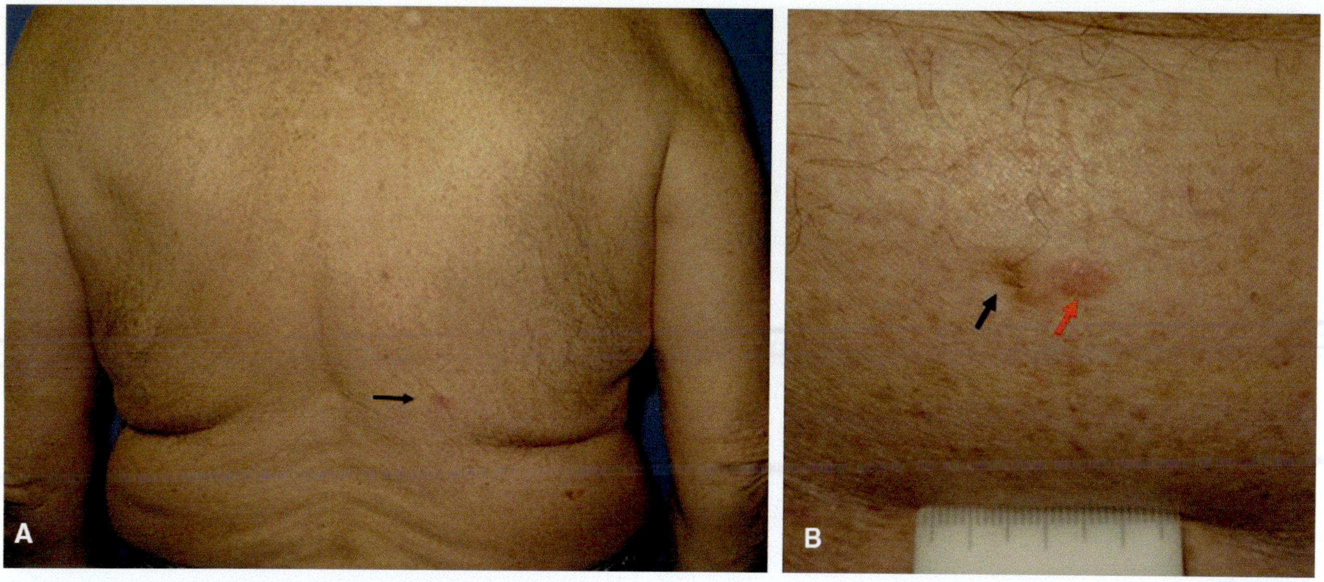

Fig. 26 A-Clinical view (black arrow); B-Clinical close up with two components can be seen, a light brown flat area (black arrow) and on the other side a pink papule (red arrow)

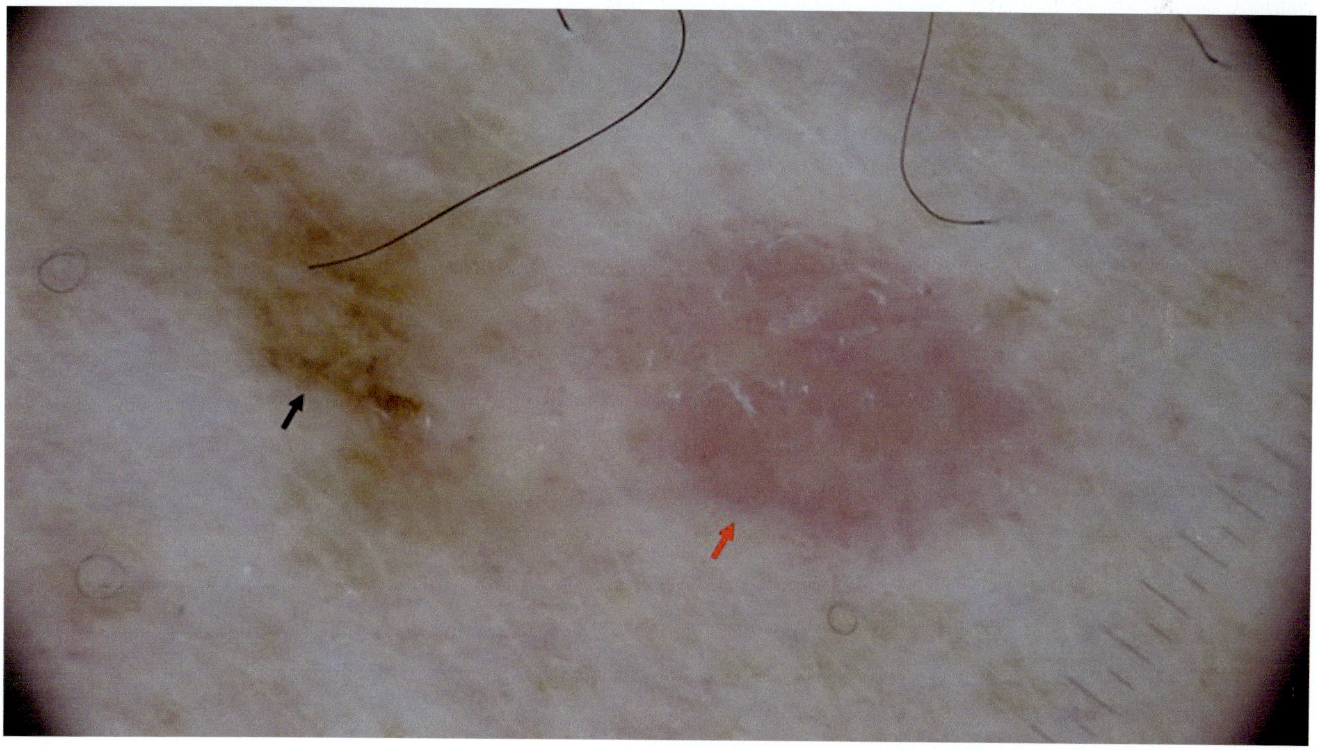

Fig. 27 Dermoscopy showing brown structureless area and atypical network on the flat component (black arrow). The amelanotic pink papule presented dotted and linear irregular vessels (red arrow)

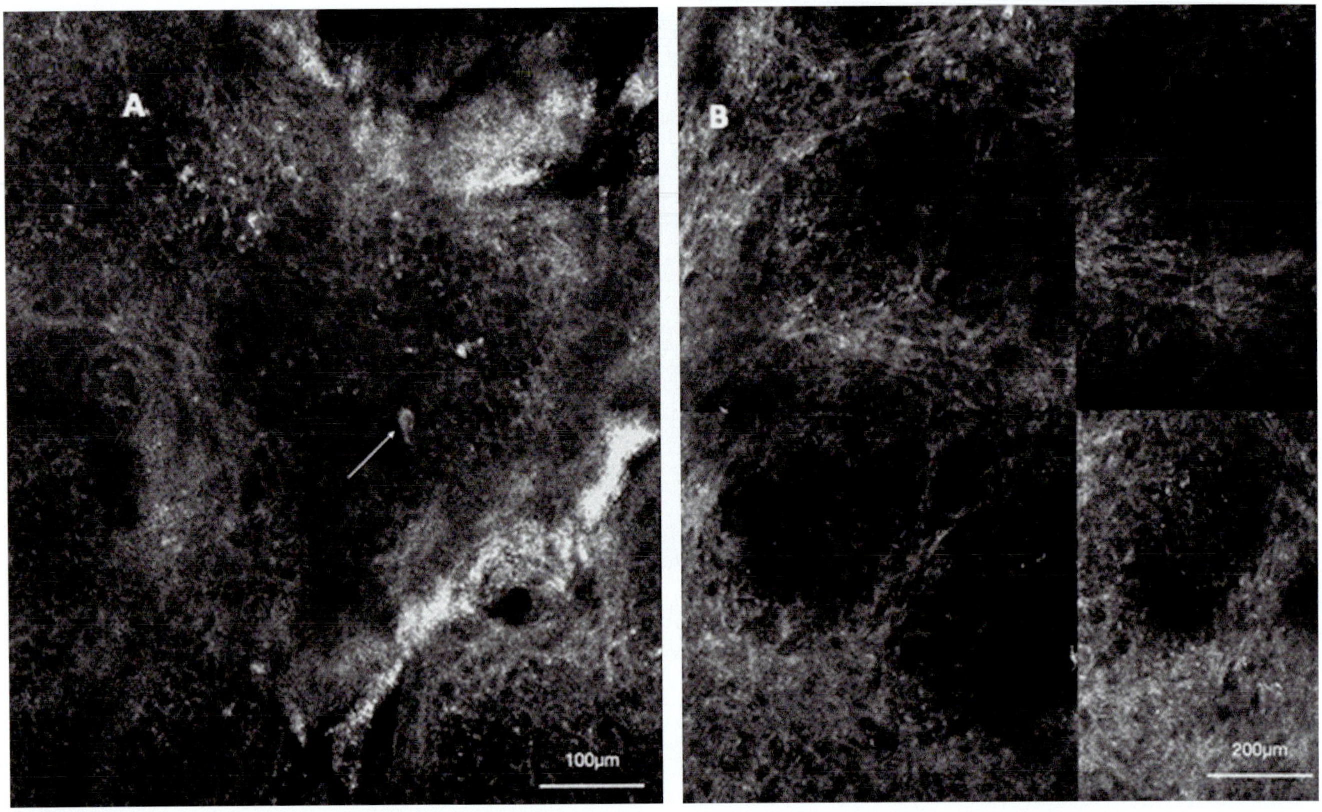

Fig. 28 Reflectance confocal microscopy imaging. A- RCM image at the level of the epidermis, presence of honeycombed pattern with some roundish nucleated cells (arrow). B- RCM mosaic at the level of the dermal epidermal junctions, showing disarray and cerebriform nests. On histology, the lesion was a 0.6 mm Breslow thickness melanoma

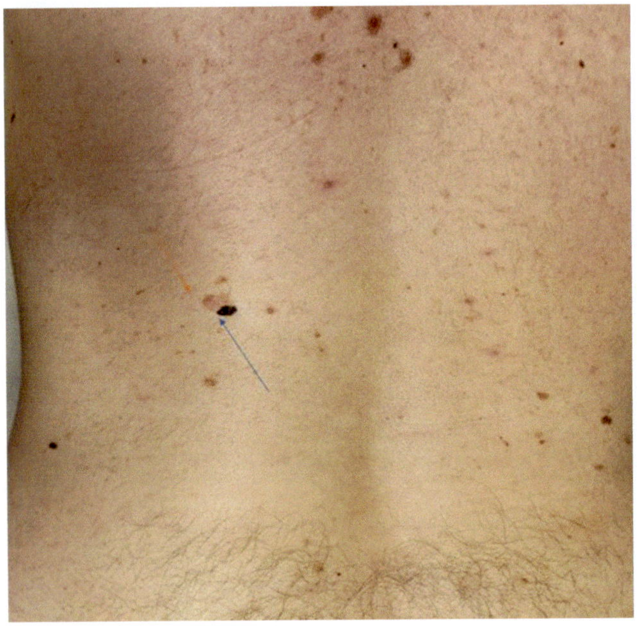

Fig. 29 Clinical image of the left lumbar area, which shows a lesion with a dark brown pigmented area in the inferomedial pole (blue arrow), which in its upper pole presents a pink area (red arrow) with some scales on its surface

Clinical description the case or the lesion: Erythematous plaque

Body site: Chest

Surface: Flat

Maximum diameter: 1 cm

Duration of the lesion: Several years

History of morphologic changes: Slowly progressive

Personal history of skin cancer: Five BCC previously excised (4 on the back and 1 on the face)

Family history of skin cancer: None

Skin Phototype: III

Clinical diagnosis: Epithelioma

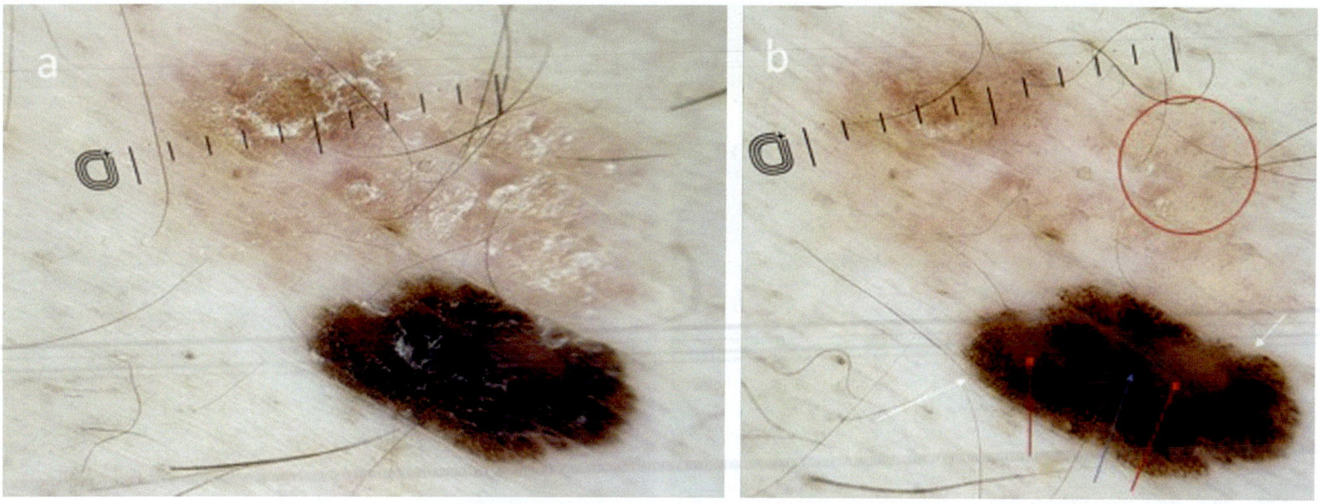

Fig. 30 (a) Dermatoscopy without cleaning the surface with alcohol allows one to see a scaly surface that predominates over the non-pigmented area. (b) Dermatoscopy with polarized contact light with surface covered with alcohol, allows to see pigmented lesion of 8 × 4 mm with atypical reticular structure at the periphery (white arrows) with brown areas without structure (red arrows) and at the central area black dots in focus that converge to form a black blotch (blue arrow). Non-pigmented zone with punctiform and curved linear vessels (red circle), some surrounded by a whitish halo distributed in a diffuse regular arrangement with isolated scales on the surface

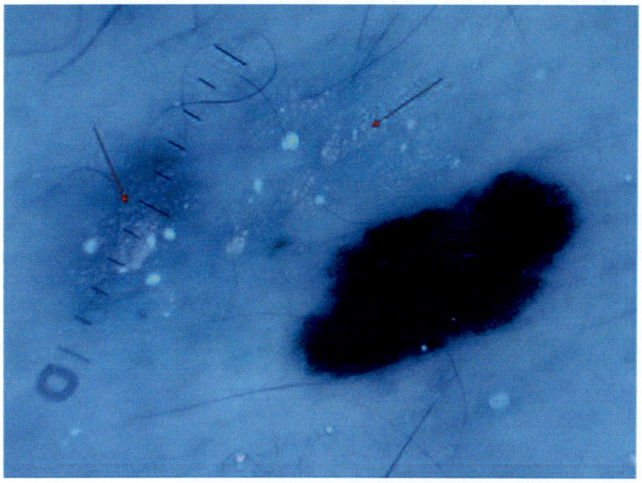

Fig. 31 Dermatoscopy with UV light: Presence of bright circular lesions that are compatible with a seborrheic keratosis stands out in the non-pigmented area (red arrows)

Dermoscopic findings: Red structureless area with coiled vessels arranged in clusters combined with scales

Other clinical findings: Asymptomatic lesion (Figs. 33, 34 and 35)

Diagnosis: Bowen disease

Key message: Examination of the vessels with dermatoscope is the clue in the diagnosis of Squamous cell carcinoma in situ (Bowen disease).

Case 11

Authors: Giuseppe Micali, Anna Elisa Verzì, Livia Liguori

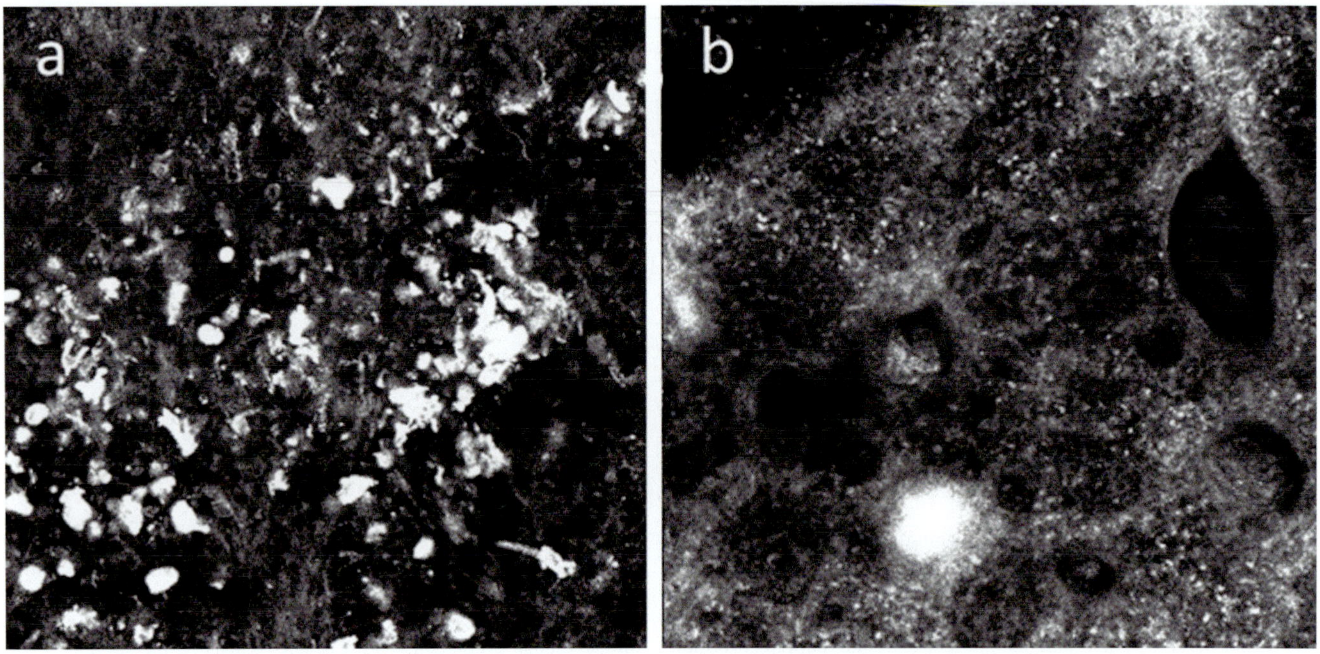

Fig. 32 Reflectance confocal microscopy (a) in the pigmented area shows in epidermis, large bright cells with prominent dark nuclei and multiple dendritic cells, in addition to epidermal disarray, concordant with the melanoma diagnosis. (b) In the non-pigmented area, multiple dendritic cells associated with hyperkeratosis and rope-like structures were observed in the epidermis, which support the diagnosis of an irritated seborrheic keratosis

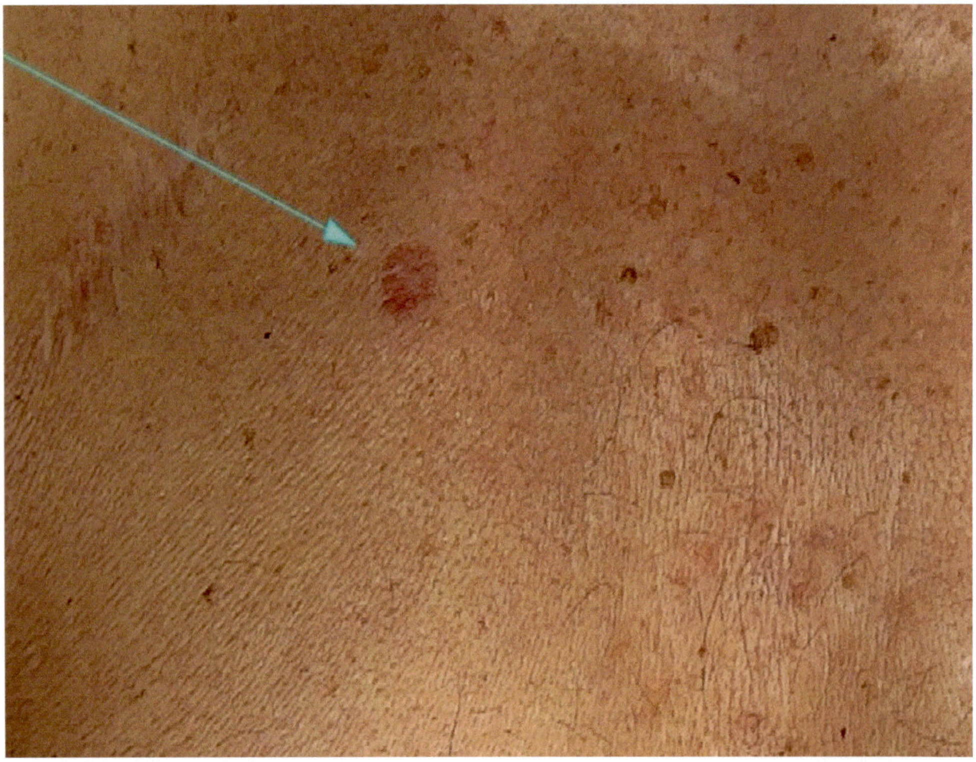

Fig. 33 Bright red, well-demarcated, scaly plaque (arrow)

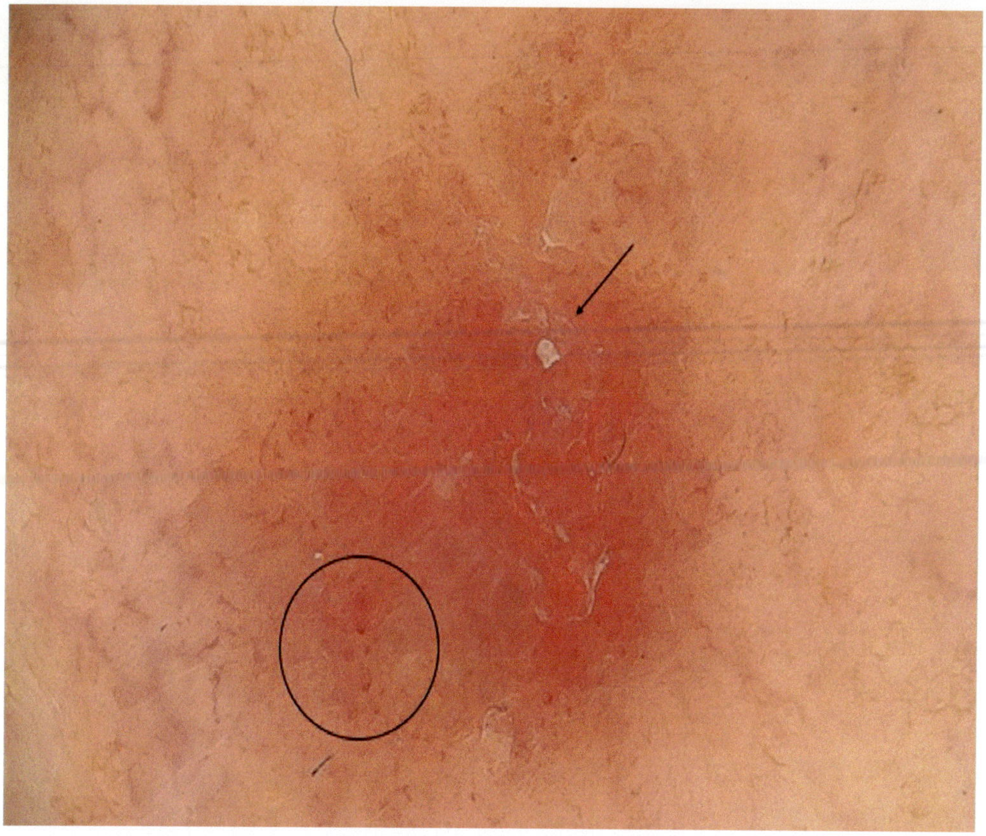

Fig. 34 Red structureless area with coiled vessels arranged in clusters (black circle), combined with scales (red arrow)

Clinical record:

Sex: Female

Age: 45-years-old

Clinical description the case or the lesion: Asymptomatic, slightly erythematous, nodular lesion of the nipple showing a smooth surface.

Body site: Breast

Surface: Nodular

Maximum diameter: 7 mm

Duration of the lesion: 6 months

History of morphologic changes: Slow enlargement

Personal history of skin cancer: No

Family history of skin cancer: Father with history of multiple basal cell carcinomas

Skin Phototype: II

Clinical diagnosis: adnexal tumour

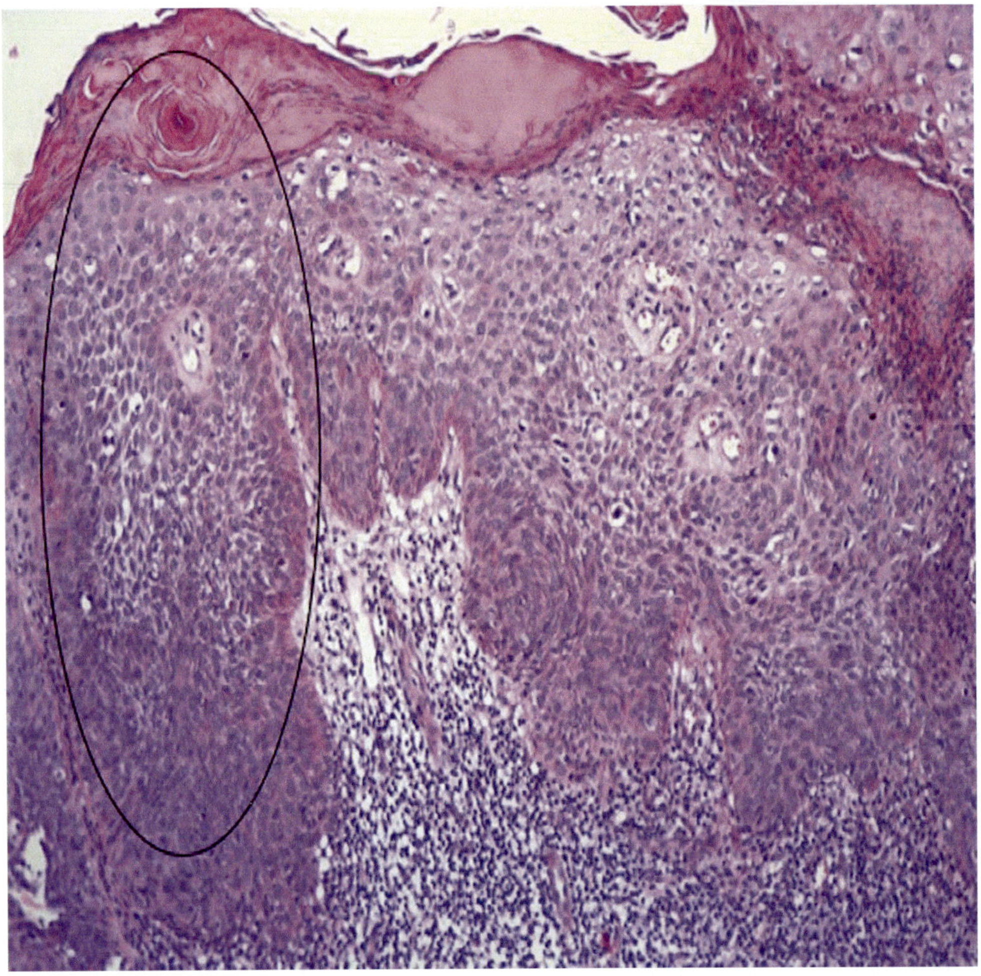

Fig. 35 Irregular epidermal hyperplasia with atypical pleomorphic keratinocytes throughout the entire epidermal thickness (black oval) (hematoxylin eosin stain; original magnification 100x)

Dermoscopic findings: Pinkish background, linear branching vessels at the periphery, and small roundish yellowish structures ("pores") in the center of the lesion

Other clinical findings: None (Figs. 36, 37 and 38)

Diagnosis: Molluscum contagiosum

Key message: In adult patients, molluscum contagiosum located outside the genital area may be clinically difficult to diagnose, especially when the characteristic umbilication is

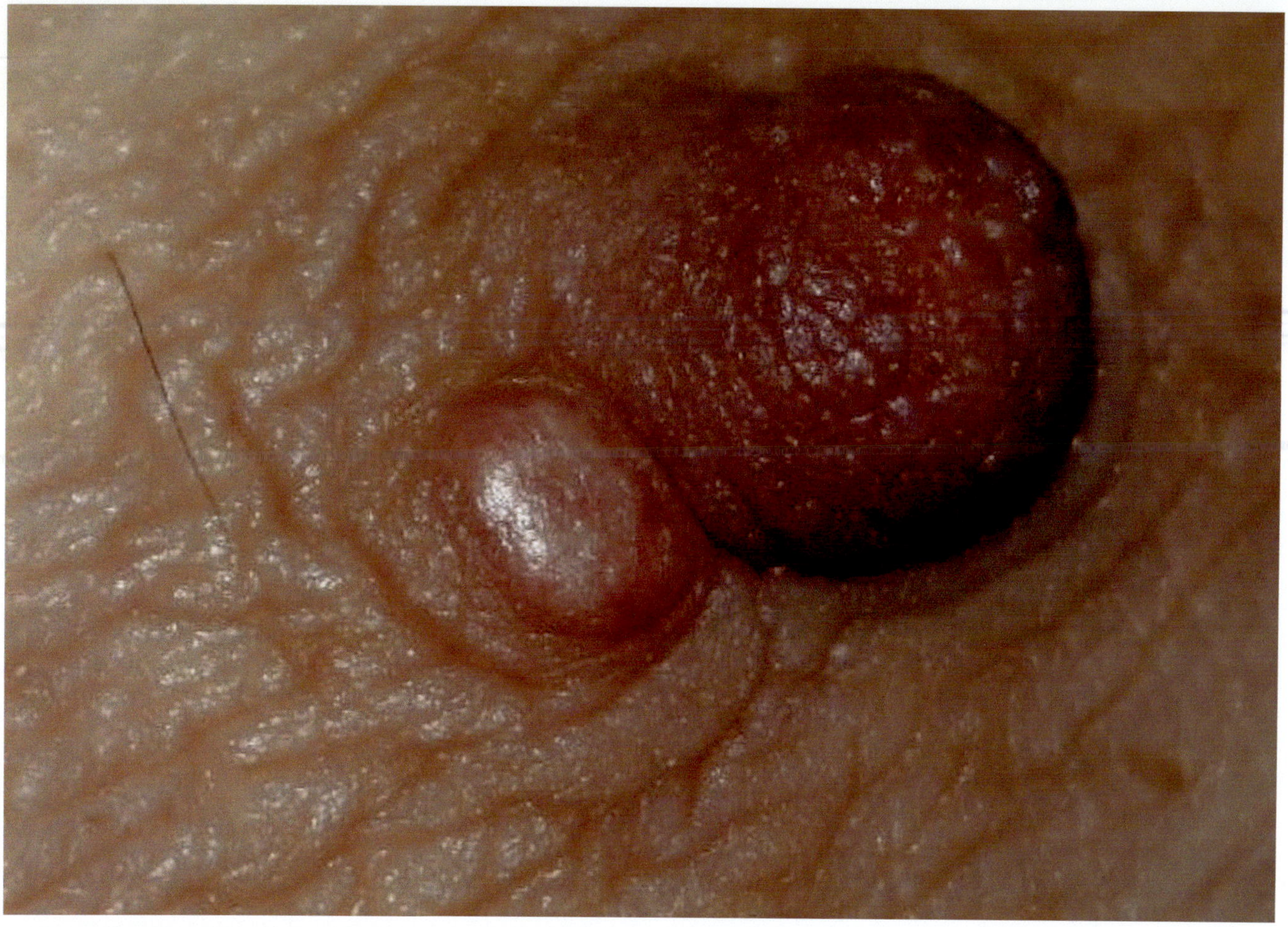

Fig. 36 Smooth, non-pigmented, nodular lesion of the nipple in a 45-year-old woman

lacking; dermoscopy may help by showing the typical features of the infection.

Case 12

Author: Roger A. González Ramírez

Clinical record:

Sex: Female

Age: 5-years-old

Clinical description the case or the lesion: the chief complaint was an itchy growing warty lesion in the last 2 weeks

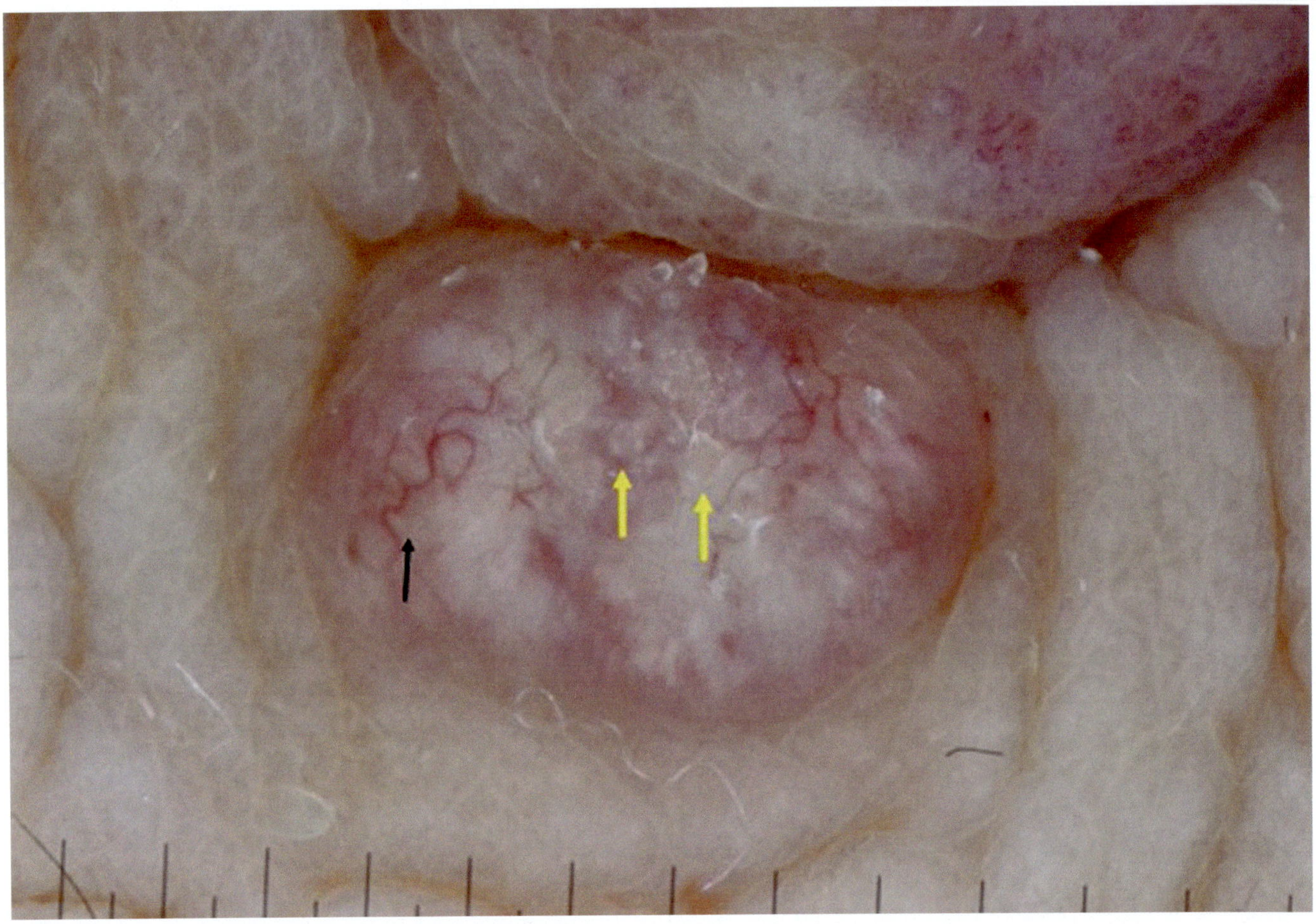

Fig. 37 Polarized dermoscopy showing a pinkish background, linear branching vessels at the periphery (black arrow), and small roundish yellowish structures ("pores") in the center of the lesion (yellow arrows)

Body site: Left hypocondrium

Surface: Palpable

Maximum diameter: 15 mm

Duration of the lesion: 3 years

History of morphologic changes: In the last 2 weeks, lesion has turned reddish

Personal history of skin cancer: None

Family history of skin cancer: None

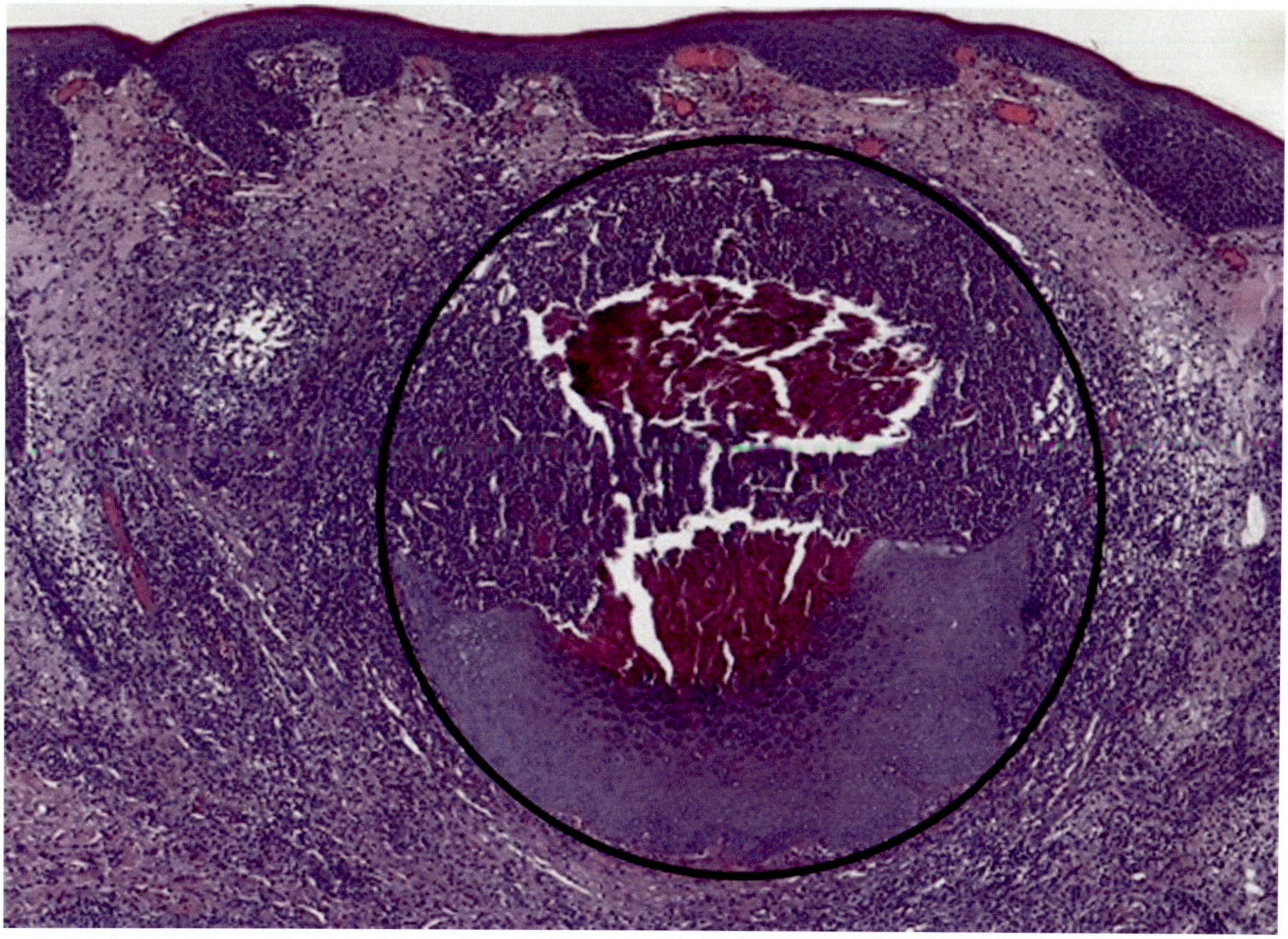

Fig. 38 Histopathology showing inverted lobules of hyperplastic squamous epithelium infiltrated by acute inflammation, expanding the superficial and medium dermis (black circle). Large intracytoplasmic eosinophilic inclusion bodies (so-called "Henderson-Paterson bodies") are visible within the lobules (H&E staining; original magnification 150x)

Skin Phototype: V

Clinical diagnosis: Lymphangioma

Dermoscopic findings: One big dark-blue lacuna, and multiple yellowish well circumscribed oval small lacunae containing blood, which was characteristically accumulated in the lowest part of the lacuna (hyphema-like structures), all of them surrounded by an erythematous halo (Figs. 39 and 40).

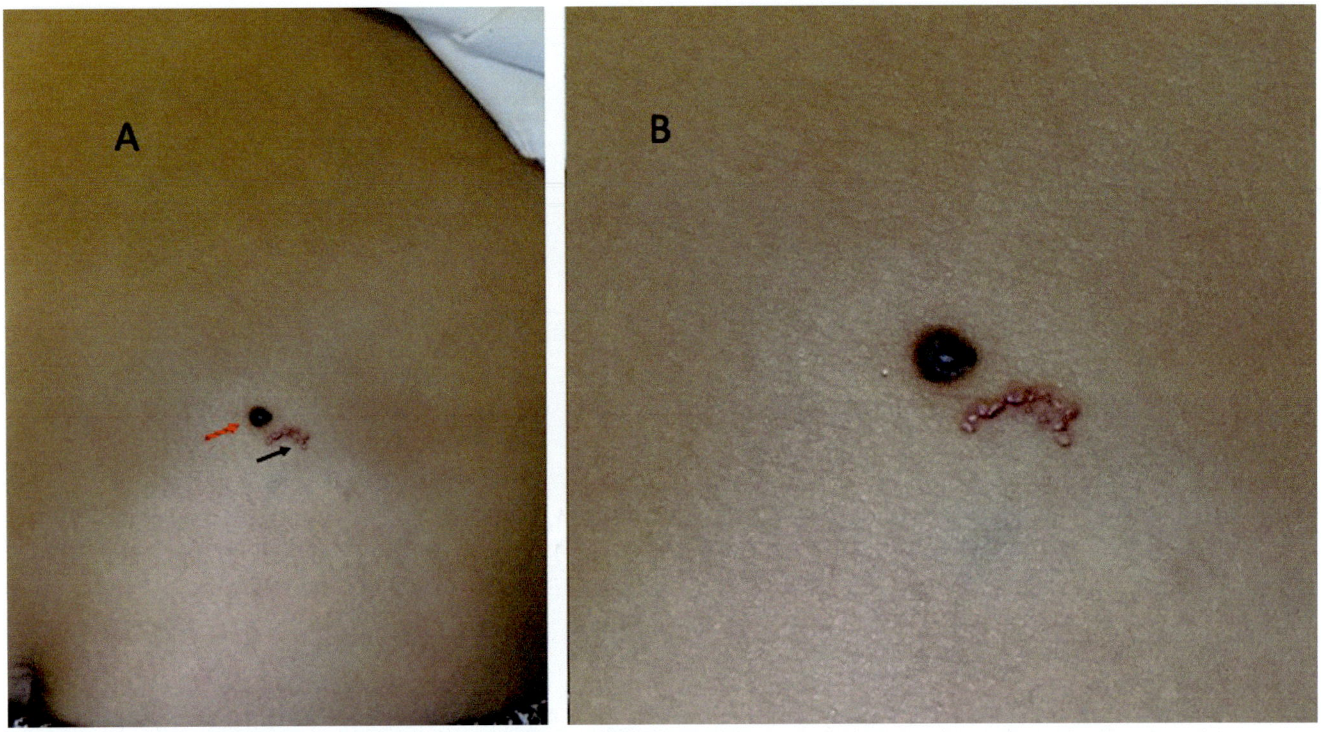

Fig. 39 A- Clinical image of a circumscribed lymphangioma, located on the left side of the trunk. A blue-black papule (red arrow) and some reddish tiny confluent papules in a linear arrangement are noticeable (black arrow). B- Close-up clinical image

Other clinical findings:

Diagnosis: Lymphangioma

Key message: Lymphangiomas can be "clean", showing a yellow content, but sometimes (after trauma), can change its aspect, presenting blood inside.

Case 13

Author: María Sofía Nicoletti Russi

Clinical record:

Sex: Male

Age: 65

Clinical description the case or the lesion: Asymptomatic solitary erythematous papule

Body site: Back

Surface: Palpable.

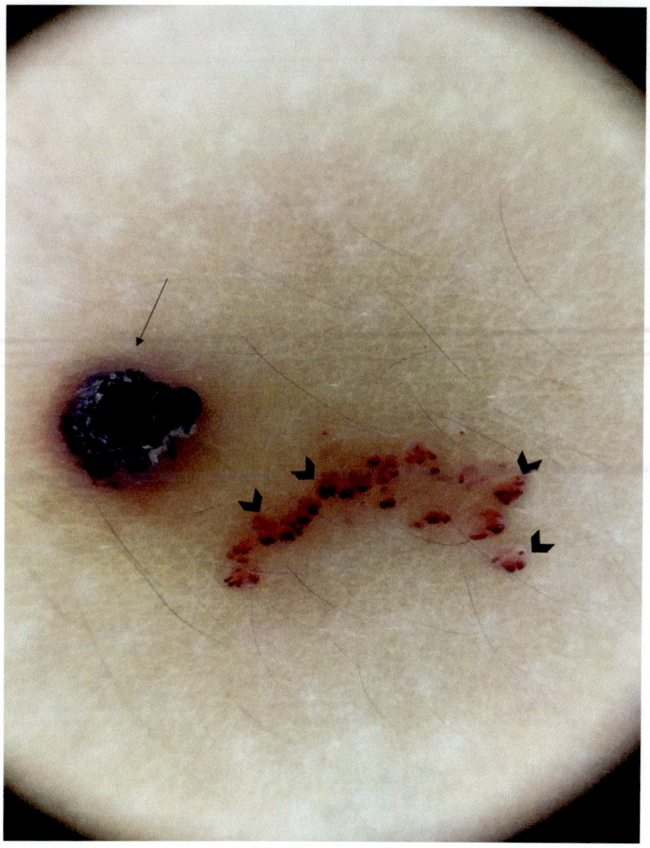

Fig. 40 Dermoscopic image shows a big dark blue lacuna (arrow), and multiple yellow little lacunae with blood on the bottom of all tiny lesions (arrowheads), mimicking hyphema-like image (in the anterior chamber of the eye). Also, an erythematous halo is present all around the whole lesion

Maximum diameter: 5 mm

Duration of the lesion: Unknown

History of morphologic changes: None

Personal history of skin cancer: Multiple basal cell carcinomas

Family history of skin cancer: None

Skin Phototype: II/III

Clinical diagnosis: Solitary erythematous papule

Dermoscopic findings: Dermoscopy with polarized light showing glomerular vessels with "pearl necklace" distribution, an image highly characteristic of clear cell acanthoma

Other clinical findings: None (Figs. 41, 42 and 43)

Diagnosis: Clear cell acanthoma

Key message: Clear cell acanthoma is a rare tumor. It presents as a slow-growing papular-nodular lesion or erythematous plaque, frequently located on the lower limbs.

Differential diagnoses include pyogenic granuloma, amelanotic melanoma, squamous cell carcinoma, Bowen's disease, basal cell carcinoma and irritated seborrheic keratosis.

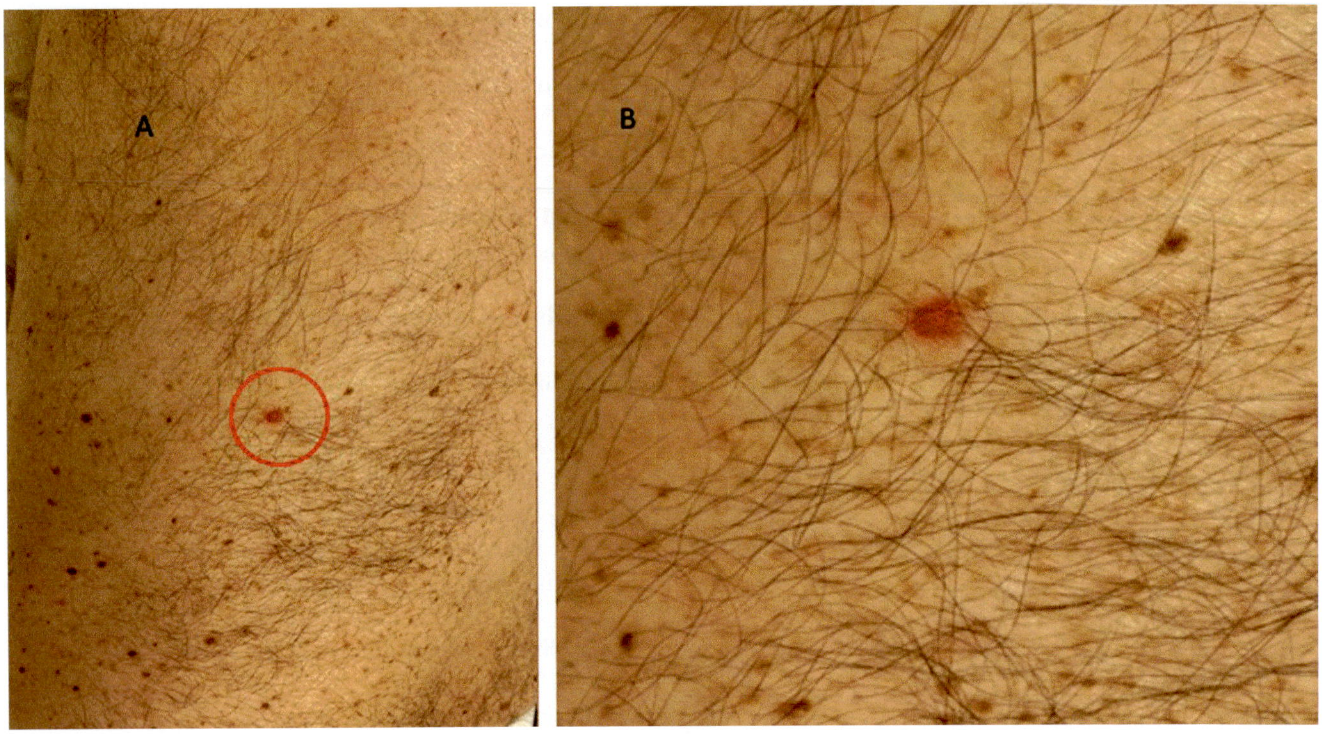

Fig. 41 A – Clinical view: solitary, well-defined erythematous papule lesion (red circle). B- Close-up of the clinical image

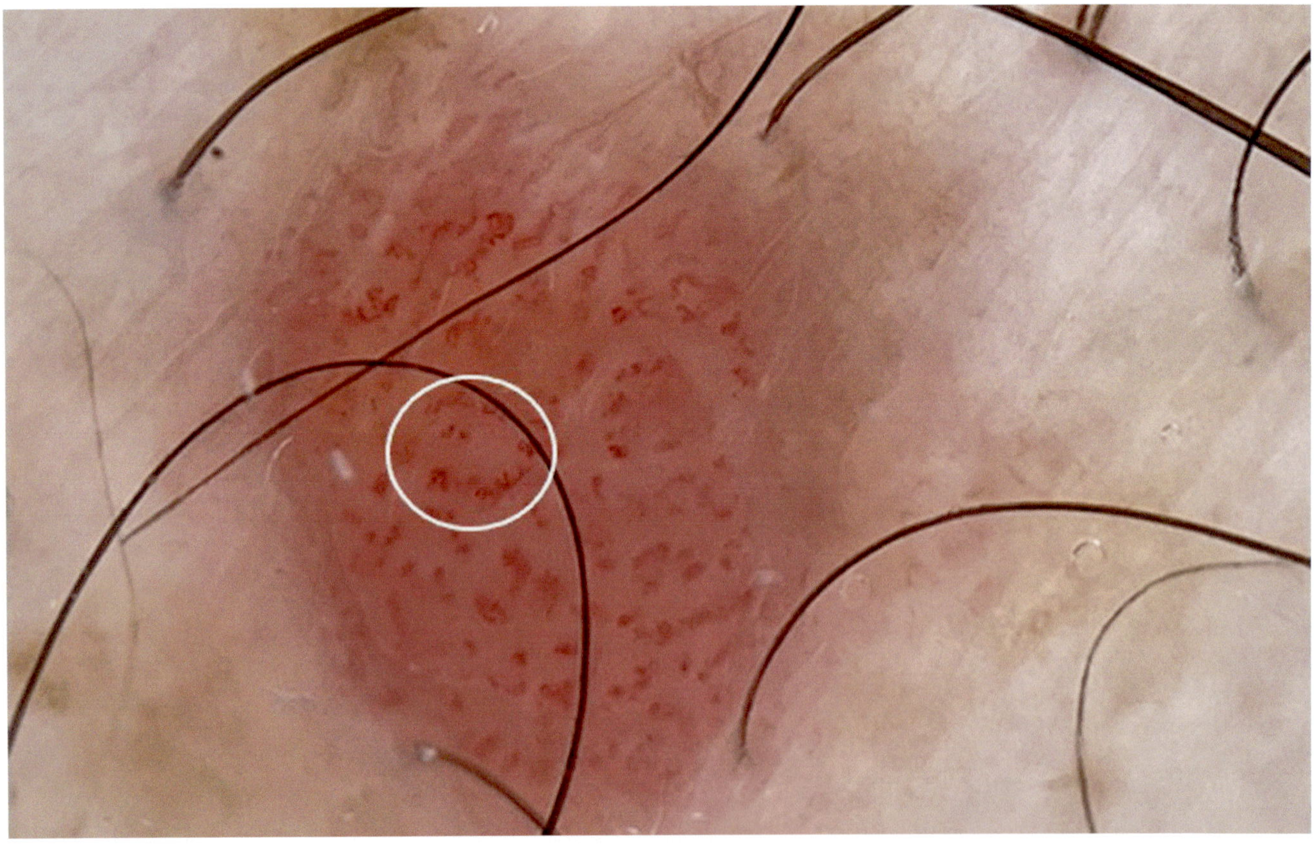

Fig. 42 Dermoscopy showed glomerular and punctiform vessels with a "pearl necklace" distribution (white circle)

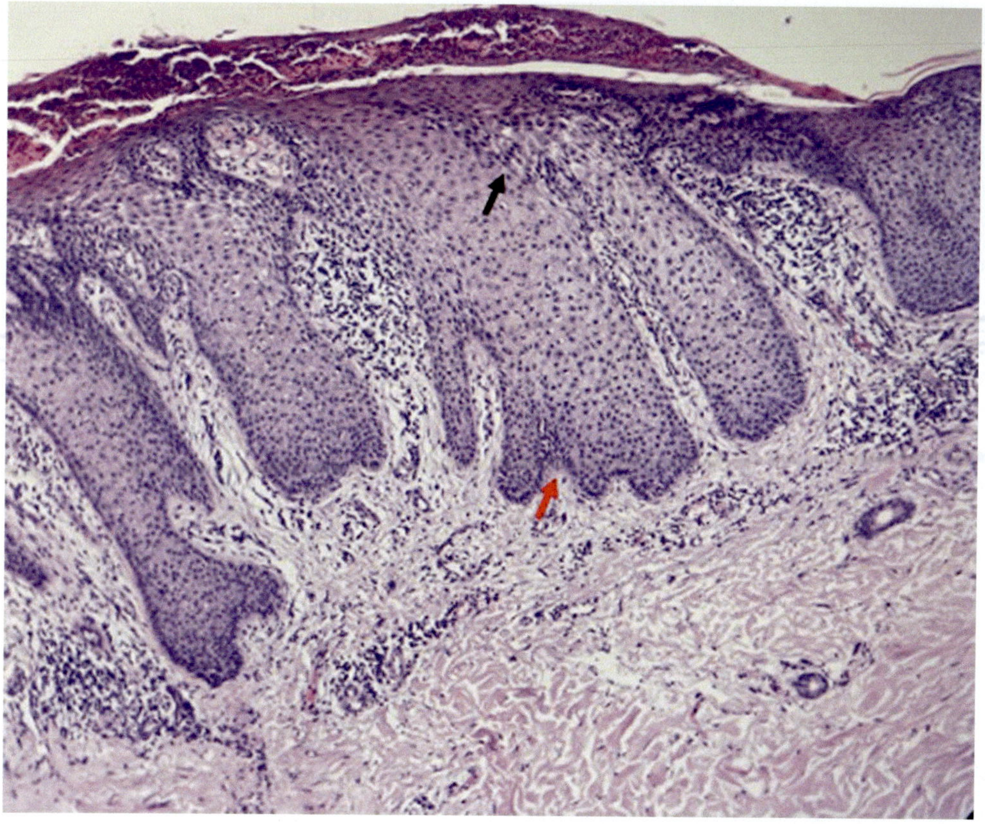

Fig. 43 Clear cell acanthoma: HE 10X. Intraepithelial tumor made up of pale keratinocytes without atypia (black arrow). Abrupt transition to normal skin. The psoriasiform pattern is characteristic, with suprapapillary thinning, hypogranulosis, and neutrophils in the epidermis and corneous layer (red arrow)

Under dermoscopy, has a unique appearance that is helpful to improve diagnostic accuracy, characterized by red dots, globules, and glomerular vessels arranged in linear or serpiginous patterns with a "pearl necklace" distribution.

Case 14

Authors: Quiñones-Venegas, Ricardo, Quiñones-Hernández, Deyanira Gabriela

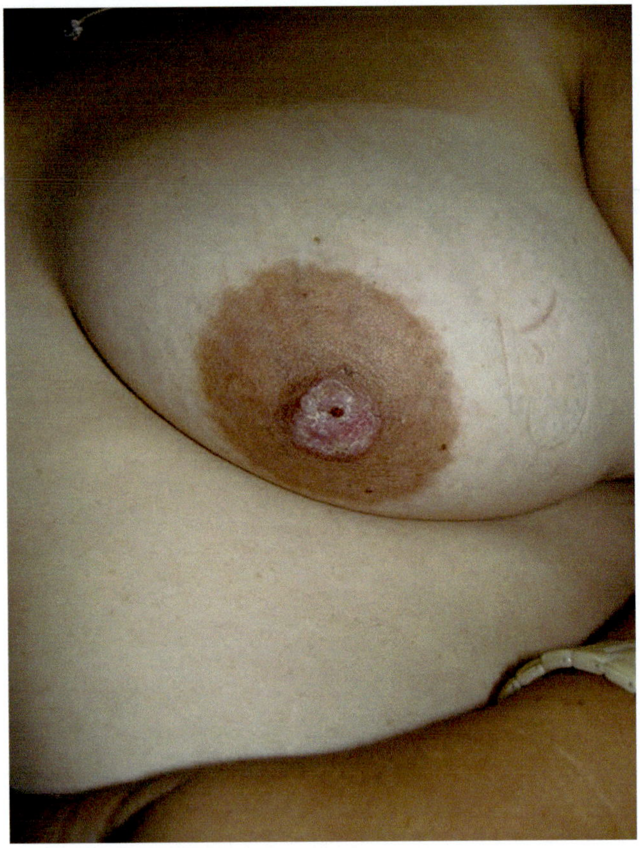

Fig. 44 Clinical appearance of lesion. Scally erythematous plaque at the center of the nipple

Clinical record:

Sex: Female

Age: 45-years-old

Clinical description: Patient presents with a 2-and-a-half-year history of a small, asymptomatic, serohematic crust on her left nipple. Previously treated with topical corticosteroids and emollients without noticeable improvement. At physical examination there were no palpable breast masses and no supraclavicular or axillary lymphadenopathy. A previous, two-years-ago mammography revealed no abnormalities.

Body site: Left nipple

Surface: flat, palpable, scally erythematous plaque

Maximum diameter: 1.8 × 1.9 × 0.1 cm

Duration of the lesion: 2-and-a-half- year

History of morphologic changes: 8 months

Personal history of skin cancer: No

Family history of skin cancer: No

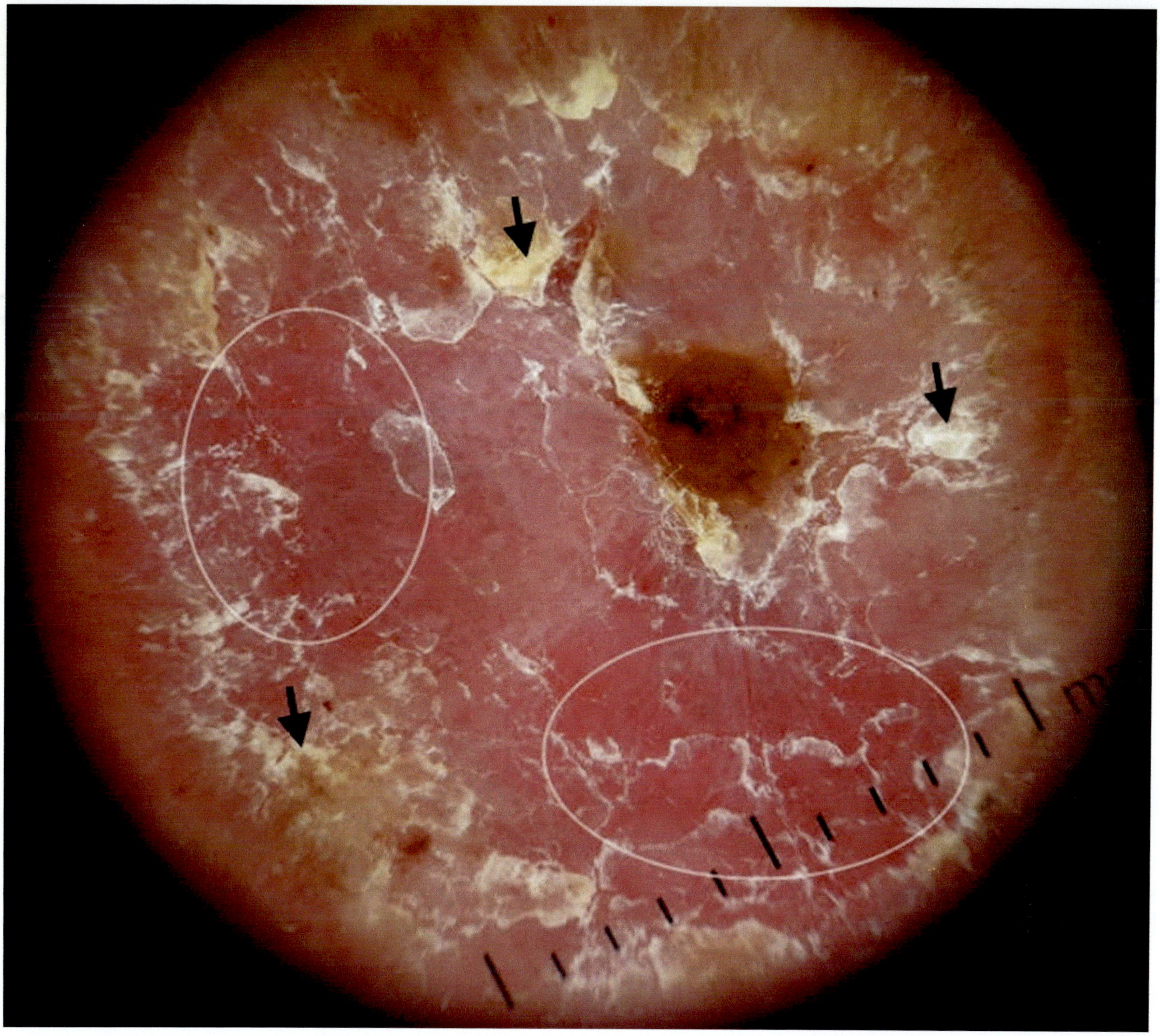

Fig. 45 Dermatoscopic appearance. Reddish-pink areas (white ovals) alternate with surface keratin as hyperkeratotic structures (black arrows)

Skin Phototype: III

Clinical diagnosis: Breast eczema

Dermatoscopic findings: reddish-pink areas alternate with hyperkeratotic structures, dotted and linear regular vessels at the center of the lesion on a pinkish-paler background

Other clinical findings: Obesity (Figs. 44, 45, 46 and 47)

Diagnosis: Paget's disease

Key message: In the diagnostic approach of a chronic and persistent erythematous lesion on the nipple or areola, accompanied by pruritus, Paget's Disease should be

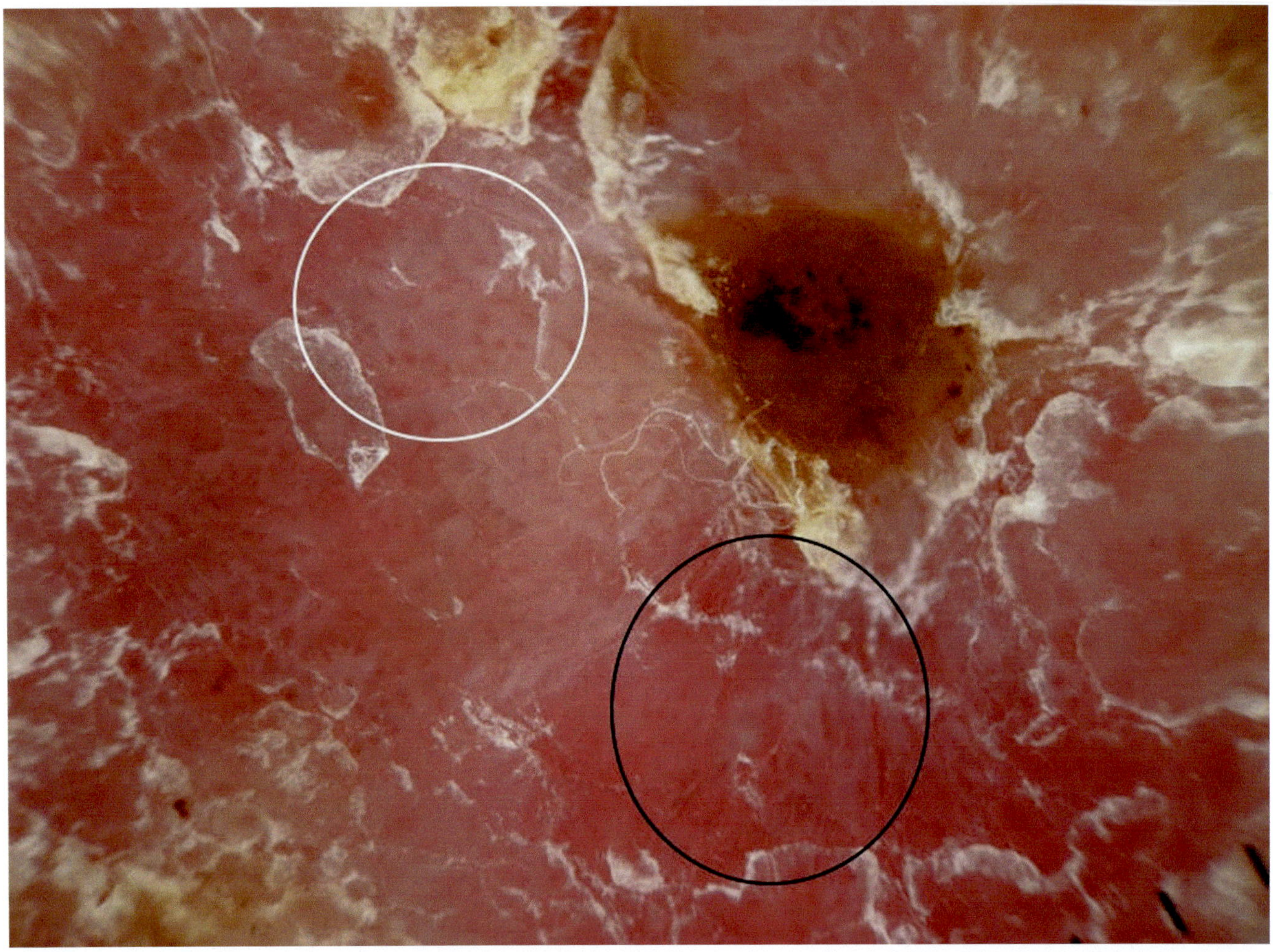

Fig. 46 Close up dermatoscopic appearance. Dotted vessels (white circle) and linear regular vessels (black circle) over a paler whitish-pink background

considered as a differential diagnosis. Dermoscopy in this entity guides and supports the diagnosis, since the dermatoscopic findings of the publications collected to date coincide with the findings that this case presents: surface keratin, red and/or pink background; dotted vessels and aggregate in this case: linear vessels, not observed in other publications.

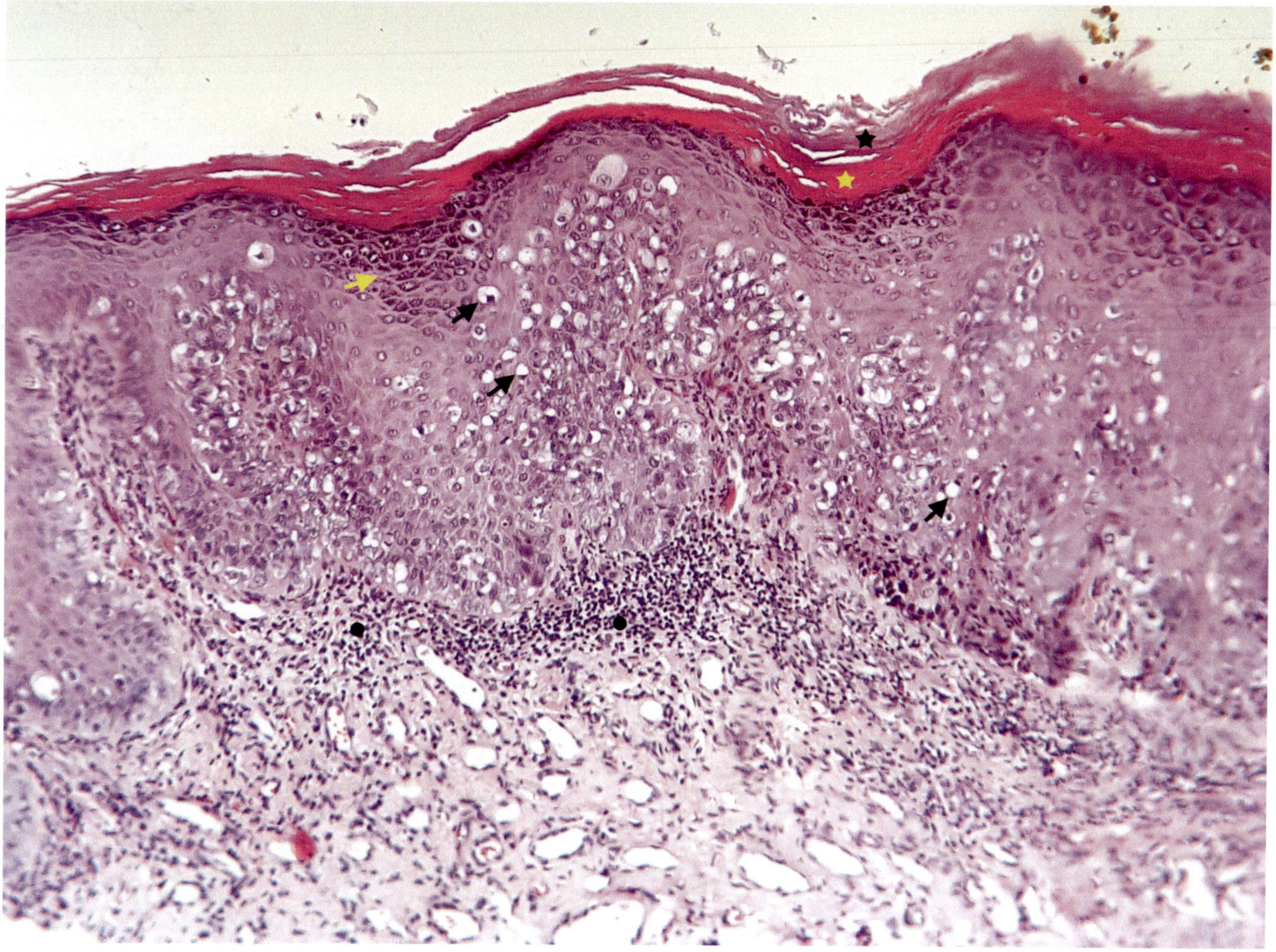

Fig. 47 Histologic examination of the lesion revealed atypical large cells with hyperchromatism, eccentric nuclei and abundant clear cytoplasm that can be seen throughout the epidermis (black arrows), as well as hyperkeratosis (yellow star) alternating with parakeratosis (black star), acanthosis and focal hypergranulosis (yellow arrow). Dense and difusse lymphocytic infiltrate in papillar dermis (black dots)

Gluteal Area Lesions

Bengu Nisa Akay, Elisa Camela, and Horacio Cabo

Abstract

This chapter is about of non-pigmented lesion in gluteal area such as eccrine porome and Spitz nevus and Squamous Cell Carcinoma in situ focusing in their dermatoscopic features.

Keywords

Eccrine porome • Spitz nevus • Squamous Cell Carcinoma in situ

Case 1

Author: Bengu Nisa Akay

Clinical record:

Sex: Female

Age: 81-year-old

Clinical description: Growing pink nodular lesion

Body site: Lateral side of the right gluteal region

Surface: Nodular

Maximum diameter: 7 mm

Duration of the lesion: 8 months

History of morphologic changes: Growth in recent months

Personal history of skin cancer: None

Family history of skin cancer: None

Skin Phototype: III

Clinical diagnosis: Rule out nodular melanoma, nodular bcc, another glandular tumor

Dermoscopic findings: Polymorphic vessels including vessels with bulbous endings (flower like vessels), serpentine and branched vessels, white interseptal lines, ulceration and blood crusts

Other clinical findings: None (Figs. 1 and 2)

Diagnosis: Eccrine Porome

Key message: Dermoscopy clues are very usefull for the diagnosis of Eccrine poroma

Case 2

Author: Elisa Camela

Clinical record:

Sex: Female

Age: 56-years-old

B. N. Akay
Faculty Department of Dermatology, Ankara University Medicine, Ankara Universitesi Tip Fak. Ibni Sina Hast, Dermatoloji ABD Akademik yerleşke binası M1 blok, 06100 Altindag Ankara, Turkey

E. Camela
Dermatology Unit, Istituto Dermopatico Dell'Immacolata, IDI IRCCS, Via Dei Monti di Creta 104, 00167 Rome, Italy

H. Cabo (✉)
University of Buenos Aires, Arenales 1446 1 °C (1061) CABA, Buenos Aires, Argentina
e-mail: cabohoracio@gmail.com

H. Cabo and A. Lallas (eds.), *Dermatoscopic Atlas of Non-Pigmented Lesions*,
https://doi.org/10.1007/978-3-031-34310-0_5

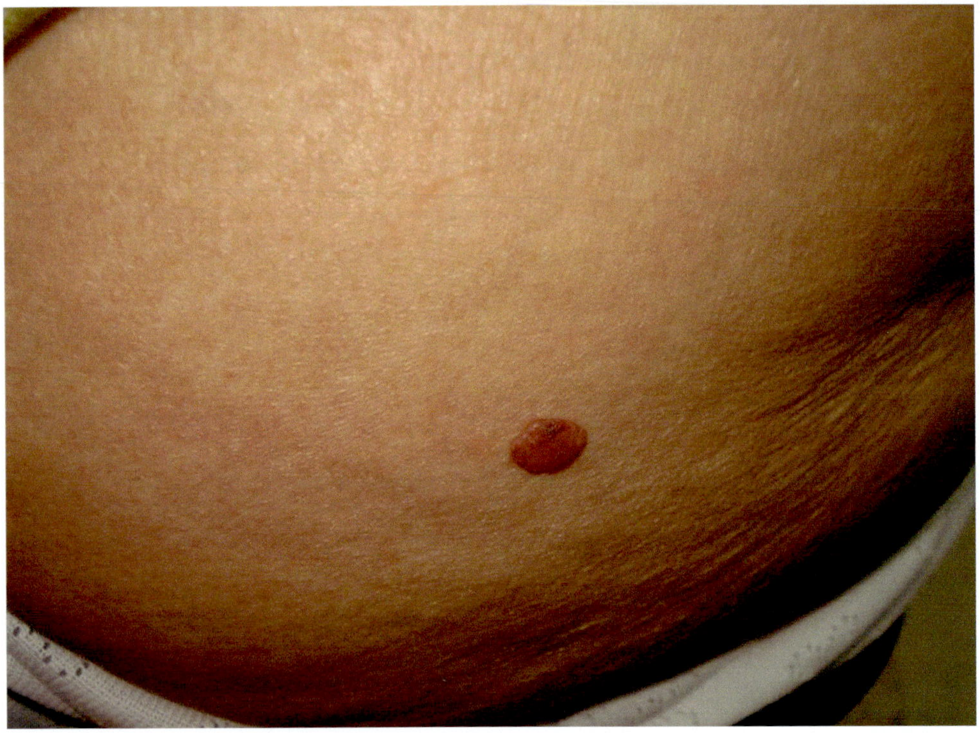

Fig. 1 Growing pink nodular lesion on lateral side of the right gluteal region

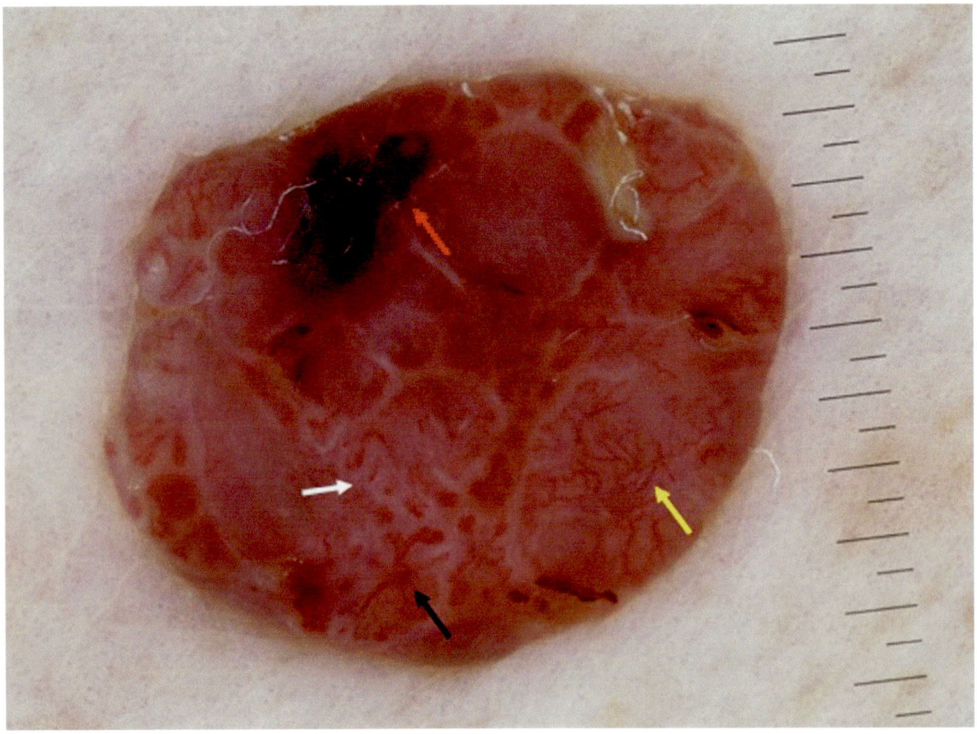

Fig. 2 Polymorphic vessels including vessels with bulbous endings (flower like vessels) (black arrow); serpentine and branched vessels /yellow arrow); white interseptal lines (white arrow); ulceration and blood crusts (red arrow)

Clinical description the case or the lesion: An otherwise healthy patient referred the occurrence a "new" lesion on the left gluteus few months earlier. She was used to perform periodic skin check (every 6 months) for the elevated number of nevi and the family history of melanoma.

Body site: Left gluteus

Surface: Palpable

Maximum diameter: 4 mm

Duration of the lesion: Few months earlier

History of morphologic changes: De novo lesion

Personal history of skin cancer: No

Family history of skin cancer: Melanoma

Skin Phototype: II

Clinical diagnosis: Spitz Nevus

Dermoscopic findings: Presence of negative pigment network and regularly distributed red dotted vessels.

Other clinical findings: N/A (Figs. 3 and 4)

Diagnosis: Spitz Nevus

Key message: Dermoscopy may help the diagnosis of pink lesions allowing differentiate benign from malignant ones and guide the management

Case 3

Author: Horacio Cabo

Sex: Female

Age: 75-year-old patient

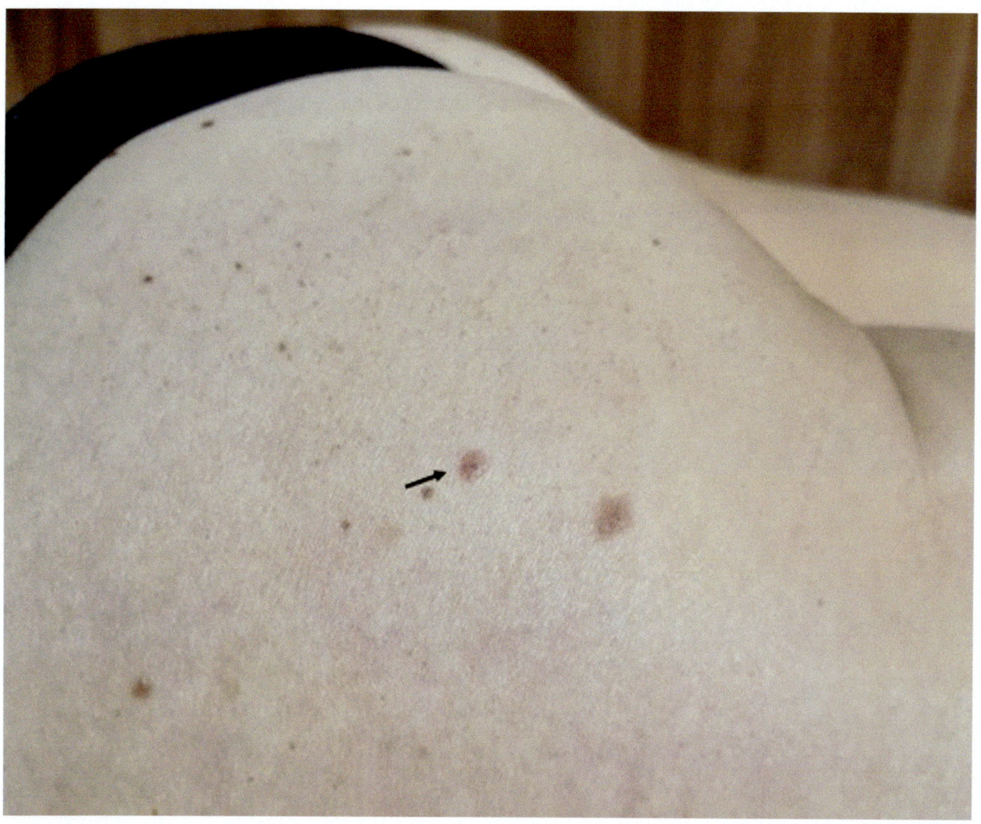

Fig. 3 Clinical aspect of Spitz Nevus: pink papule (black arrow)

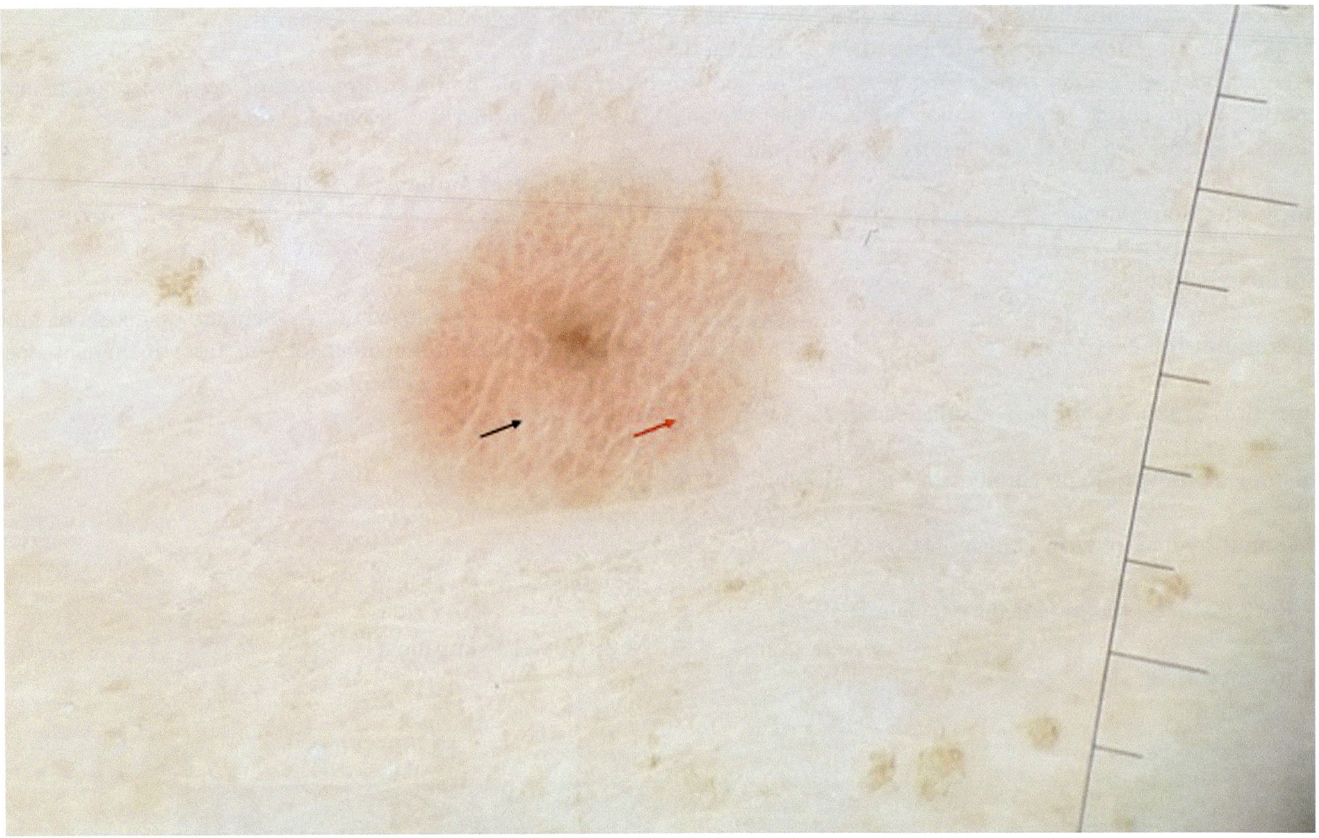

Fig. 4 Dermoscopic pattern of Spitz Nevus: negative pigment network (black arrow); and regularly distributed red dotted vessels (red arrow)

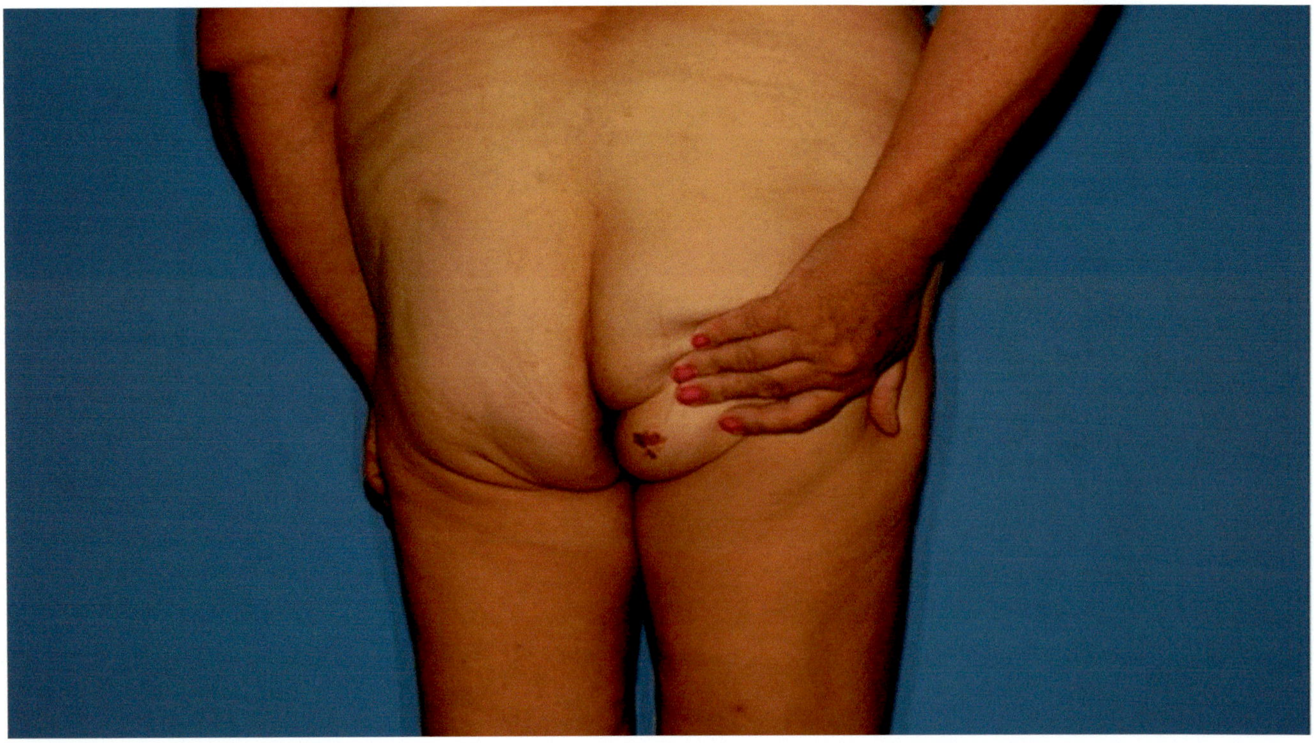

Fig. 5 Clinical view

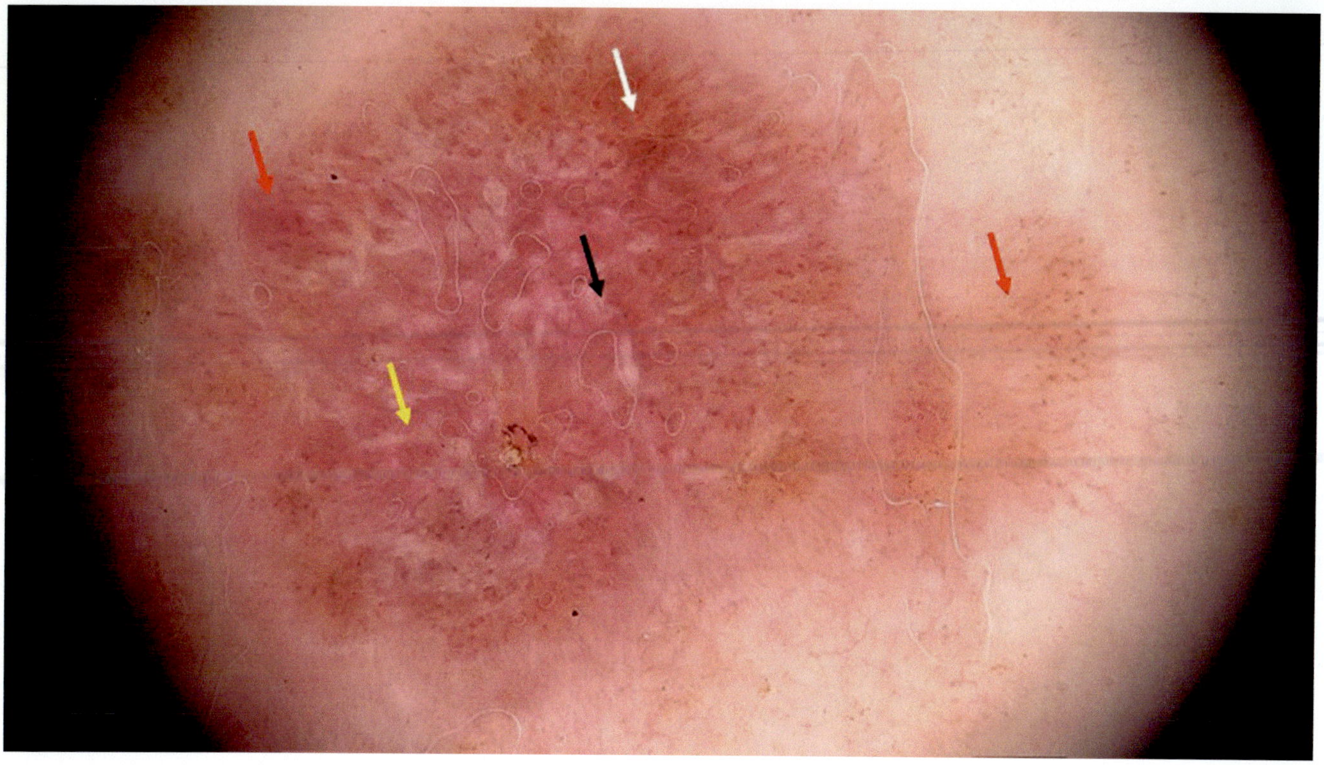

Fig. 6 Dermatoscopy view: dotted vessels in linear distribution

Clinical description the case or the lesion: Asymptomatic non pigmented lesion

Body site: Gluteal area

Surface: Palpable

Maximum diameter: 15 mm

Duration of the lesion: Unknown

History of morphologic changes: Unknown

Personal history of skin cancer: No

Family history of skin cancer: No

Skin Phototype: III

Clinical diagnosis: Psoriasis, Lichen Plano, Saquamos cell carcinoma

Dermoscopic findings: Dotted vessels in linear distribution

Other clinical findings: None (Figs. 5 and 6)

Diagnosis: Squamous Cell Carcinoma in situ

Key message: When we realize total body skin examination, we have to include genital areas.

In this way we were able to make the diagnosis of squamous cell carcinoma in situ

Upper Limbs Lesions

Gabriella Brancaccio, Raimonds Karls, Laura Freiberga, Horacio Cabo, and Emilia Noemi Cohen Sabban

Abstract

Some non-pigmented lesion localized in the upper limbs are described in this chapter. Between them, Basal cell carcinoma, superficial acral fibromyxoma, Bowen's disease and Pigmented Squamous cell carcinoma in situ are foucusing specialy their dermoscopic features.

Keyword

Basal cell carcinoma • superficial acral fibromyxoma • Bowen's disease • Pigmented Squamous cell carcinoma in situ

Case 1

Author: Gabriella Brancaccio

G. Brancaccio
Dermatology Unit, University of Campania "Luigi Vanvitelli", Via Sergio Pansini, 5, 80131 Naples, Italy
https://www.dermatologs.lv
https://www.adasvezis.lv

R. Karls
SIA "Derma Clinic Riga" Valdes priekšsēdētajs, International Dermoscopy Society Neanglisko aktivitāšu komitējas vadītājs, Grebenščikova ielā 1, Rīga, 1003, Latvia

Chair of Non-English Activities Committe of International Dermoscopy Society, Derma Clinic Riga, Ltd., Grebenscikova Str. 1, Rīga, 1003, Latvia

L. Freiberga
Derma Clinic Riga Ltd., University of Latvia, Riga, Latvia

H. Cabo (✉)
Clinical Dermatology, University of Buenos Aires, Arenales 1446 1 °C (1061) CABA, Buenos Aires, Argentina
e-mail: cabohoracio@gmail.com

E. N. C. Sabban
Chief of Dermatology Division of the "Instituto de Investigaciones Médicas A. Lanari", University of Buenos Aires, Arenales 1446 1 °C, Buenos Aires, Argentina

Clinical record:

Sex: Female.

Age: 55-years-old

Clinical description the case or the lesion: Reddish papule on the right shoulder

Body site: Right shoulder (trapezius area)

Surface: Palpable

Maximum diameter: 9 mm

Duration of the lesion: <6 months

History of morphologic changes: This patient undergoes routinary Total Body Photography and Sequential digital Dermoscopy images. At the previous visit (6 months before) the lesion was

Personal history of skin cancer: Melanomas stage IA of the back (0.3 and 0.5 before 2014), melanoma in situ of the abdomen (2021), multiple basal cell carcinoma of the trunk

Family history of skin cancer: Father, multiple squamous and basal cell carcinomas of limbs, trunk and head and neck

Skin Phototype: II

Clinical diagnosis:Basal cell carcinoma vs amelanotic melanoma

Dermoscopic findings: On-focus sharply demarcated fine arborizing vessels, homogenously distributed, and the presence of a yellow component, may aid in the diagnosis of basal cell carcinoma (Figs. 1, 2, and 3)

H. Cabo and A. Lallas (eds.), *Dermatoscopic Atlas of Non-Pigmented Lesions*,
https://doi.org/10.1007/978-3-031-34310-0_6

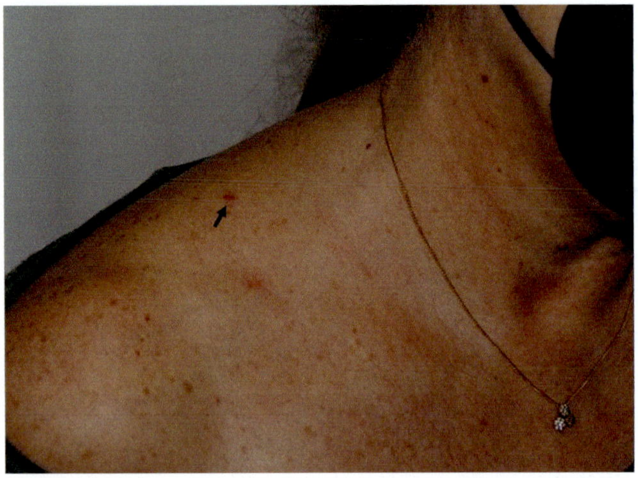

Fig. 1 In 55-year-old women, on a severe photodamaged skin, a reddish papule is visible on the right shoulder (arrow)

Diagnosis: Basal Cell Carcinoma

Key message: The presence of on-focus, fine, arborizing telangiectasias and of yellow-orange color aids the diagnosis of basal cell carcinoma. However, to rule out nodular amelanotic melanoma histopathology is mandatory.

Case 2

Author: Raimonds Karls, Laura Freiberga

Clinical record:

Sex: Male

Age: 24-years-old

Clinical description the case or the lesion: Erythematous round plaque, shiny surface, diameter 12 × 13 mm. Slight scaling ring around the lesion

Body site: right elbow

Surface: Palpable

Maximum diameter: 12 × 13 mm

Duration of the lesion: Lesion for more than 3 years

History of morphologic changes: Slow growing in diameter and elevation. No topical treatment before. For last 4–6 weeks' patient used bandage due to increased wetting.

Personal history of skin cancer: No dysplastic nevus syndrome, no previous skin cancers. Some severe sunburns during lifetime. There are some solar lentigo lesions on the patients' shoulders, melanocytic nevi total number up to 150.

Fig. 2 At a close-up image the firm papule exhibits both red and yellow colors

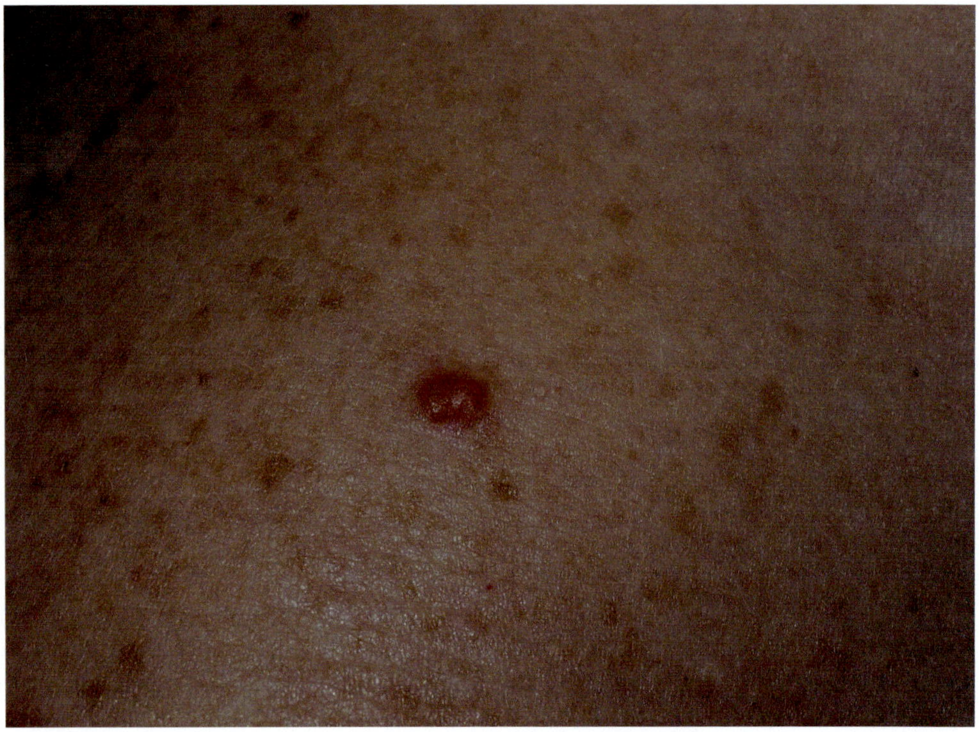

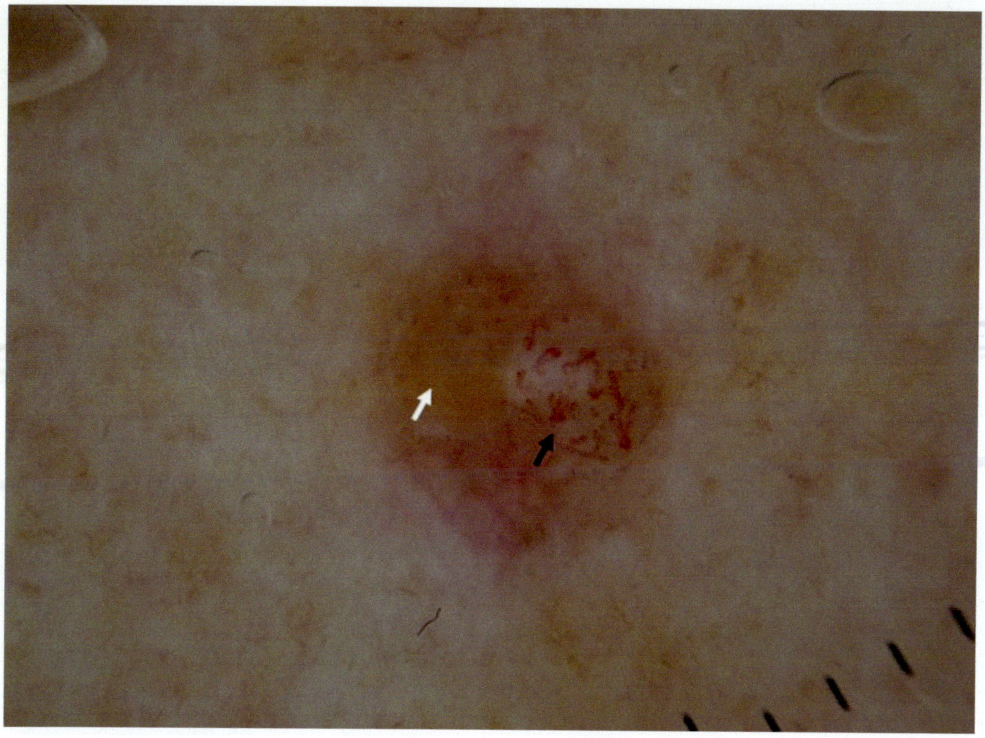

Fig. 3 Dermoscopically the lesion is composed by sharply demarcated, on-focus and homogeneously distributed fine arborizing vessels on the right (black arrow), and by a yellow-orange homogeneous component on the left side (white arrow)

Family history of skin cancer: No data about skin cancer in family relatives

Skin Phototype: Skin type II

Clinical diagnosis: Amelanotic melanoma

Dermoscopic findings: Milky-red background, structureless whitish areas. Multiple vessels, different in diameter and pattern—polymorphous vessels. Under polarized light structureless areas reveals slight shiny crystalline phenomena.

Other clinical findings: None (Figs. 4, 5 and 6)

In subepidermal tissue, proliferation of spindle-shaped cells in a collagenous and myxoid stroma (4) without cell atypia, without mitoses, without necrosis, no nuclear pleomorphism

Diagnosis: Superficial acral fibromyxoma

Key message: Diagnosis of non-pigmented lesion is always a challenge for practicing doctors with any level of experience. In addition to more common non-pigmented lesions with clear dermatoscopic features, malignant tumors, rare and appendage tumors are observed.

Case 3

Authors: Horacio Cabo; Emilia Noemi Cohen Sabban

Clinical record:

Sex: Female

Age: 62- years-old

Clinical description the case or the lesion: Asymptomatic pink lesion

Body site: Left arm

Surface: Flat

Maximum diameter: 12 mm

Duration of the lesion: More than one year

History of morphologic changes: Growing in the last months

Personal history of skin cancer: None

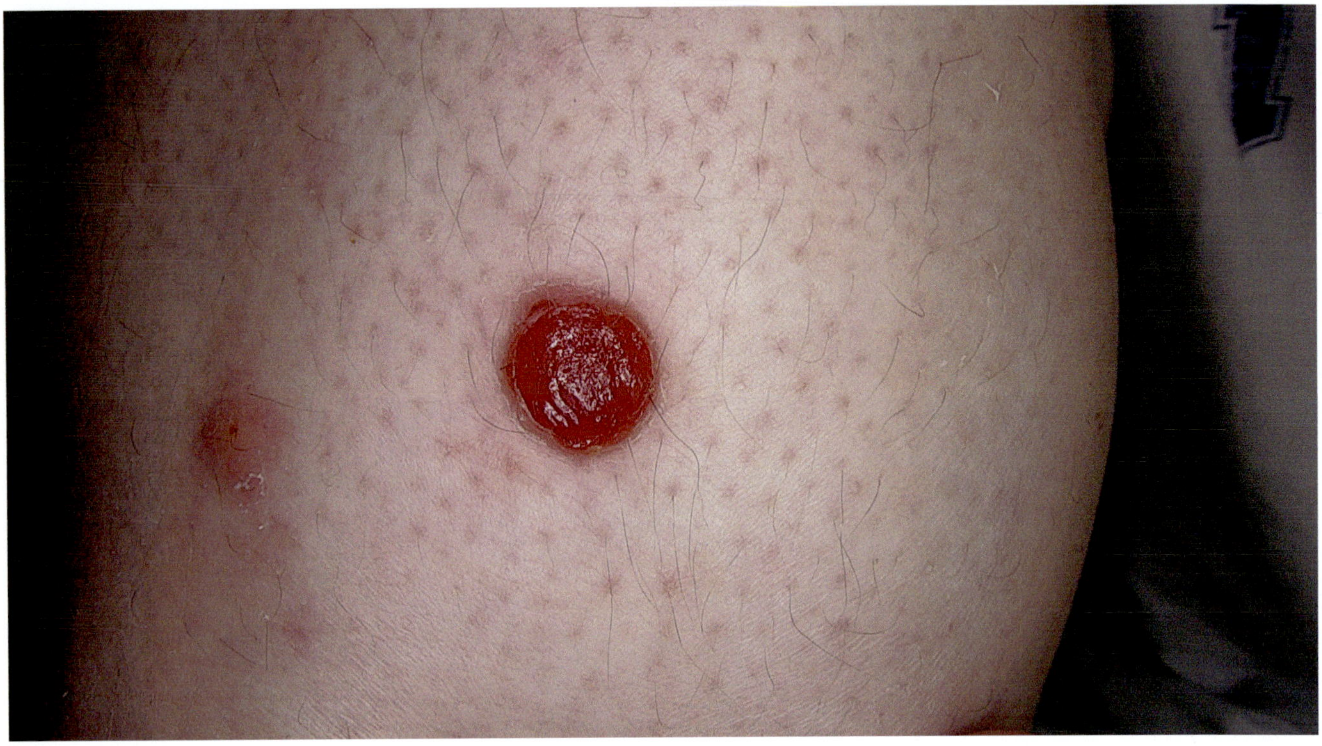

Fig. 4 Clinical view

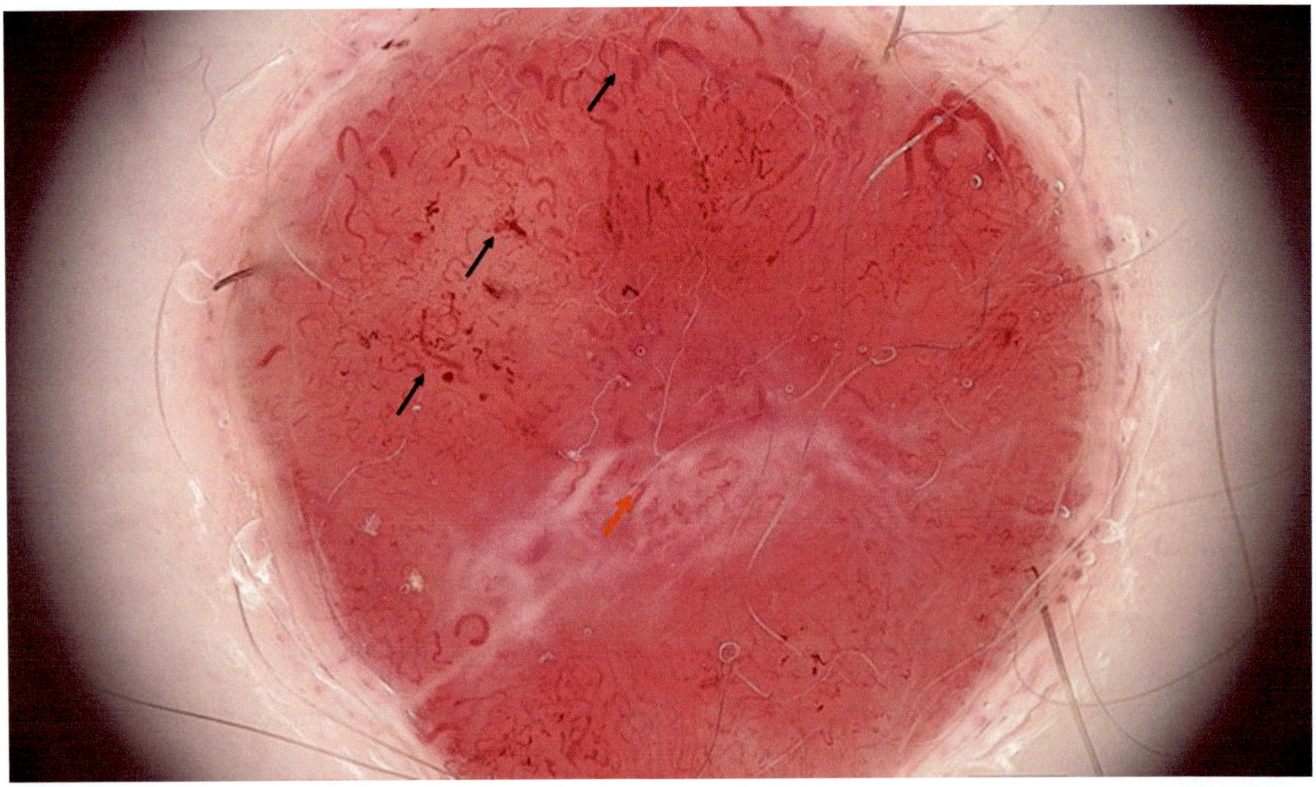

Fig. 5 Polarized dermatoscopy. Magnification 20x. Milky-red background, structureless whitish areas. Multiple vessels, different in diameter and pattern – polymorphous vessels (black arrows). Under polarized light structureless areas reveals slight shiny white crystalline phenomena. (red arrow)

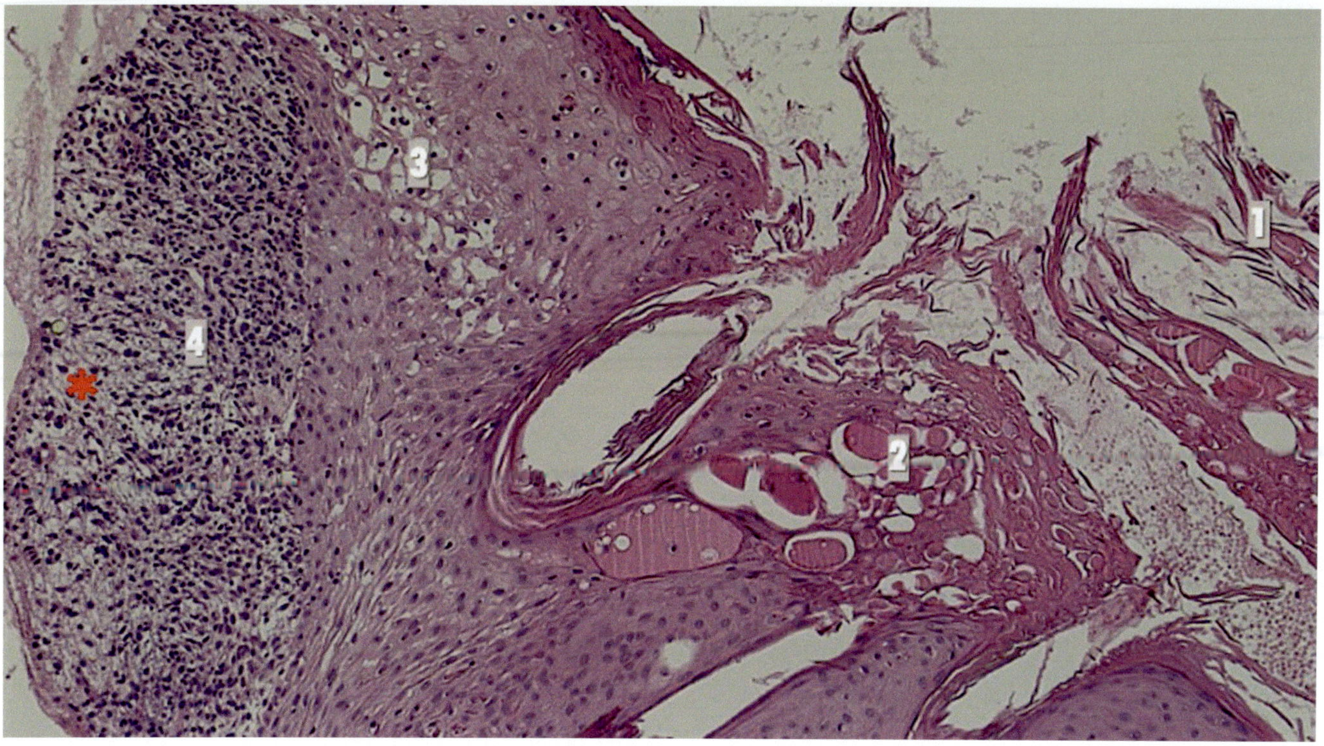

Fig. 6 Skin fragment with parakeratosis (1), plasma clots (2), epidermal secondary hypoplasia, spongiosis (3)

Family history of skin cancer: None

Skin Phototype: II

Clinical diagnosis: Basal Cell carcinoma

Dermoscopic findings: white scales and glomerular vessels with cluster distribution

Other clinical findings: None (Figs. 7 and 8)

Diagnosis: Bowen's disease

Key message: No pigmented squamous cell carcinoma in situ (Bowen's disease) is sometimes a differential diagnosis from no pigmented superficial basal cell carcinoma.

Case 4

Authors: Horacio Cabo; Emilia N. Cohen Sabban

Clinical record:

Sex: Male

Age: 68-years-old

Clinical description the case or the lesion: Large asymptomatic scaly erythematous plaque on the right arm

Body site: Upper limbs

Surface: Flat

Maximum diameter: 20 mm

Duration of the lesion: More than one year

History of morphologic changes: Growing

Personal history of skin cancer: None

Family history of skin cancer: None

Skin Phototype: III

Clinical diagnosis: Squamous cell carcinoma

Dermoscopic findings: Focal distribution of glomerular vessels on a brown, pink, white scaly background. In some peripheral areas red dots with linear arrangement are seen.

Other clinical findings: None (Figs. 9 and 10)

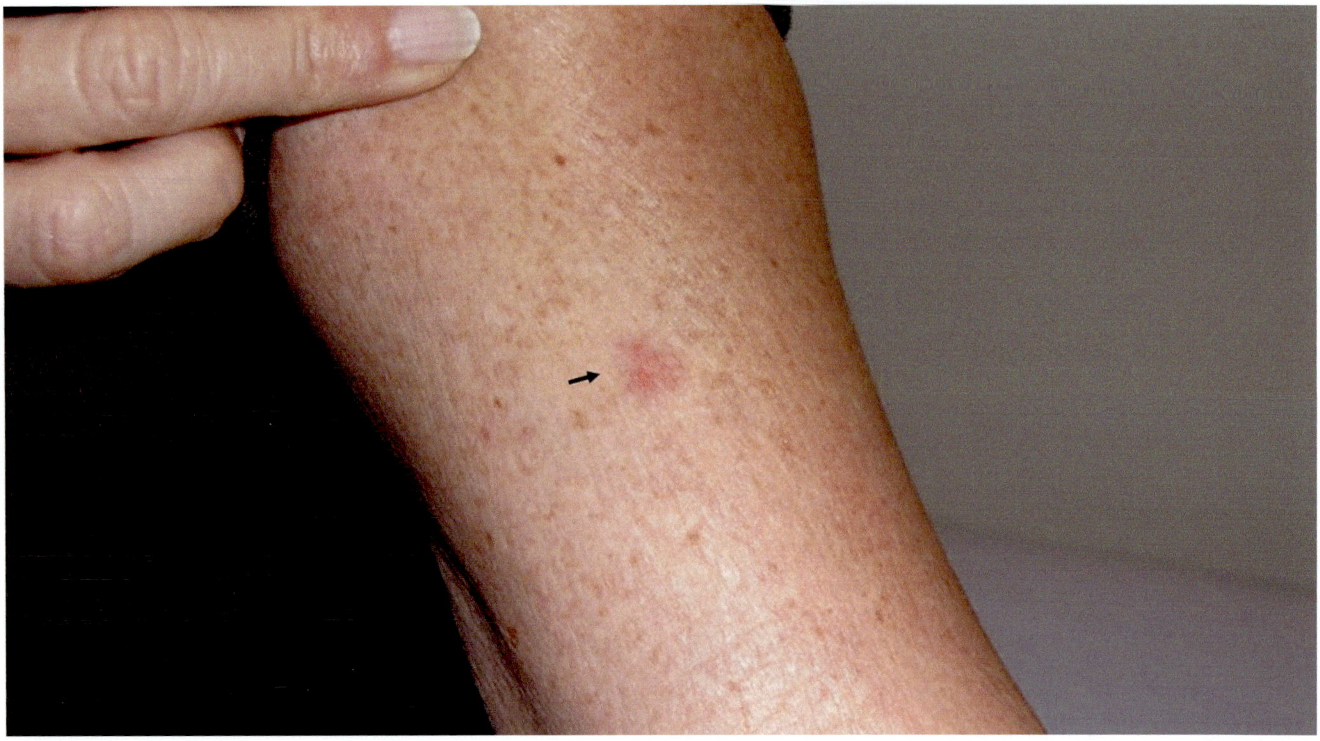

Fig. 7 Clinical view (black arrow)

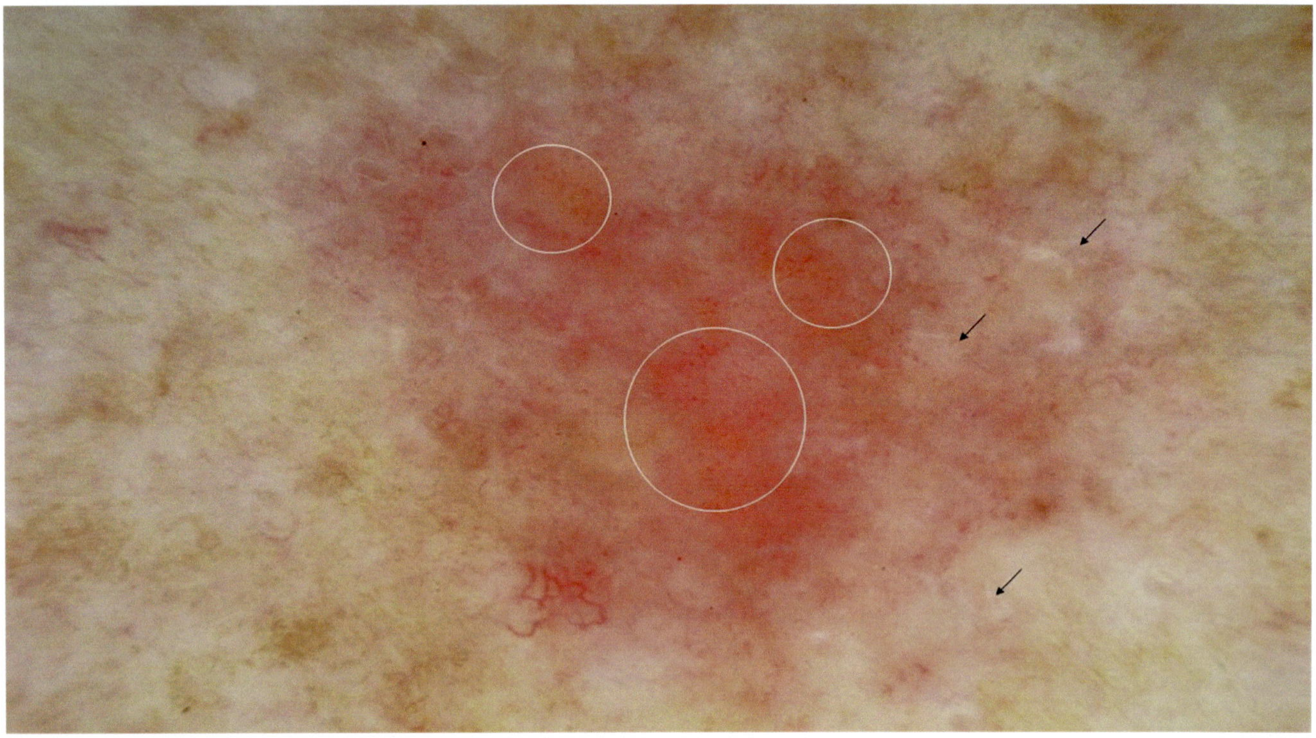

Fig. 8 White scales (black arrows) and glomerular vessels with cluster distribution (white circles)

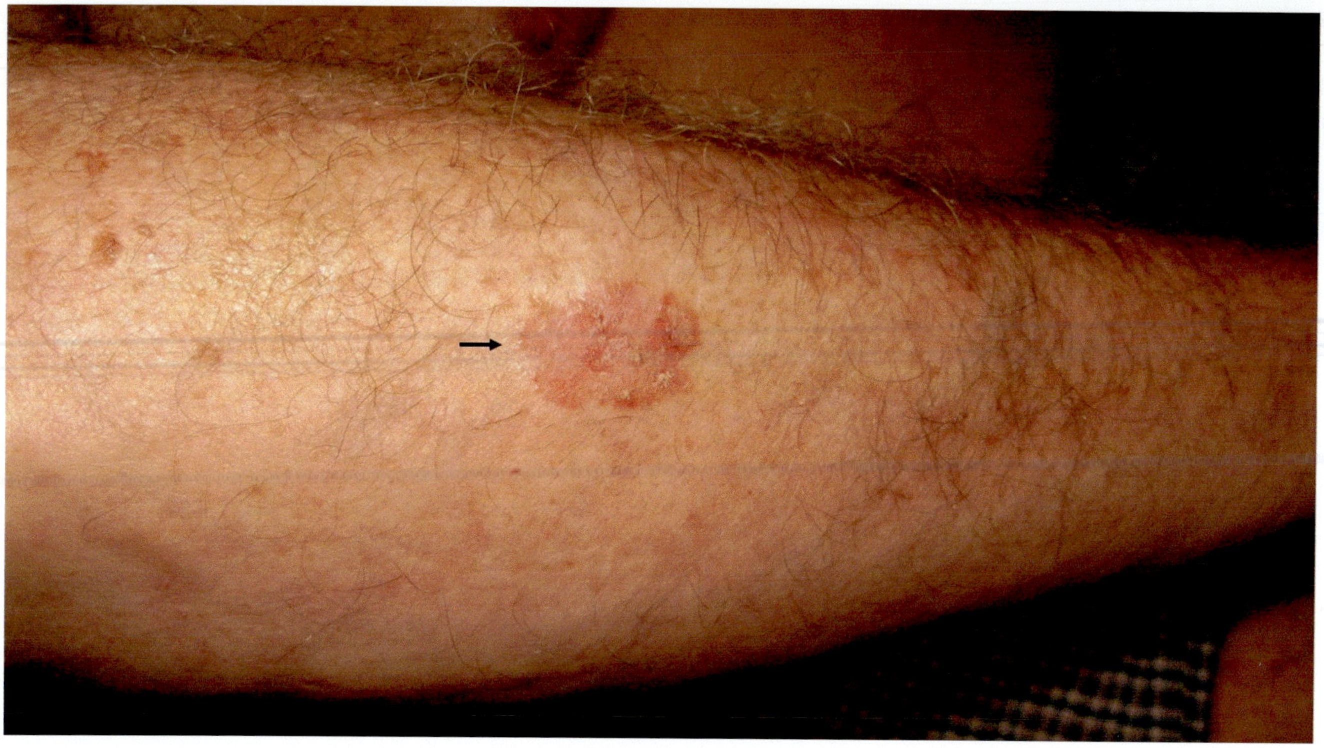

Fig. 9 Clinical image: large asymptomatic scaly erythematous plaque on the right arm (arrow)

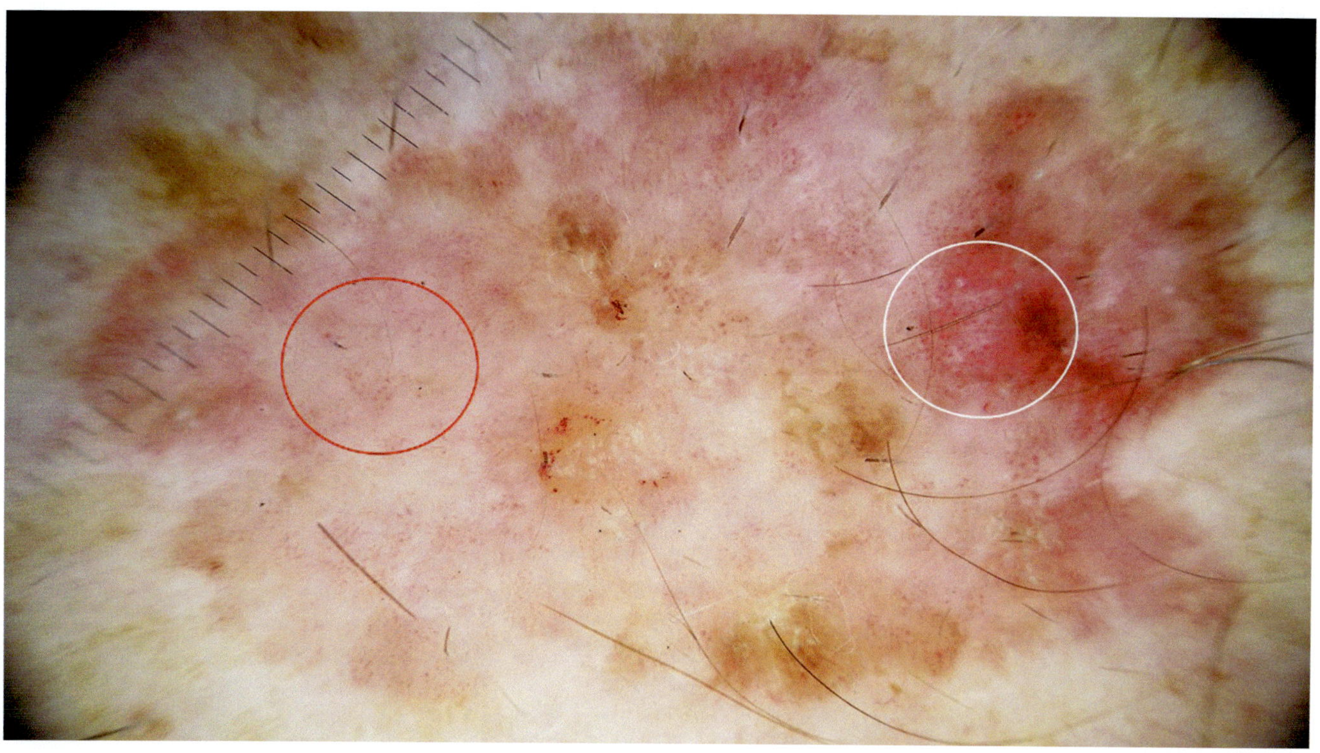

Fig. 10 Dermoscopic image: focal distribution of glomerular vessels (red circle) on a brown, pink, white scaly background. In some peripheral areas red dots with linear arrangement are seen (white circle)

Diagnosis: Pigmented squamous cell carcinoma in situ

Key message: On occasion pigmented Bowen disease shows a pink, skin color, light brown and white background under dermoscopic examination. In these cases, the clinical image is a hypopigmented lesion.

The vascular pattern with glomerular vessels is the clue

Lower Limb Lesions

Ana Maria Forsea, Andre Oliveira, Francisca Donoso, Dominga Peirano, Cristián Navarrete Dechent, Pablo Uribe, Elisa Camela, Konstantinos Liopyris, Mónica Ramos Álvarez, Angelica Ruiz Dueñas, Rosario Peralta, Virginia Mariana Gonzales, Horacio Cabo, and Emilia Cohen Sabban

Abstract

Different pink lesion on lower limbs such as Basal cell carcinoma, Tattooed skin, Clear cell acanthoma, Tinea incognita, Spitz nevus, Eccrine porome, Molluscum contagiosum, Porokeratosis, Amelanotic Melanoma, Psoriasis with their dermoscopic features.

Keywords

Basal cell carcinoma • Tattooed skin • Clear cell acanthoma • Tinea incognita • Spitz nevus • Eccrine porome • Molluscum contagiosum • Porokeratosis • Amelanotic Melanoma • Psoriasis

Case 1

Author: Ana Maria Forsea

Clinical record:

Sex: Male

A. M. Forsea
Carol Davila University of Medicine and Pharmacy Bucharest, Elias University Hospital Bucharest, Bucharest, Romania

A. Oliveira
Department of Dermatology, Hospital Particular do Algarve, Sítio Cruz da Bota Estrada de Alvor, 8500-322 Alvor, Algarve, Portugal
e-mail: andre.oliveira@sapo.pt

F. Donoso · D. Peirano · C. Navarrete Dechent · P. Uribe
Department of Dermatology, Escuela de Medicina, Pontificia Universidad Católica de Chile, Diagonal Paraguay 362, 6th Floor, 8330077 Santiago, Chile
e-mail: fdonoso4@uc.cl

D. Peirano
e-mail: dpeirano@miuandes.cl

E. Camela
Dermatology Unit, Istituto Dermopatico dell'Immacolata, IDI IRCCS, Via dei Monti di Creta 104, 00167 Rome, Italy

K. Liopyris
Andreas Sygros Hospital for Cutaneous and Venereal Diseases, University of Athens, Memorial Sloan Kettering Cancer Center. Chairman of Communications, International Dermoscopy Society, Athens, Greece

M. R. Álvarez
Dermatology, Dermika Centro Dermatológico Láser, Diag. Golfo de Cortés 3002, Vallarta Nte., 44690 Guadalajara, Jalisco, México
e-mail: monica.ramos@dermika.com.mx

A. R. Dueñas
Dermatology, Dermatology Dermika Centro Dermatológico Láser, Diag. Golfo de Cortés 3002 Vallarta Nte. 44690 Guadalajara, Jalisco, México
e-mail: angelica.ruiz@dermika.com.mx

R. Peralta
Dermatology Department, Medical Research Institute "A. Lanari", University of Buenos Aires, 3150 Combatientes de Malvinas, CP 1427, Ciudad Autónoma de Buenos Aires, Argentina

V. M. Gonzales
Head of Dermato-Oncology and Dermoscopy Section, Hospital Aleman, Pueyrredon A. 1640 Postal Code, C1118AAT- Buenos Aires, Argentina

H. Cabo (✉)
Clinical Dermatology, University of Buenos Aires, Arenales 1446 1 °C (1061) CABA, Buenos Aires, Argentina
e-mail: cabohoracio@gmail.com

E. C. Sabban
Chief of Dermatology Division of the "Instituto de Investigaciones Médicas A. Lanari", University of Buenos Aires, Arenales 1446 1 °C, Buenos Aires, Argentina

H. Cabo and A. Lallas (eds.), *Dermatoscopic Atlas of Non-Pigmented Lesions*,
https://doi.org/10.1007/978-3-031-34310-0_7

Age: 53-years-old

Clinical description the case or the lesion: Asymptomatic, erythematous, slightly rough plaque, 1.3 cm maximal diameter, polygonal shape, geographic contour, noticed by the patient as increasing in dimension and roughness, on the lateral aspect of the left calf.

Body site: Lateral aspect of the left lower limb.

Surface: Flat, moderately rough

Maximum diameter: 1.3 cm

Duration of the lesion: Observed by the patient 2–3 months prior to the presentation, A small pigmented macula on the same site was identified on earlier clinical total-body-photography pictures taken 2 years prior to the presentation.

History of morphologic changes: Patient reported increased in size and roughness for several months prior to the presentation. From presentation time (Fig. 1) to excision time (2.5 months) (Fig. 2) slightly increased erythema and scaling.

Personal history of skin cancer: Melanoma Stage III right ankle (diagnosis 2003); melanoma in situ posterior thorax (diagnosis 2020), status post -chemotherapy adjuvant (2014), post adjuvant immunotherapy Nivolumab + Ipilimumab (2017), immunotherapy-related pituitary insufficiency under glucocorticoid and thyroid hormone substitution.

Family history of skin cancer: Not known

Skin Phototype: II

Clinical diagnosis: suspicion: Bowen disease/Actinic keratosis

Dermoscopic findings: Red-white structureless areas, peripheral polymorphous vessels (cork-screw, hairpin, dotted), shiny white lines (chrysalids) and blotches on polarized dermoscopy.

Suggested diagnosis: basal cell carcinoma

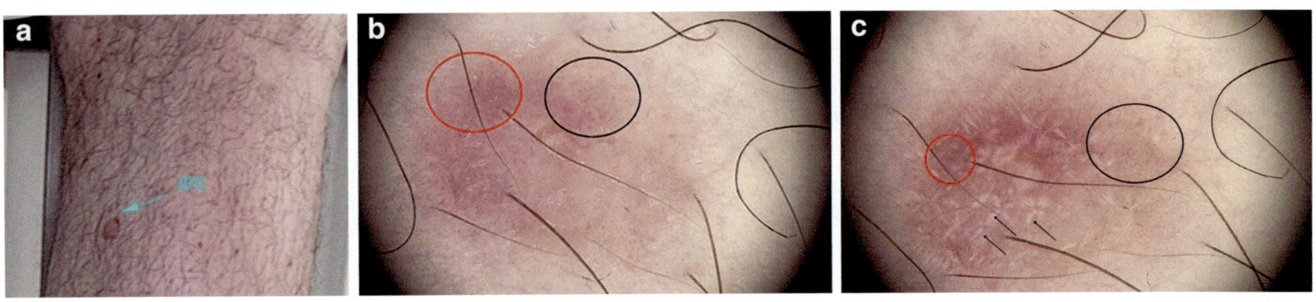

Fig. 1 Aspect on first presentation. 1a Clinical aspect (green line 01). 1b Dermoscopy non-polarized: Red-white structureless areas (red circle), peripheral polymorphous vessels (cork-screw, hairpin, dotted) (black circle). 1c Dermoscopy polarized: Red-white structureless areas (red circle), peripheral polymorphous vessels (cork-screw, hairpin, dotted) (black circle), and shiny white lines (black arrows)

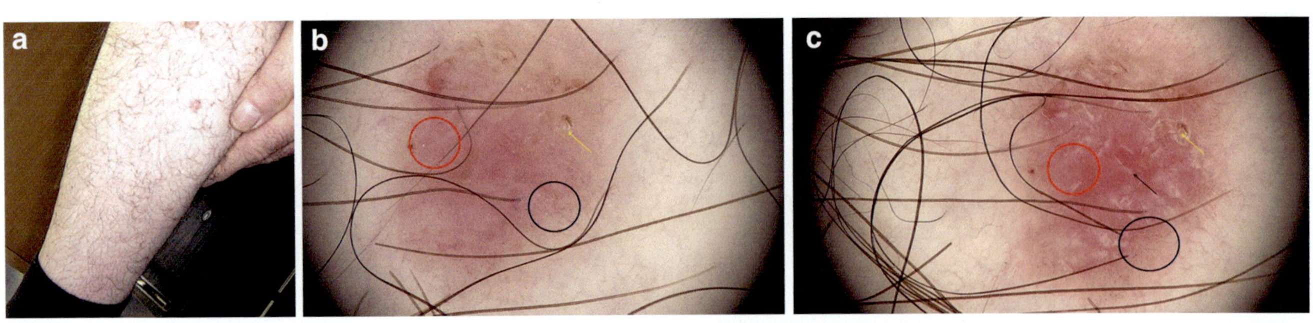

Fig. 2 Aspect 3 months after the initial presentation, before excision: 1a Clinical aspect. 1b dermoscopy non-polarized: Red-white structureless areas (red circle), peripheral polymorphous vessels (cork-screw, hairpin, dotted) (black circle). 1c dermoscopy polarized: Red-white structureless areas (red circle), peripheral polymorphous vessels (cork-screw, hairpin, dotted) (black circle), and shiny white lines (black arrows); small erosion (yellow arrow)

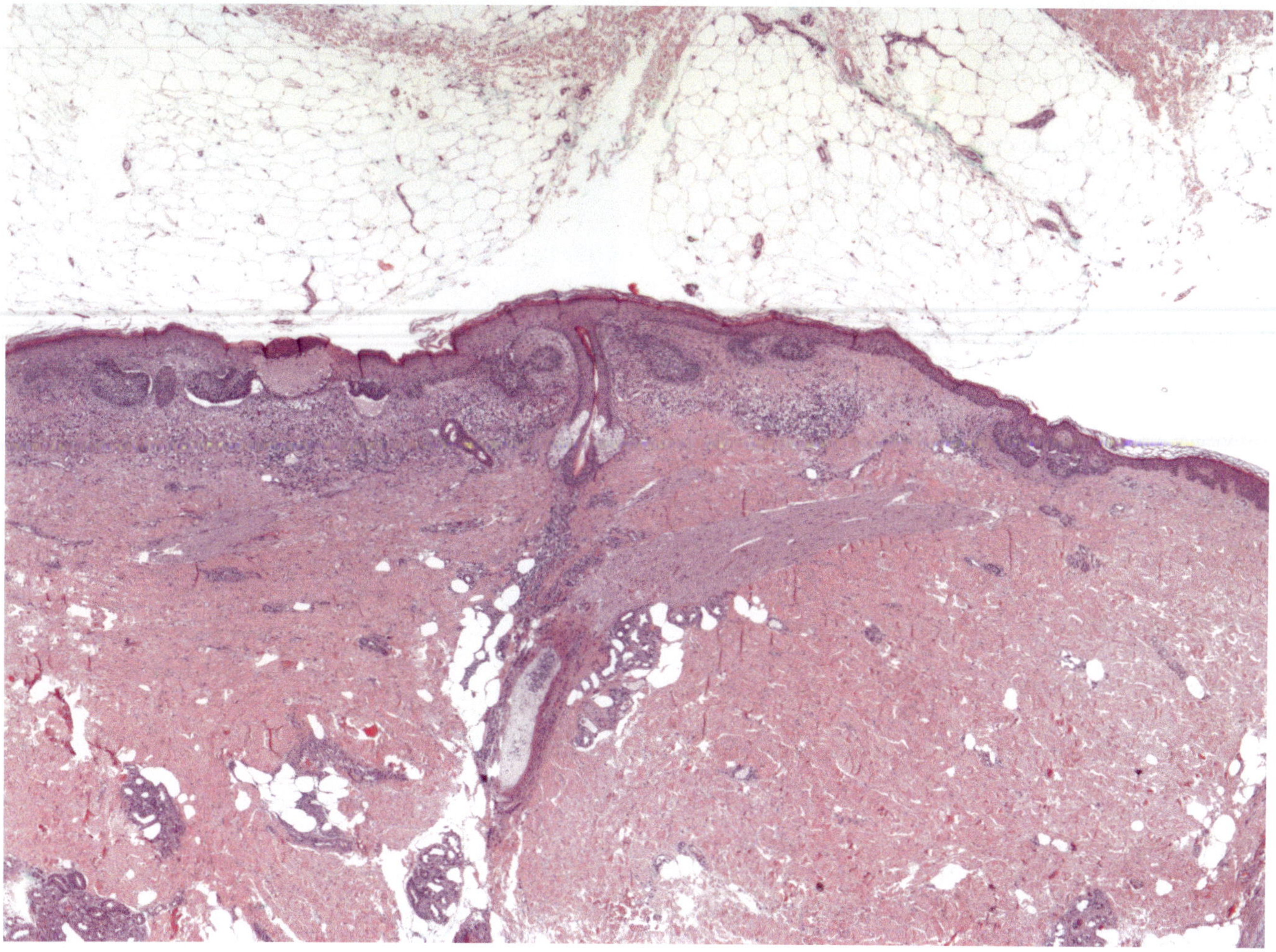

Fig. 3 Histopathology after in toto excision (Hematoxylin–eosin, 50 × magnification): Germinal epithelial (basaloid) tumor proliferation emanating multicentrically from beneath the epidermis and penetrating the superficial dermis in the form of variably-sized tumoral aggregates, with peripheral palisading and retraction artefact from adjacent stroma

Other clinical findings: None

Histopathological examination: Superficial Basal Cell Carcinoma (Fig. 3)

Diagnosis: Superficial Basal Cell Carcinoma

Key message: Dermoscopy, especially combination of polarized and non-polarized dermoscopy is helpful in suggesting the diagnosis in clinically equivocal lesions, in patients at high risk for skin cancer.

Superficial basal cell carcinoma may lack most characteristic clinical/dermoscopic features for BCCs such as arborizing vessels or pigment-relates features. Polarized dermoscopy showing shiny white structures is helpful in these cases.

Acknowledgement: Histopathological image provided by Dr. Irina Margaritescu, Oncoteam Diagnostics, Bucharest

Case 2

Author: André Oliveira

Clinical record:

Sex: Female

Age: 47-years old

Surface: Pink palpable papule on underlying multicolored decorative tattoo located on the right thigh

Maximum diameter: 5 mm of maximum diameter

Duration of the lesion: Less than 6 months

History of morphologic changes: The patient presented for her regular 6-month screening. A pink papule was observed on the left thigh. The patient did not give it any relevance as she considered it as a "normal" change of her 1-year-old tattoo, even if a sustained growth was admitted

Personal history of skin cancer: The patient has had several basal cell carcinomas and squamous cell carcinomas removed. She was under regular skin screenings every 6 months. Her previous examination was unremarkable

Family history of skin cancer: No

Skin phototype: Skin type II

Clinical diagnosis: Basal cell carcinoma;

Dermoscopic findings: Arborizing vessels, shiny-white strands, pink homogeneous areas with underlying and adjacent dark black and gray ink corresponding to **basal cell carcinoma**.

Other clinical findings: None (Figs. 4, 5, 6 and 7)

Diagnosis: Superficial Basal Cell crcinoma on tattooed skin

Key message: Decorative tattoos are becoming progressively popular among all age groups. The diagnosis of skin cancer on tattooed skin can be challenging: 1) the usual clinical and dermoscopic findings are masked by the tattoo's ink; 2) patients are not aware of such changes (including the number of colors, size, shape or elevation) many times considering it as a "normal part of the tattoo"; 3) tattooed skin is often skipped from office skin examinations.

Basal cell carcinomas on tattooed skin have been infrequently reported. Again, the observation of arborizing vessels as the main dermoscopic vascular pattern facilitated the diagnosis, which was confirmed both in confocal microscopy and histologic examinations.

Case 3

Authors: Francisca Donoso, Dominga Peirano, Cristián Navarrete Dechent, Pablo Uribe

Clinical record:

Sex: Male

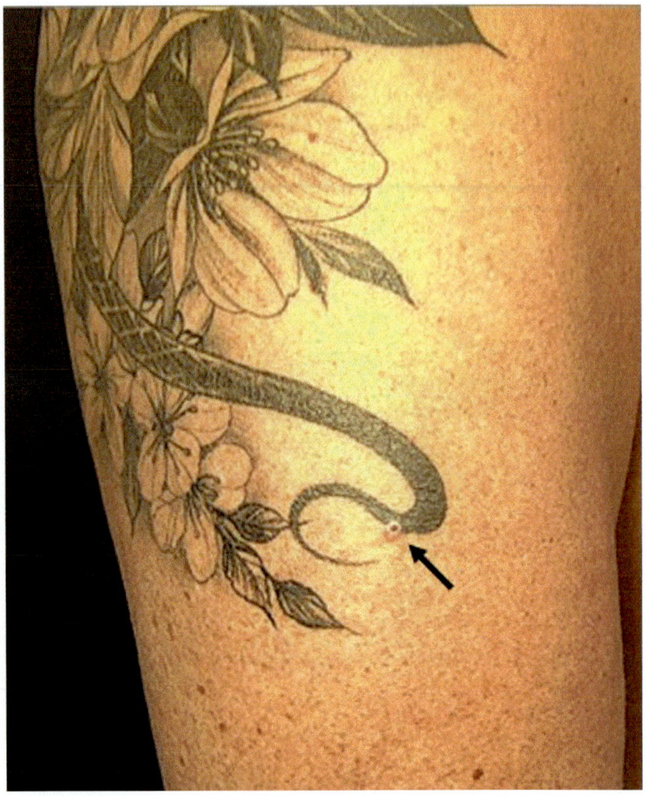

Fig. 4 Basal cell carcinoma on tattooed skin. Clinical appearance. Pink papule with 5 mm of maximum diameter on the right thigh. (black arrow)

Age: 59

Clinical description of the case or the lesion: Patient with personal history of invasive melanoma. During his physical examination, an asymptomatic pink papule of 4 × 5 mm was incidentally found on physical examination.

Body site: Left medial knee

Surface (flat/palpable/nodular): Palpable

Maximum diameter: 5 mm

Duration of the lesion: Unknown

History of morphologic changes: The patient was not aware of this lesion. No history of changes, bleeding or ulceration.

Personal history of skin cancer: Yes, prior history of superficial spreading melanoma in the left shoulder.

Family history of skin cancer: None

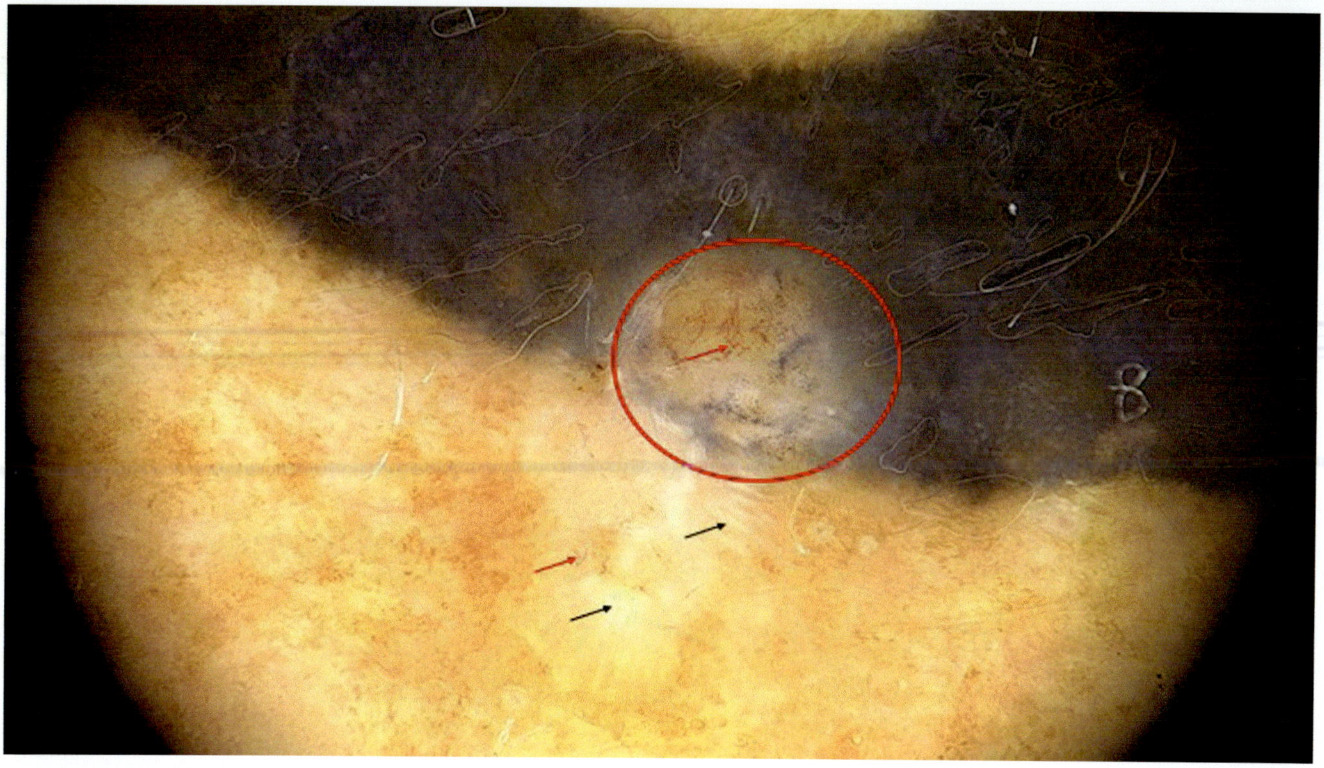

Fig. 5 Basal cell carcinoma on tattooed skin. Dermoscopic presentation. Arborizing vessels (red arrows); shiny-white lines (black arrows); pink homogeneous areas with underlying and adjacent dark black and gray ink corresponding to the on tattooed skin (red circle). (contact, polarized)

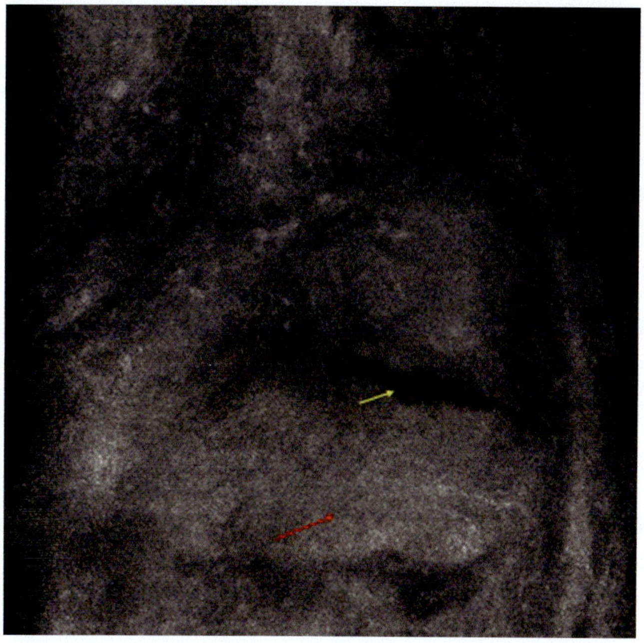

Fig. 6 Basal cell carcinoma on tattooed skin. Reflectance confocal microscopic presentation. Bright tumor islands (red arrow); cleft-like dark spaces (yellow arrow) dendritic and plump-bright cells at the dermal-epidermal and superficial dermal level. (basic image, 0.5 × 0.5 mm)

Skin Phototype: II

Clinical diagnosis: Clear Cell Acanthoma

Dermoscopic findings: Dermoscopy showed a pink background with glomerular blood vessels arranged in a serpiginous pattern with a "strings of pearls" appearance

Other clinical findings: (-) (Figs. 8 and 9)

Diagnosis: Clear Cell Acanthoma

Key message: Clear Cell Acanthoma (CCA) is a rare benign epidermal tumor also known as "Degos acanthoma". It classically presents as a solitary, slow growing, well demarcated, pink to brown, dome-shaped lesion on the lower extremities of middle-aged adults. Under dermoscopy, CCA shows a highly characteristic pattern of a serpiginous arrangement of dotted or coiled vessels, with a "string of pearls" appearance. Nevertheless, this feature is not seen in all cases of CCA and could be confused with the vascular pattern of other malignant lesions, such as the dotted or coiled vascular pattern seen iin Bowen´s disease. Other differential diagnosis includes irritated seborrheic keratosis,

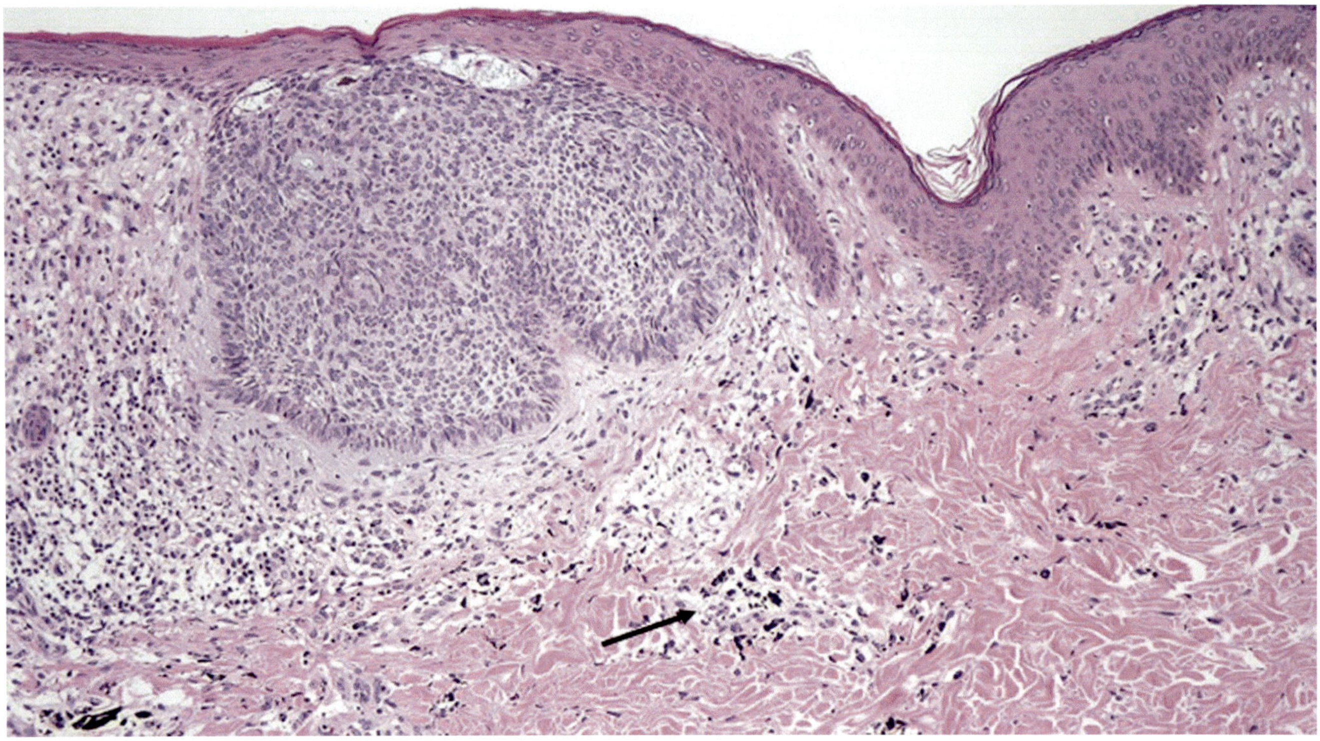

Fig. 7 Basal cell carcinoma on tattooed skin. Histologic diagnosis. Nodular and superficial basal cell carcinoma with abundant dark ink on the dermis corresponding to the underlying tattoo (black arrow). **(H&E, x100)**

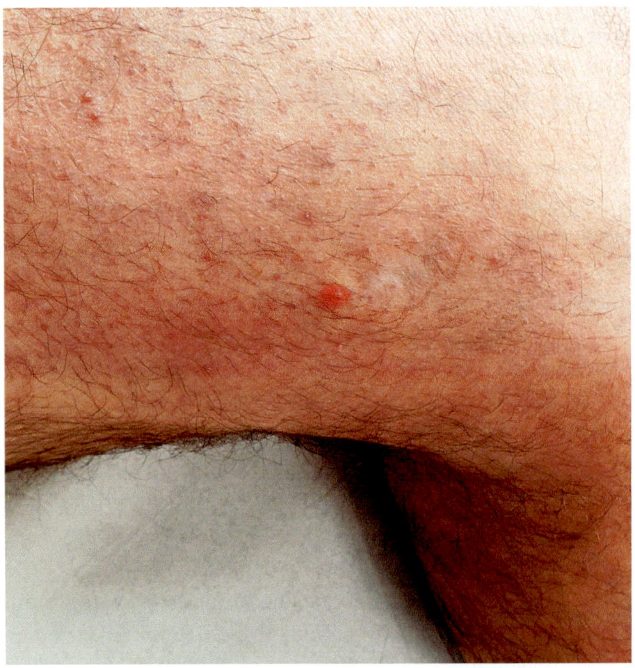

Fig. 8 **Clinical Image**: A pinkish papule with an erythematous background located on the left medial knee

hemangioma, pyogenic granuloma, irritated dermatofibroma, and Amelanotic melanoma. Most of the time, histopathology is required to confirm the diagnosis, showing characteristically a compact acanthosis that is sharply demarcated from the surrounding epidermis.

Case 4

Author: Elisa Camela

Clinical record:

Sex: Female

Age: 53-years-old

Clinical description the case or the lesion: An otherwise healthy patient referred the occurrence of an erythematous-violaceous lesion on the lateral aspect of the right leg four months earlier. For this reason, she visited a dermatologist that prescribed a topical corticosteroid/antibiotic treatment with no improvement. An incisional biopsy showed the

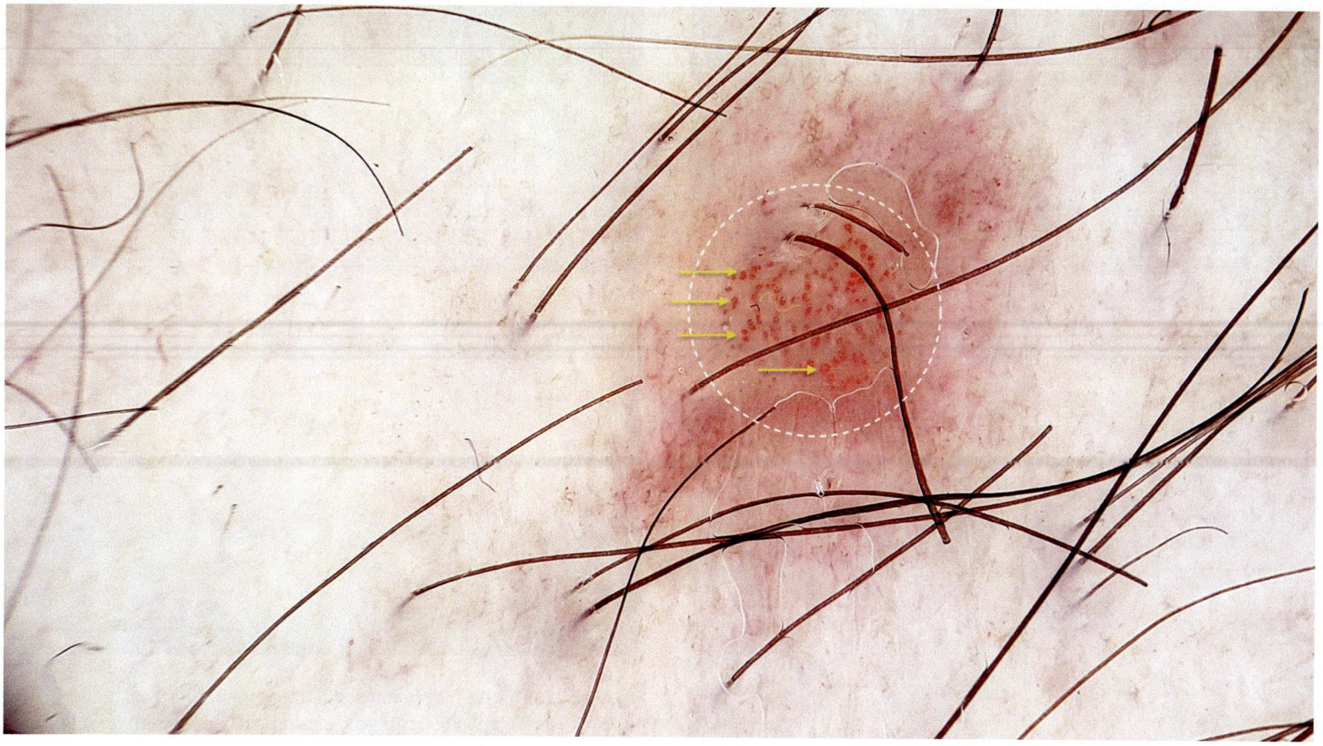

Fig. 9 **Dermoscopy image (polarized light)**: Dermoscopy showed a papule with a pink background (white dotted circle) and coiled/glomerular blood vessels arranged in a linear/serpiginous pattern with a "string of pearls" appearance (yellow arrow)

presence of unspecific findings, ruling out Bowen's disease and psoriasis. Then, she was prescribed topical corticosteroid/vitamin D analogue with partial modification of the clinical pictures. When she presented to my attention, the lesion displayed partial peripheral clearing with areas of infiltration and desquamation. Occasional itch was reported.

Body site: Lateral aspect of the right leg

Surface: Palpable

Maximum diameter: 5.5 cm

Duration of the lesion: 4 months

History of morphologic changes: Slow enlargement and partial peripheral clearing after treatment with topical corticosteroid/vitamin D analogues.

Personal history of skin cancer: No

Family history of skin cancer: No

Skin Phototype: II

Clinical diagnosis: Tinea incognita

Dermoscopic findings: Presence of scattered micropustules on an erythematous background, white scales that peel outwards, and regularly distributed red dotted vessels (Figs. 10, 11 and 12).

Other clinical findings: N/A

Diagnosis: Tinea incognita

Key message: Dermoscopy may help diagnosis of inflammatory conditions, also when the clinical pictures is altered by topical treatment.

Case 5

Author: Konstantinos Liopyris

Clinical record:

Sex: Female

Age: 40

Clinical description the case or the lesion: Patient started presenting multiple nevi, mainly on her torso, in her early thirties with an atypical appearance. The patient has

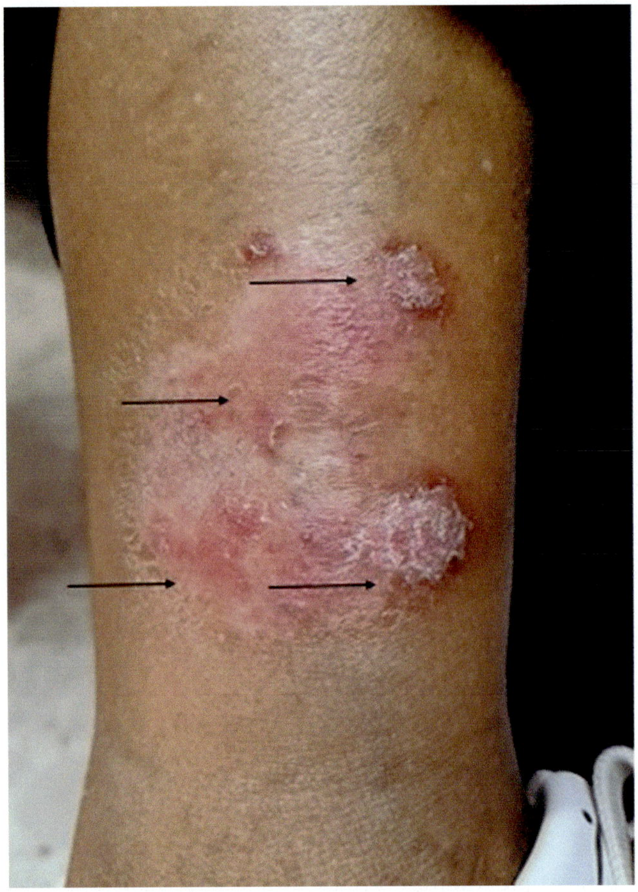

Fig. 10 Clinical picture of tinea incognita: erythematous-violaceous plaque with peripheral clearing and areas of infiltration and desquamation (black arrows)

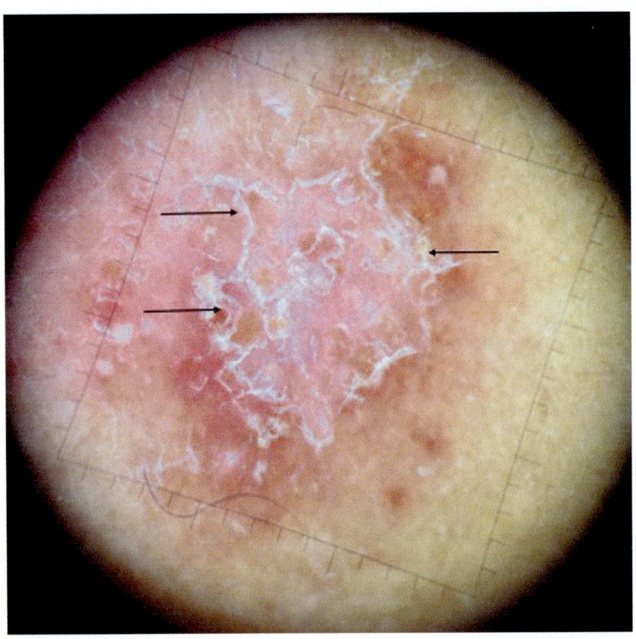

Fig. 11 Dermoscopic picture of tinea incognita: prominent white scales with outwards peeling (black arrows)

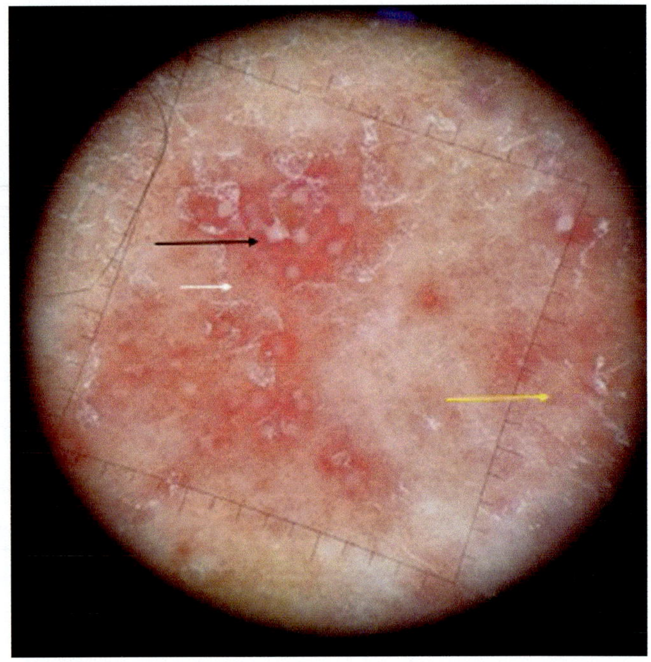

Fig. 12 Dermoscopic picture of tinea incognita: scattered micropustules (black arrow); regularly distributed red dotted vessels (white arrow); superficial white scales (yellow arrow)

undergone several excisions, as we can also see from the clinical image and all lesions were histopathologically, Spitz and atypical Spitz nevi, along with a lesion that was read out as a melanoma. Eruptive Disseminated Spitz Nevi is a rare entity with very few cases in the literature. Herein we present the clinical and dermoscopic presentation of a non-pigmented such lesion

Body site: Left Upper Anterior Thigh

Surface: Palpable

Maximum diameter: 4 mm

Duration of the lesion: Months

History of morphologic changes: Abrupt presentation and change in size

Personal history of skin cancer: History of melanoma at the age of 35

Family history of skin cancer: None

Skin Phototype: III

Clinical diagnosis: Spitz Nevus, as part of Eruptive Disseminated Spitz Nevus Syndrome

Dermoscopic findings: Pink papule with a negative network as the predominating feature and shiny white lines on Polarized Dermoscopy, lost on Non-Polarized Dermoscopy.

Other clinical findings: None (Figs. 13, 14 and 15)

Diagnosis: Spitz Nevus, as part of Eruptive Disseminated Spitz Nevus Syndrome

Key message: A very atypical lesion out of the context of the patient, however we always need to do comparative dermoscopy and keep in mind patient's personal history.

Case 6

Authors: Mónica Ramos Álvarez, Angelica Ruiz Dueñas

Clinical record:

Sex: Male

Age: 75-years-old

Clinical description the case or the lesion

Body site: Knee

Surface: Nodular

Maximum diameter: 10 mm

Duration of the lesion: 3 months

History of morphologic changes: Rapidly growing lesion that started to bleed

Personal history of skin cancer: multiple basal cell carcinomas and actinic keratosis

Family history of skin cancer: None

Skin Phototype: III

Clinical diagnosis: eccrine porome

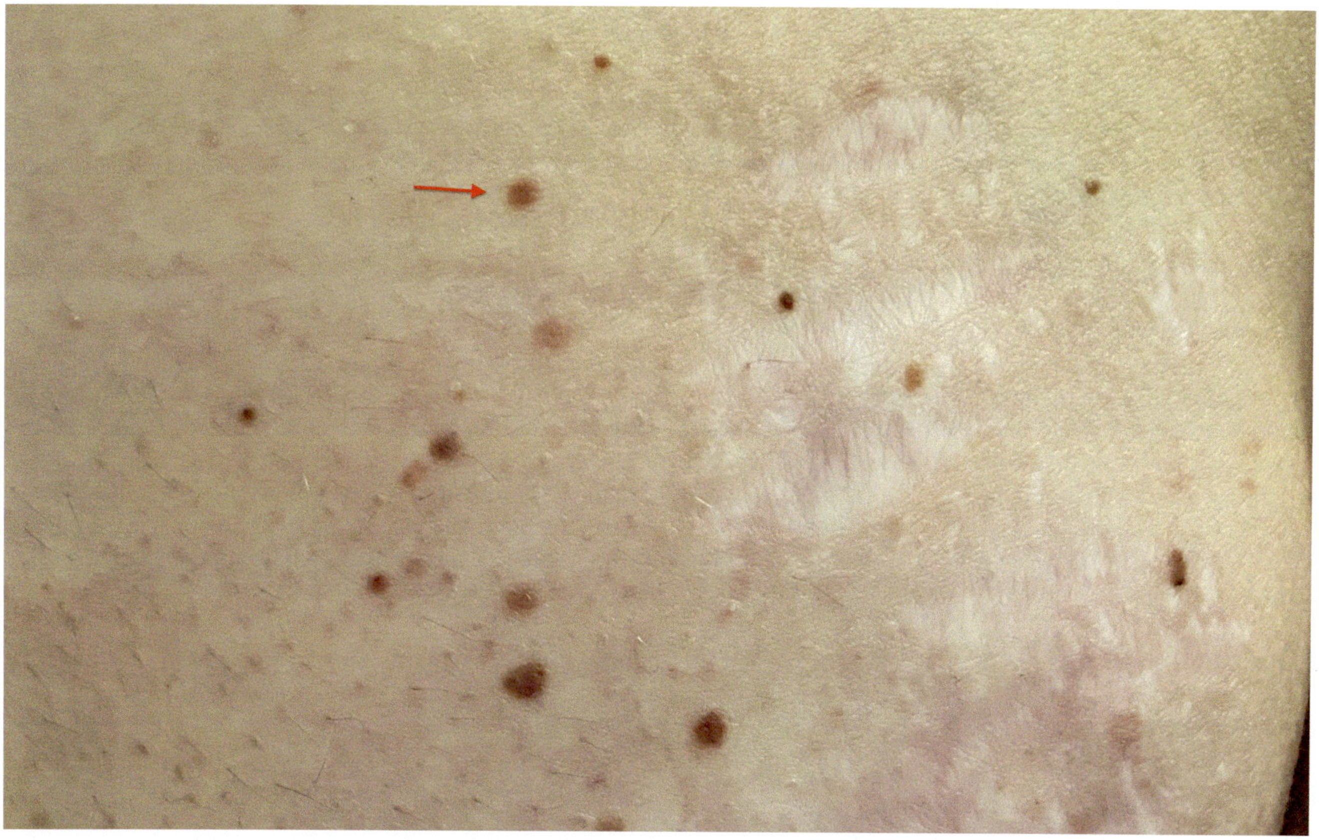

Fig. 13 Clinical image of a pink lesion on the left, upper, anterior thigh, along with several other pigmented and non-pigmented lesions, which in context are all Spitz and Atypical Spitz Nevi

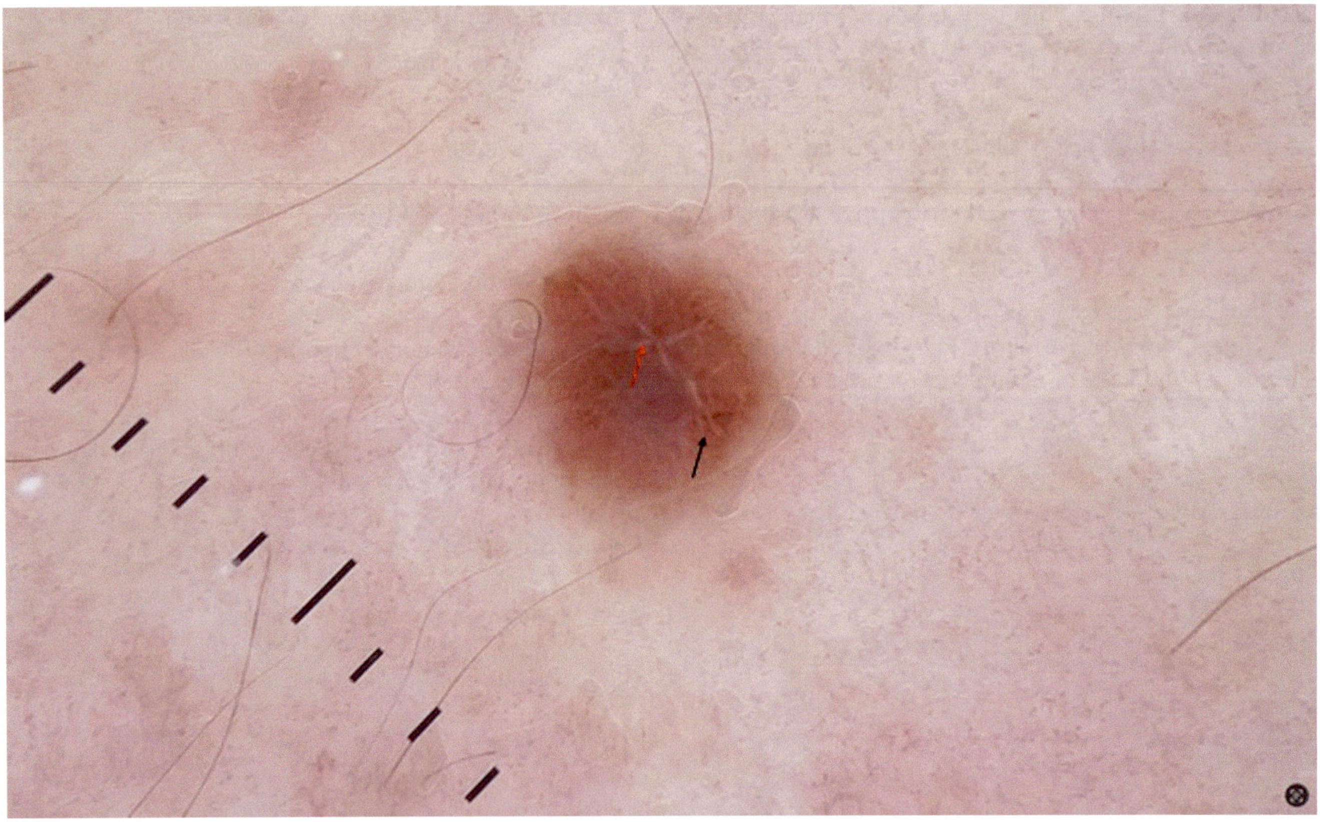

Fig. 14 Polarized Dermoscopy: negative network (black arrow); shiny white lines (red arrow)

Dermoscopic findings: Polarized light dermoscopy showing a pink nodule with ulcerated surface. Multiple glomerular vessels and red lacunes surrounded by a white halo

Other clinical findings: No (Figs. 16 and 17)

Diagnosis: Eccrine porome

Key message: Eccrine porome is a rare benign sweat glands tumor that mainly affects the distal extremities. Typically appears as a pink-to-red smooth nodule with a polymorphic vascular pattern on dermoscopy.

Flower-like vessels morphology is typical of this lesion

Case 7

Author: Rosario Peralta

Clinical record:

Sex: Female

Age: 39-years-old

Clinical description the case or the lesion: Single pearly pink papular lesion with smooth surface

Body site: Right thigh

Surface: Nodular

Maximum diameter: 7 mm

Duration of the lesion: 3 months

History of morphologic changes: An enlarging asymptomatic papular lesion

Personal history of skin cancer: None

Family history of skin cancer: None

Skin Phototype: II

Clinical diagnosis: Molluscum contagiosum

Dermoscopic findings: Round structures with a central pore, polylobular amorphous white-yellow structures, linear

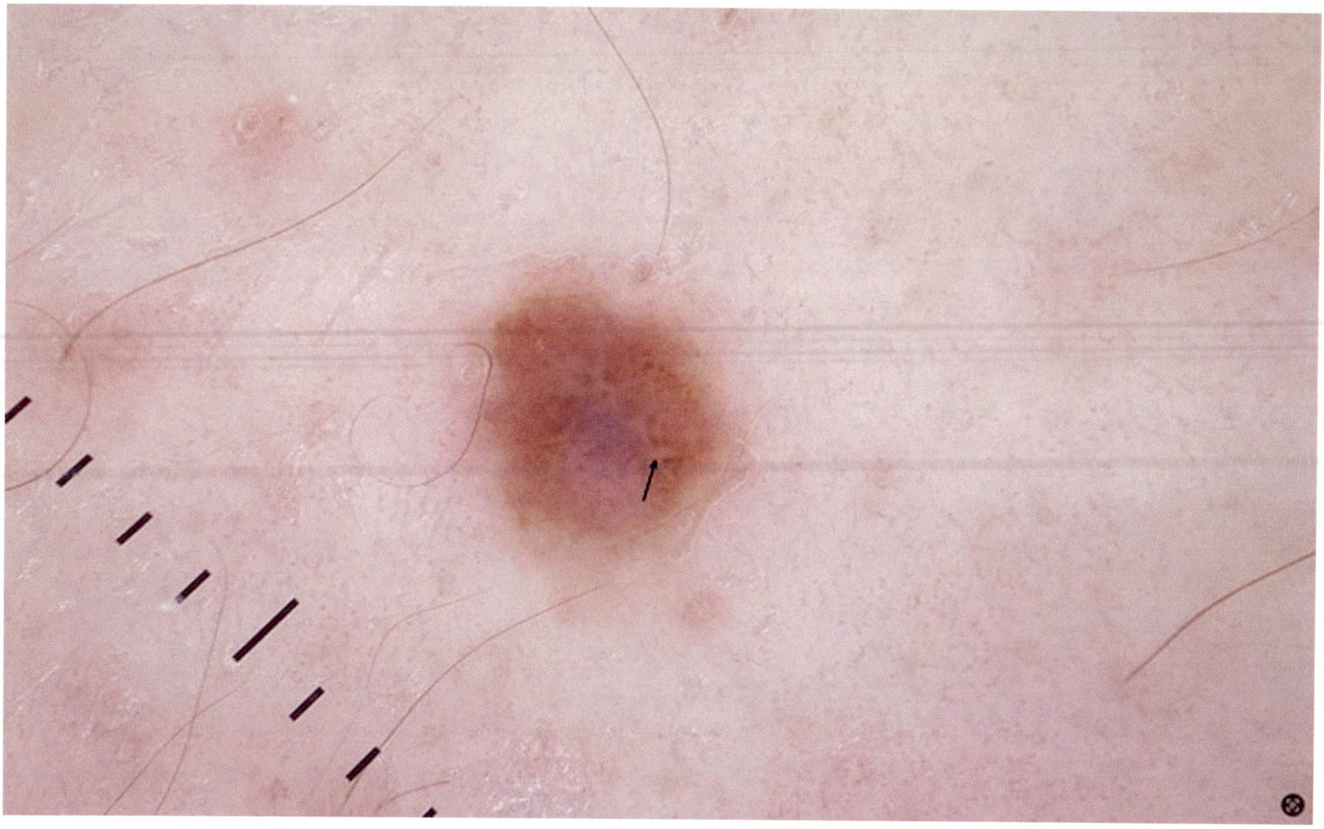

Fig. 15 Non-Polarized Dermoscopy of the Lesion: negative network (black arrow)

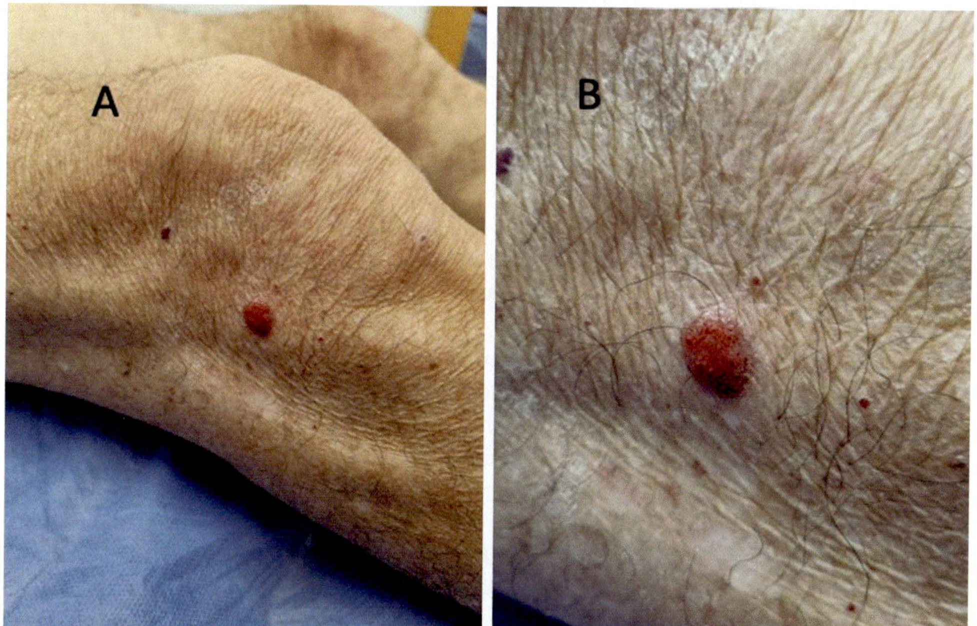

Fig. 16 Clinical image.
A- Erythematous and ulcerated nodule on the right knee;
B – Close-up of clinical view

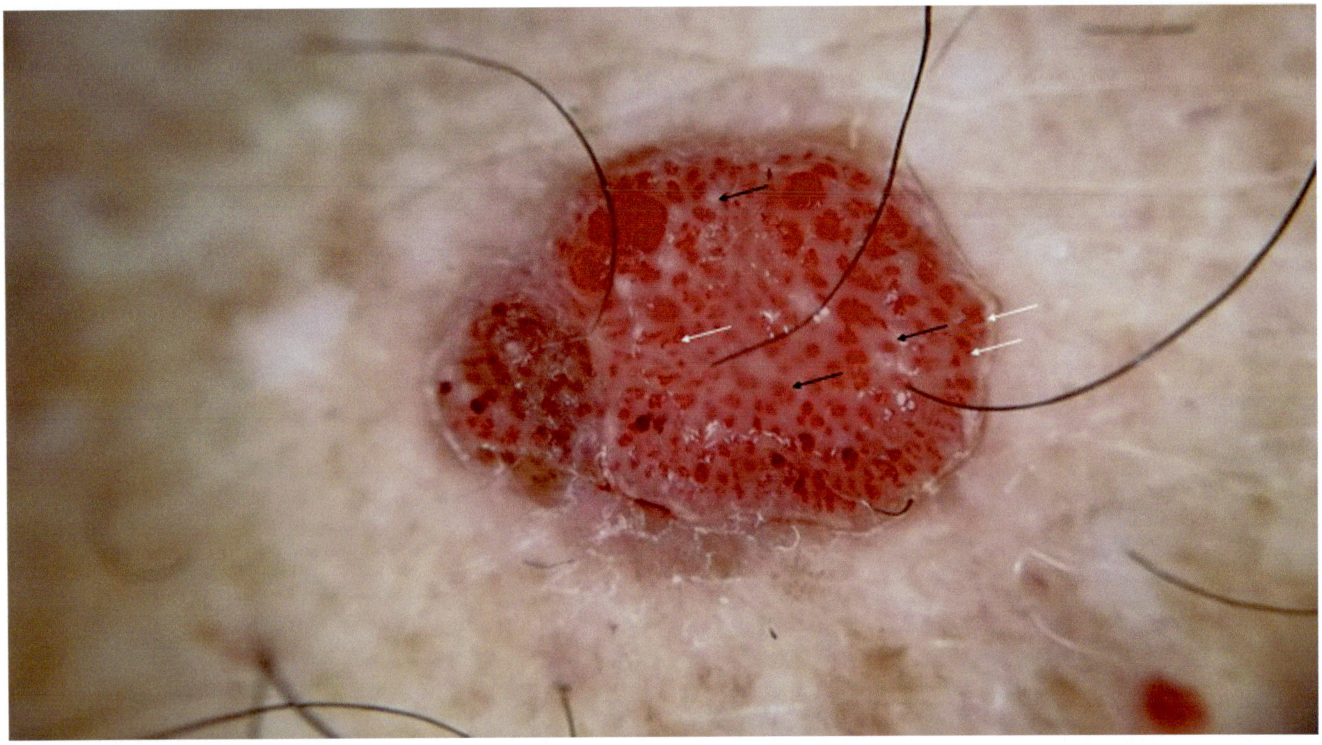

Fig. 17 Dermoscopy. Multiple glomerular vessels and red lacunes surrounded by a white halo (black arrows); Flower-like vessels (white arrows)

("radial") vessels arranged perpendicularly without crossing the central pore

Other clinical findings: None (Figs. 18, 19 and 20)

Diagnosis: Molluscum contagiosum

Key message: **Molluscum contagiosum** are usually multiple, small and umbilicated lesions caused by a poxvirus. Generally, the clinical diagnosis is simple, but some cases might be challenging and dermoscopy can also lead to a correct evaluation, especially when they are in an unusual location, have an atypical clinical presentation, or are a solitary lesion.

Dermoscopic features are characterized of round structures with a central pore also known as "fried egg" pattern, polylobular amorphous white-yellow structures, peripheral hairpin vessels in "red crown" arrangement, linear ("radial") vessels arranged perpendicularly without crossing the central pore, and dotted vessels.

Most frequently, the central pore has radial and crown vessels. When these vessels surround the lesion completely, the lesion is called "mixed flower-like pattern".

Case 8

Author: Virginia Mariana González

Clinical record:

Sex: Female

Age: 68 years

Clinical description of the lesion: Solitary, asymptomatic, annular plaque with keratotic border. No family history of similar lesions was reported.

Body site: Left ankle

Surface: Flat with slightly palpable and scaly border

Maximum diameter: 17 mm

Duration of the lesion: More than 10 years

History of morphologic changes: None reported

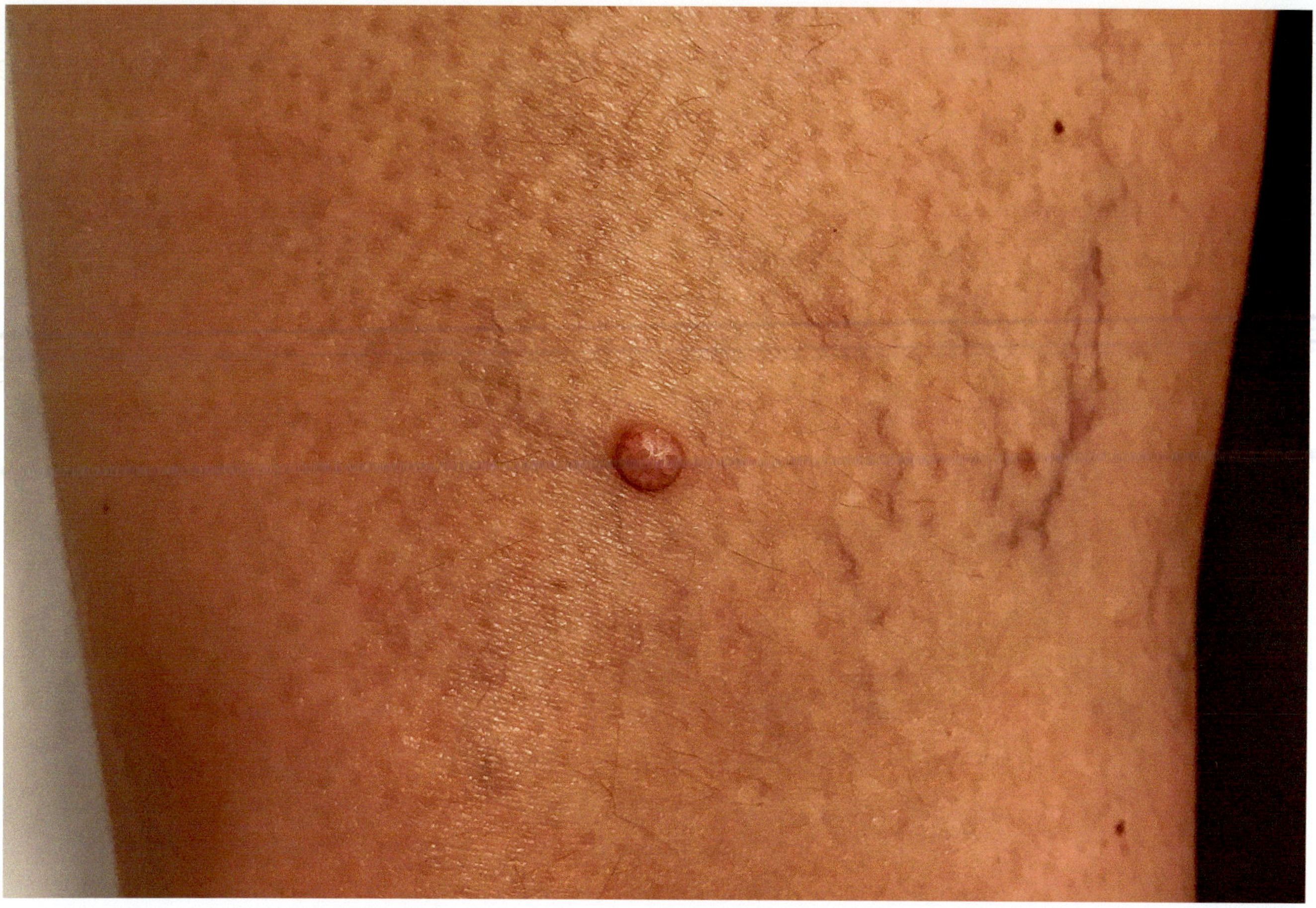

Fig. 18 Clinical image. Pearly pink round dome-shaped papule with smooth surface, measuring 7 mm in diameter, located on the right thigh

Personal history of skin cancer: Squamous cell carcinoma

Family history of skin cancer: None reported

Skin Phototype: II

Clinical diagnosis: Annular lichen planus, Porokeratosis

Dermoscopic findings: Dermoscopic examination revealed a lesion with keratin rim which is the hallmark of Porokeratosis, structureless skin-colored center with non-peripheral scales, shiny-white areas and vascular pattern with predominance of dotted vessels located on both sides of the rim.

Other clinical findings: None related (Figs. 21, 22 and 23)

Diagnosis: Porokeratosis

Key message: Porokeratosis (PK) is a keratinization disorder of uncertain etiology, related to ultraviolet radiation exposure and genetic factors, sometimes with autosomal dominant inheritance. Several clinical variants of PK have been described, with solitary or multiple annular lesions with peripheral keratotic ridge which histologically corresponds to coronoid lamella.

Sometimes the diagnosis of PK can be challenging but dermoscopy increases diagnostic accuracy by improving visualization of the characteristic keratin rim, which is the most frequent dermoscopic feature, present in more than 90% of the cases. The rim is usually double-margined and may have light-brown pigmentation, especially in Porokeratosis of Mibelli. In doubtful cases can be clearly visualized by applying marker pen ink or iodine solution. Other dermoscopic findings of PK are dotted, linear coiled ("glomerular") or linear-irregular vessels, non-peripheral

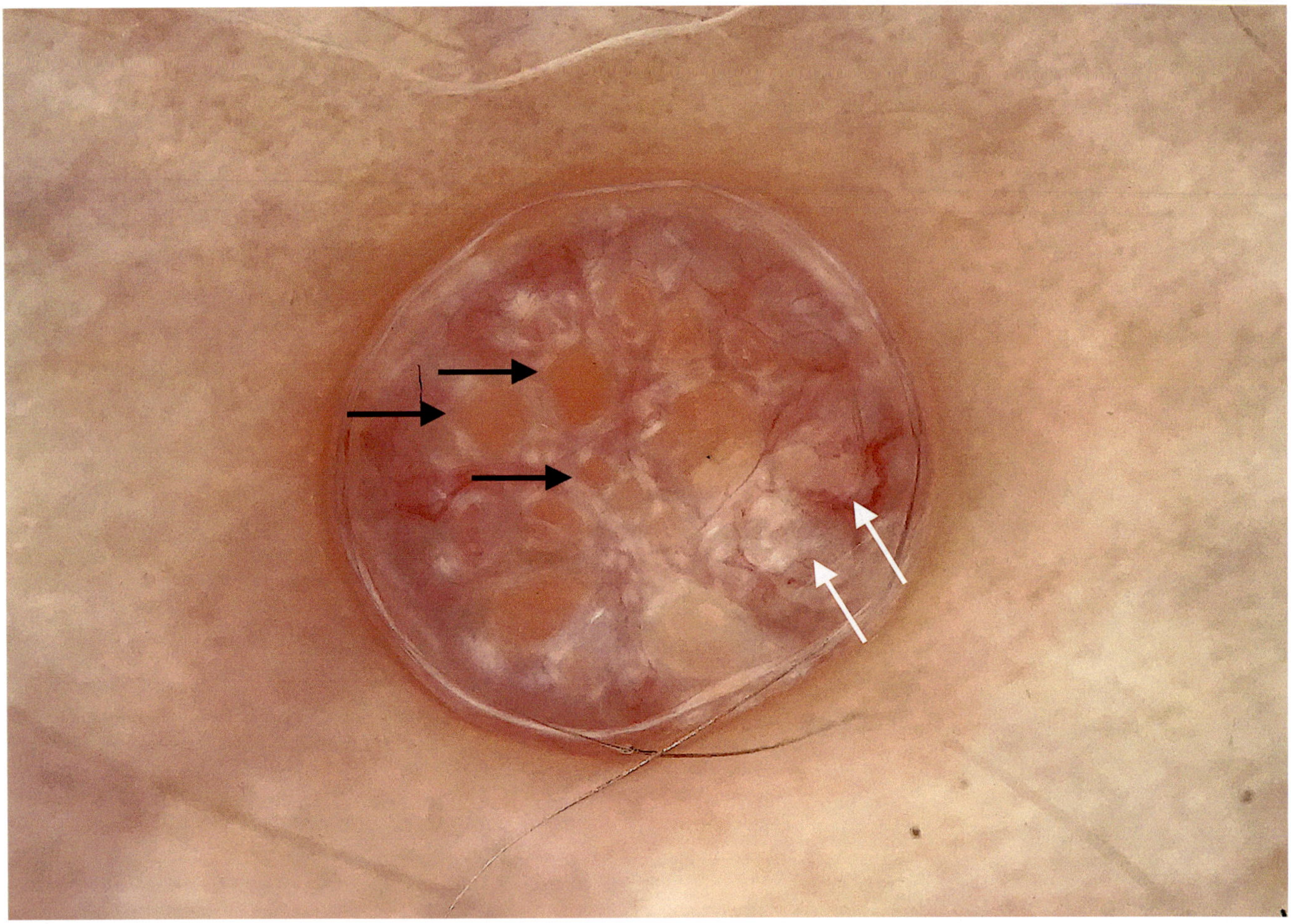

Fig. 19 Dermatoscopic examination with polarized light revealed the presence of a pinkish background with round structures with a central pore (black arrows), polylobular amorphous white-yellow structures of different sizes (white arrows), distributed over its entire surface

scales, grey-brown or reddish-brown dots, and the recently described shiny white structures, blood spots and erosions along the keratin rim.

The case presented is clinically and dermatoscopically a clear-cut example of Porokeratosis of Mibelli.

Case 9

Authors: Horacio Cabo, Emilia Noemi Cohen Sabban

Clinical record:

Sex: Male

Age: 54-years-old

Clinical description the case or the lesion: Asymptomatic non-pigmented flat macule

Body site: Right thigh

Surface: Flat

Maximum diameter: 16 mm

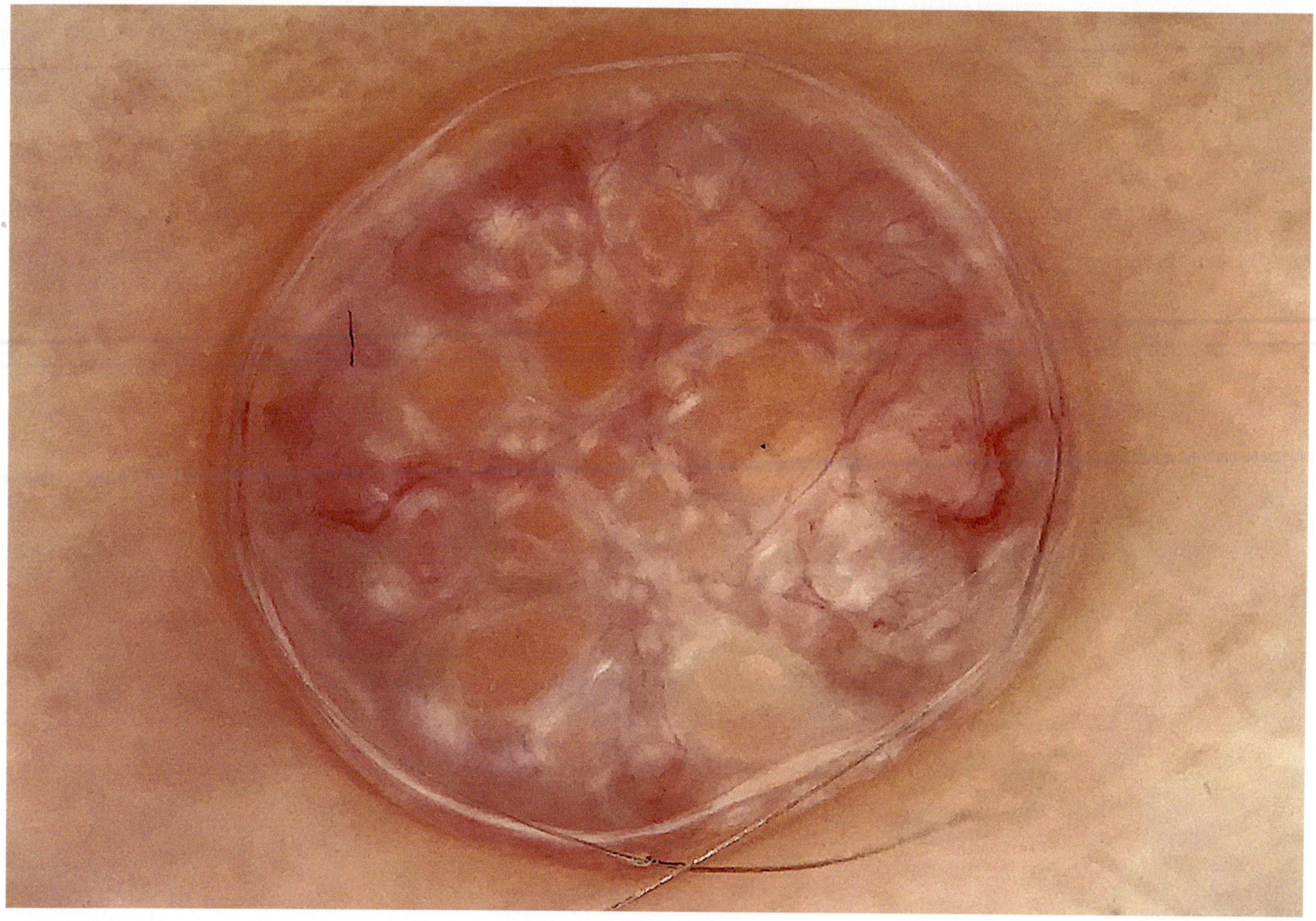

Fig. 20 At higher magnification, linear (radial) vessels arranged perpendicularly without crossing the central pore are also observed

Duration of the lesion: Unknown

History of morphologic changes: Growing in the last months

Personal history of skin cancer: None

Family history of skin cancer: None

Skin Phototype: III

Clinical diagnosis: Squamous cell carcinoma, amelanotic melanoma, psoriasis

Dermoscopic findings: Atypical polymorphous vascular pattern with dotted, linear irregular and hairpin vessels. Traces of pigmentation, erosion and white shiny areas are also seen.

Other clinical findings: Psoriasis for 10 years ago (Figs. 24 and 25)

Diagnosis: Amelanotic melanoma

Key message: This patient had psoriasis since many years ago and under clinical examination this lesion could have been a psoriasis plaque more, but here under dermoscopy the diagnosis of amelanotic melanoma is easy. Remenber that psoriasis has two major dermoscopic signs, white scales and dotted vessels with uniform distribution

Case 10

Authors: Horacio Cabo; Emilia Noemi Cohen Sabban

Clinical record:

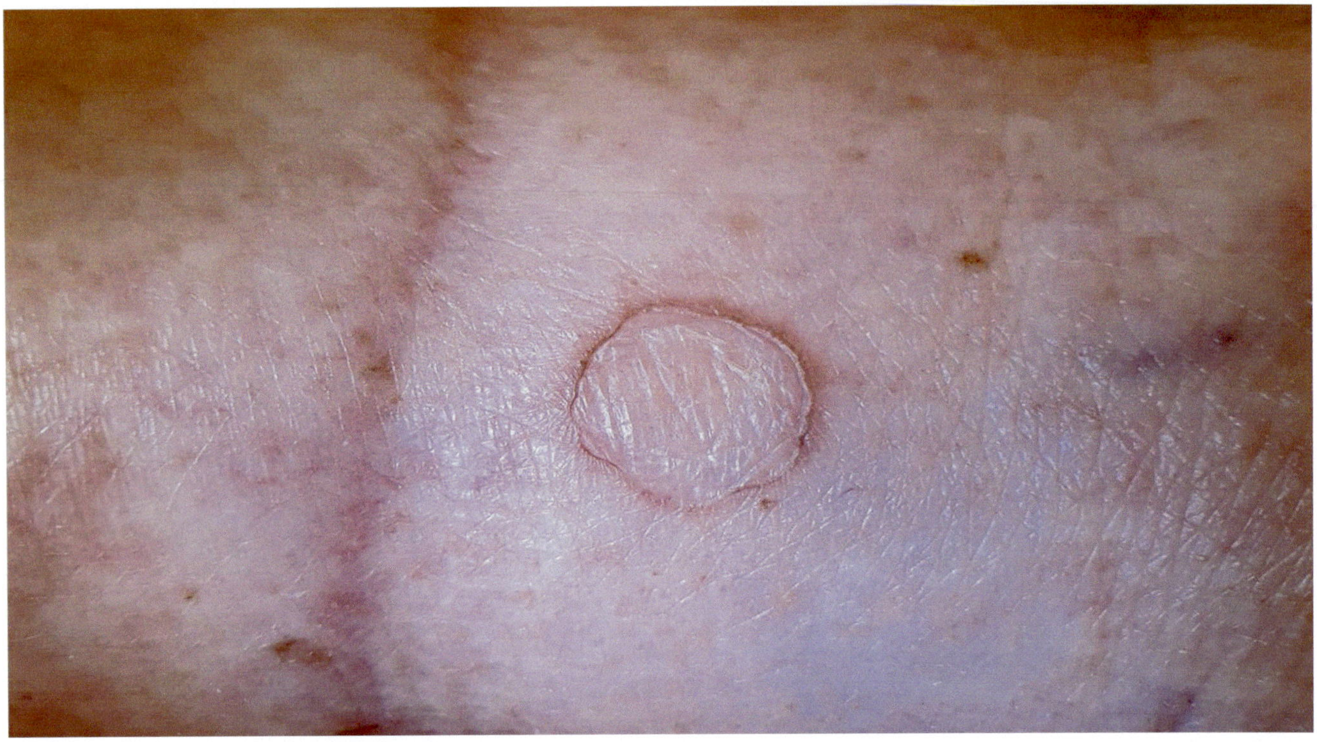

Fig. 21 Clinical image. Single sharply demarcated plaque with a brownish keratotic border and skin-colored scaly atrophic center, located on the posterior part of the left ankle

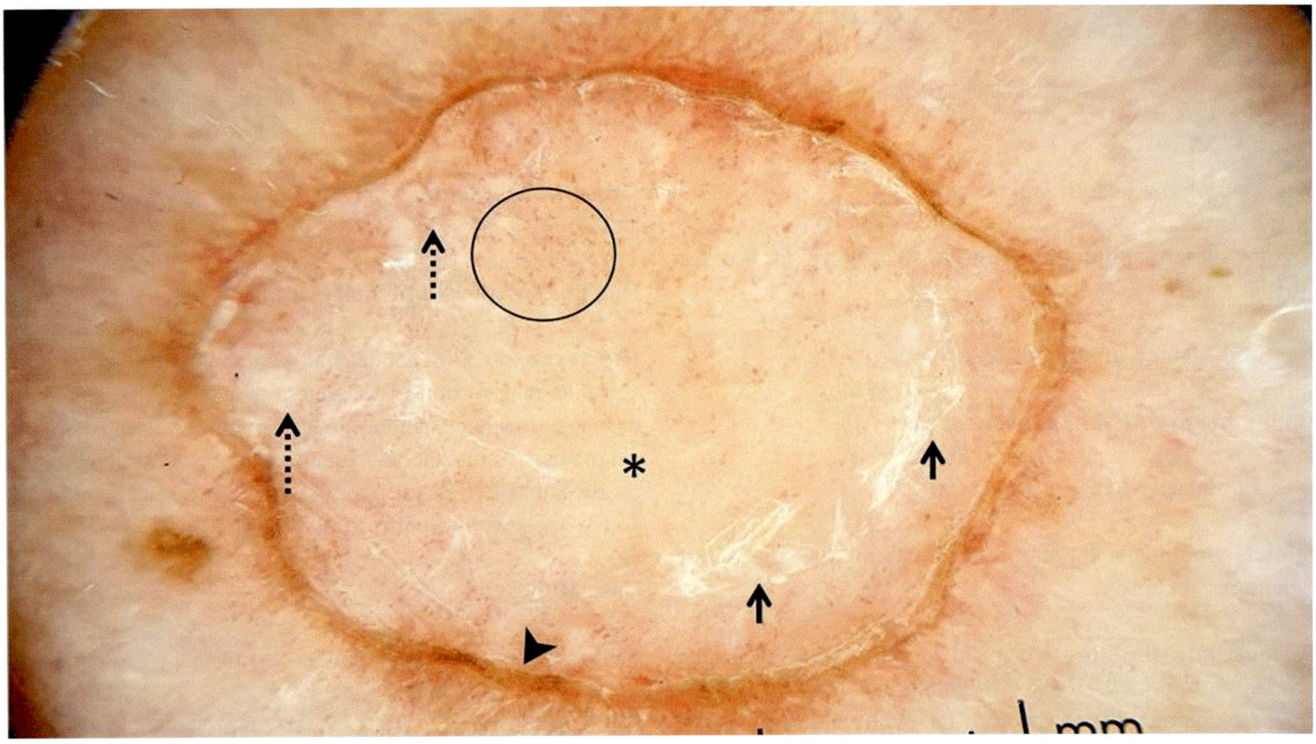

Fig. 22 Polarized dermatoscopic image (Dermlite DL200; original magnification 10x). Annular plaque with light-brown pigmented keratin rim (arrowhead), skin-colored structureless center (black asterisk), polymorphous vascular pattern composed of dotted and some short linear-irregular vessels (circle), shiny-white areas (dotted arrow) and fine non-peripheral white scales (black arrows)

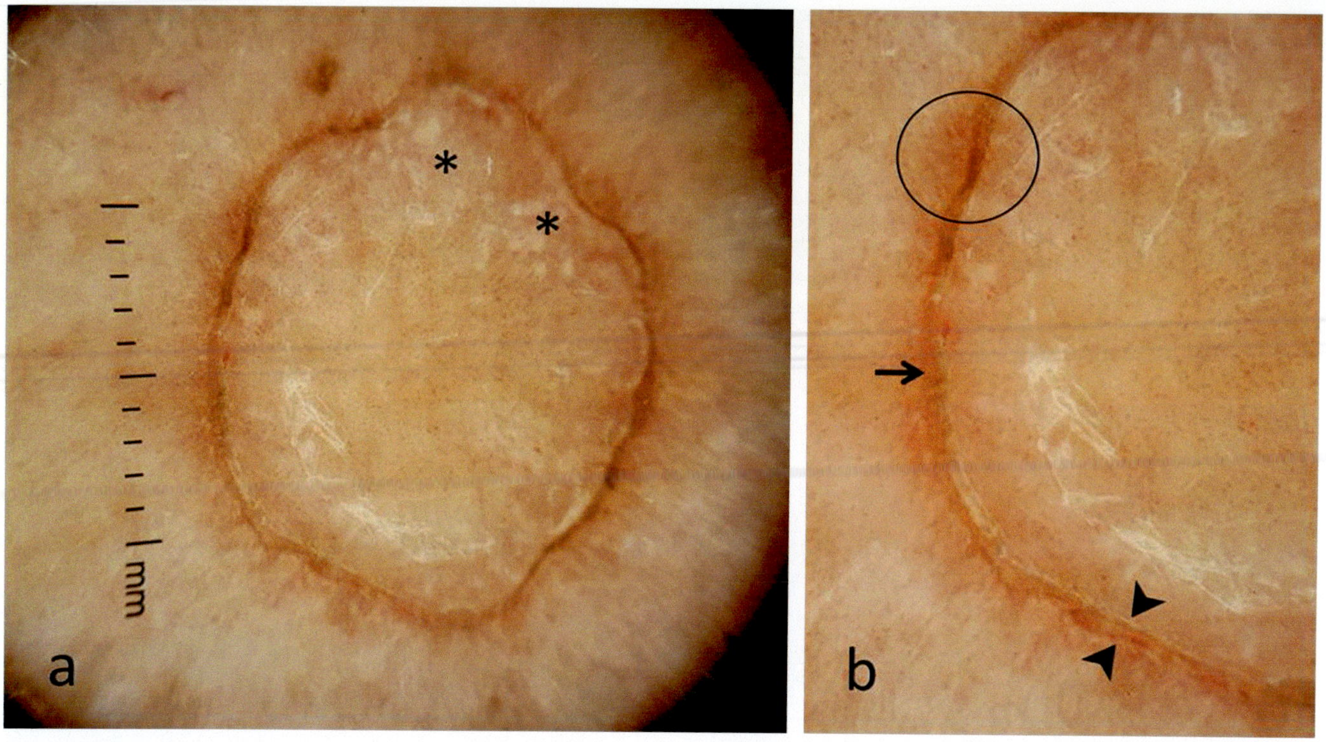

Fig. 23 Polarized dermatoscopic images without contact. a. Shiny-white areas (asterisks) and vascular structures with predominance of dotted vessels with homogeneous distribution. b. Closer view of double-edged keratin rim (arrowheads) with light-brown pigmentation along the rim (black arrow) and multiple dotted vessels on both sides (circle)

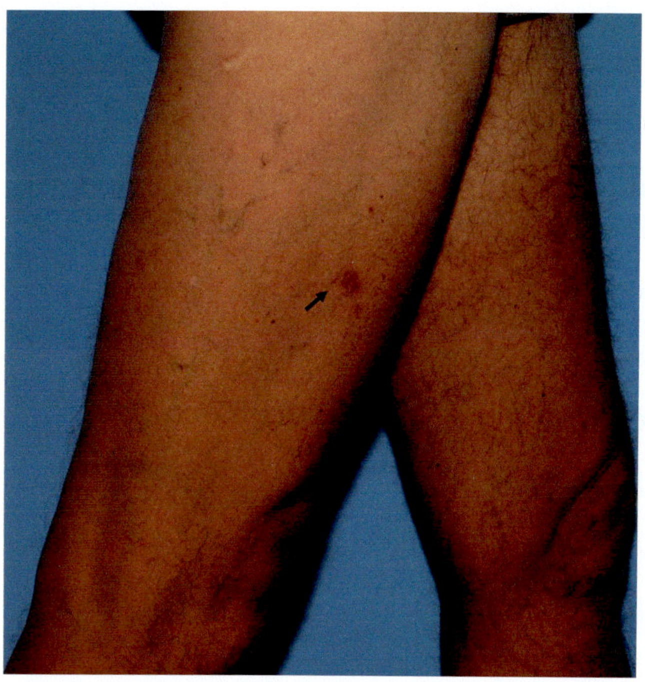

Fig. 24 Clinical image: asymptomatic non-pigmented flat macule (arrow)

Sex: Female

Age: 49-years-old

Clinical description the case or the lesion: Asymptomatic pink lesion

Body site: Right knee

Surface: Palpable

Maximum diameter: 10 mm

Duration of the lesion: 1 year

History of morphologic changes: Slow growing

Personal history of skin cancer: Yes, Melanoma ten years ago

Family history of skin cancer: None

Skin Phototype: II

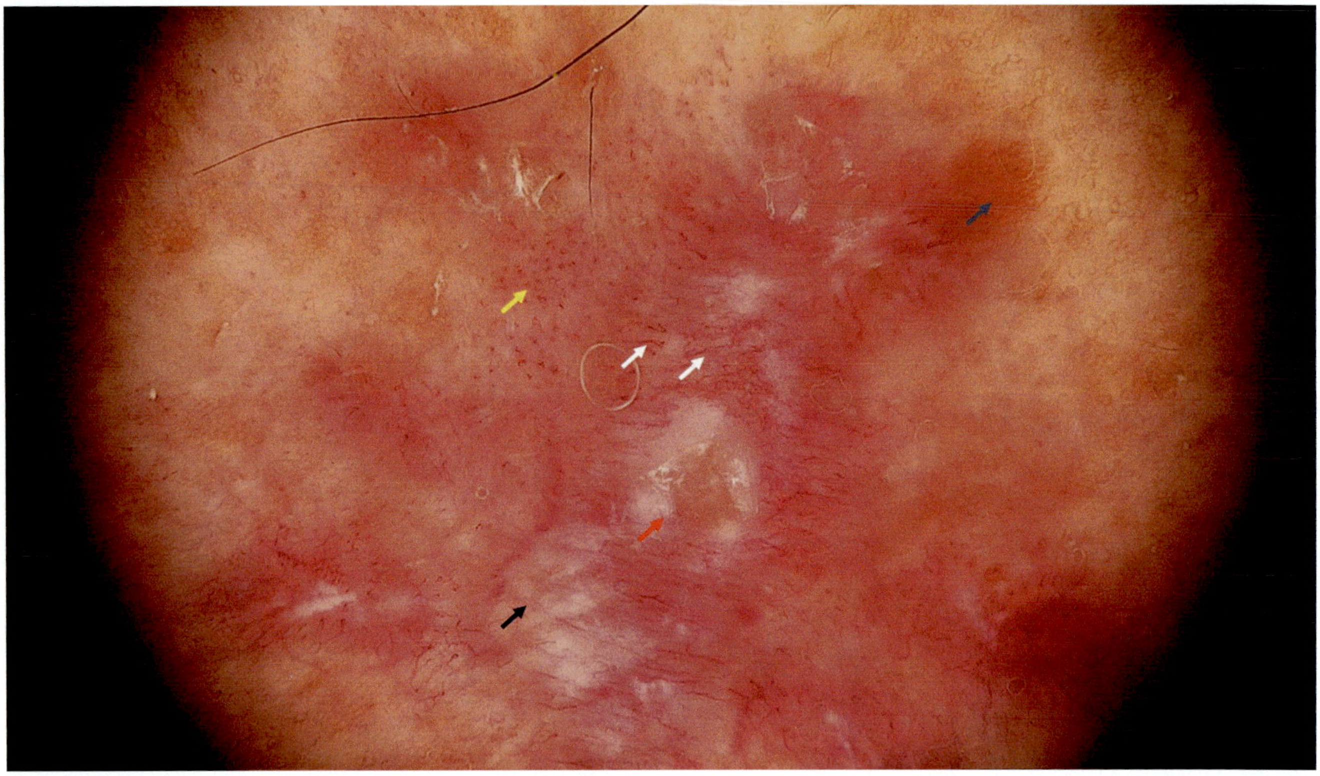

Fig. 25 Dermoscopic image: atypical polymorphous vascular pattern with dotted (yellow arrow), linear irregular and hairpin vessels (white arrows); traces of pigmentation (blue arrow), erosion (red arrow) and white shiny areas (black arrow) are also seen

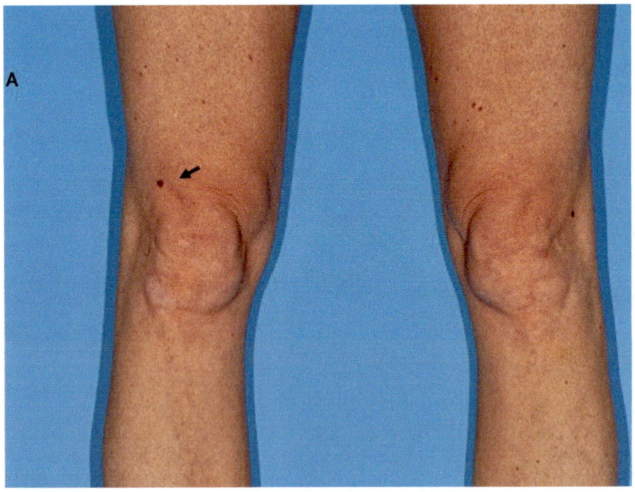

Fig. 26 Clinical image (arrow)

Clinical diagnosis: Spitz nevus

Dermoscopic findings: Red dots evenly distributed throughout the lesion

Other clinical findings: None (Figs. 26, 27 and 28)

Diagnosis: Spitz nevus, confirmed with the histopathology

Key message: sometimes the dermoscopic images of Spitz nevus and Melanoma can be very similar and we have to rule out the melanoma with the histopathology examination.

Case 11

Authors: Horacio Cabo – Emilia Noemi Cohen Sabban

Clinical record:

Sex: Male

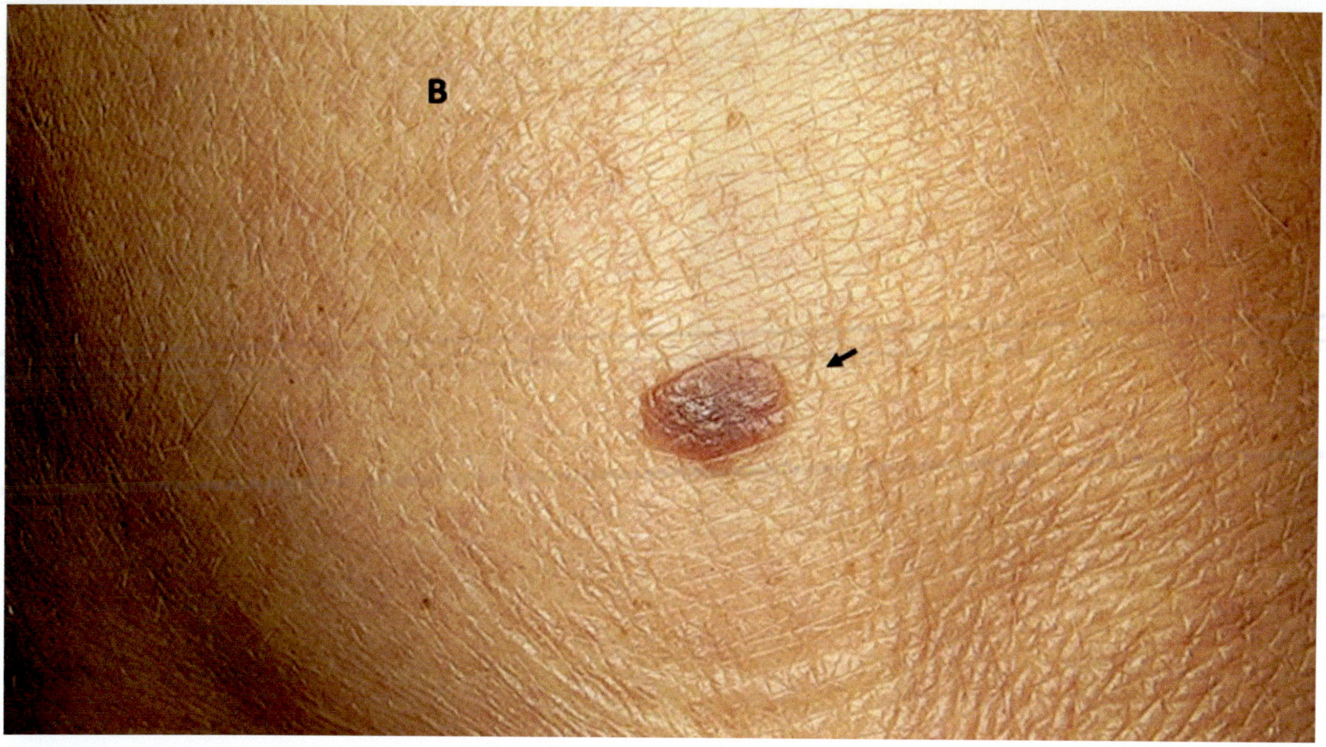

Fig. 27 Close-up clinical image (arrow)

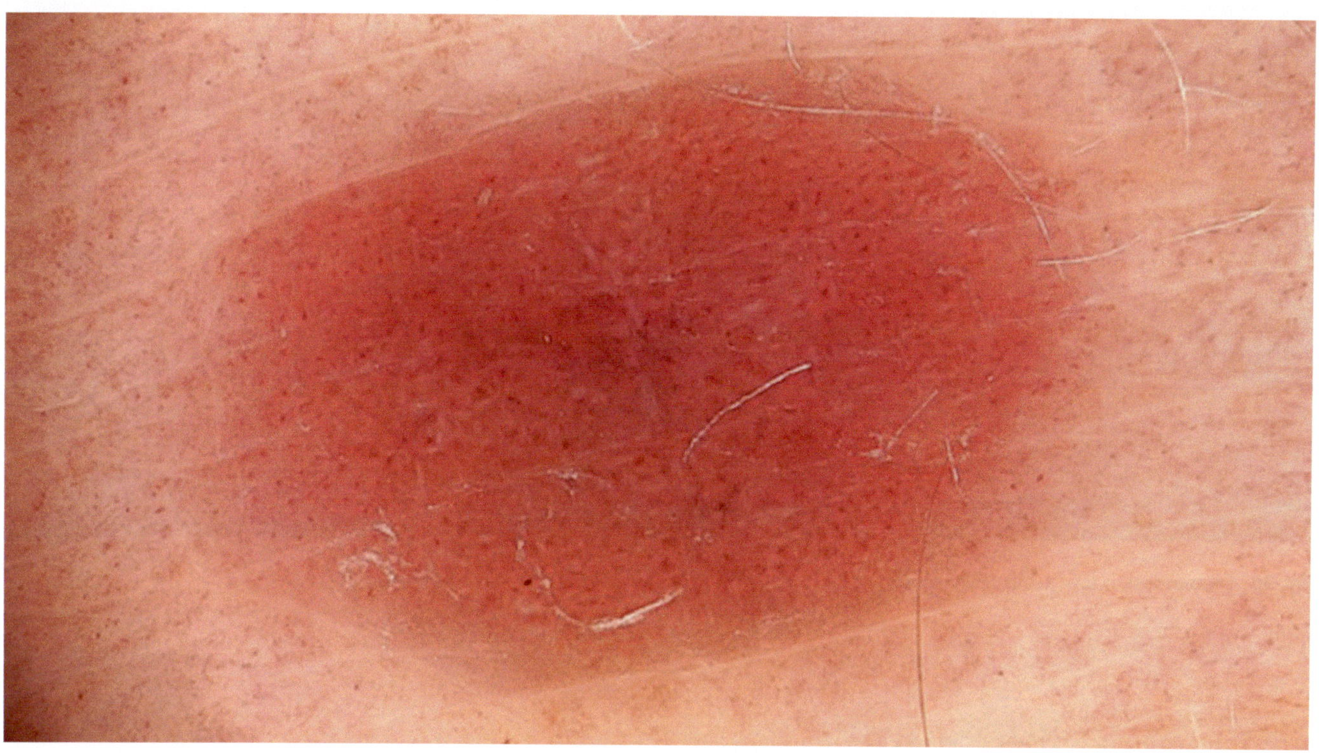

Fig. 28 Dermoscopic image showing multiple red dots evenly distributed throughout the lesion

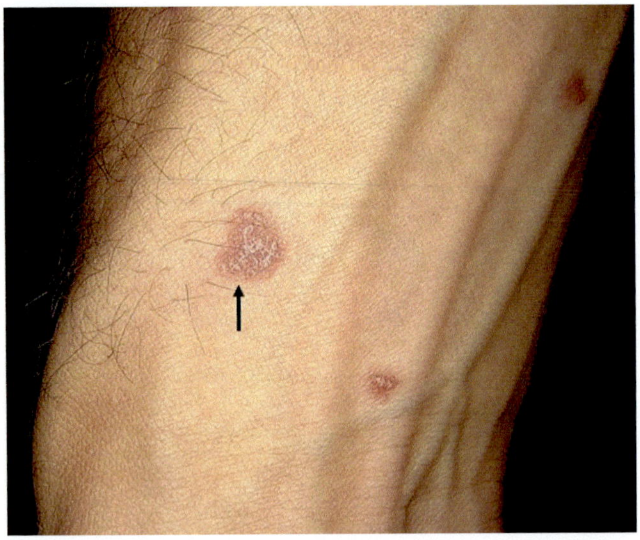

Fig. 29 Clinical image: erythematous scaly pink plaque (arrow)

Age: 45-years-old

Clinical description the case or the lesion: Pruritic erythematous scaly pink plaque of months of evolution

Body site: Left posterior thigh

Surface: Palpable

Maximum diameter: 12 mm

Duration of the lesion: More than six months

History of morphologic changes: None

Personal history of skin cancer: None

Family history of skin cancer: None

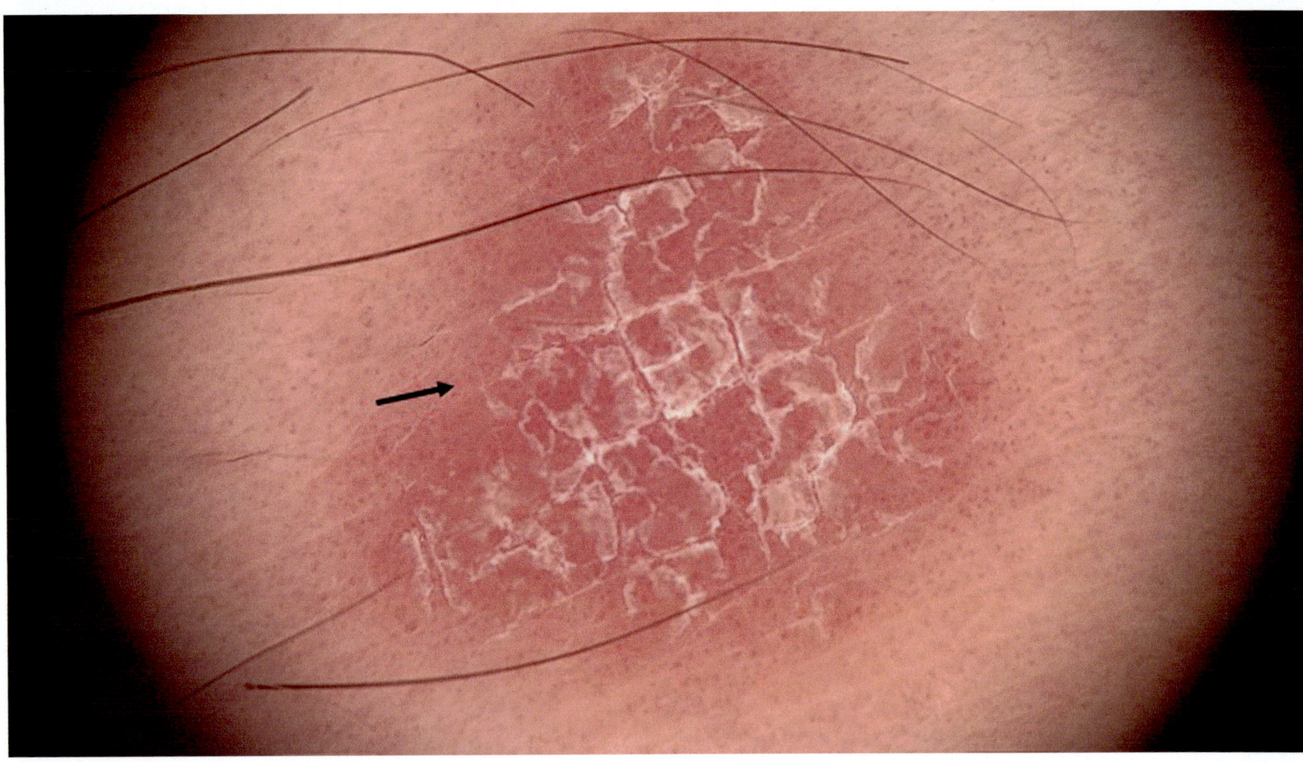

Fig. 30 Dermoscopic view: white scales covering the surface of the lesion (arrow)

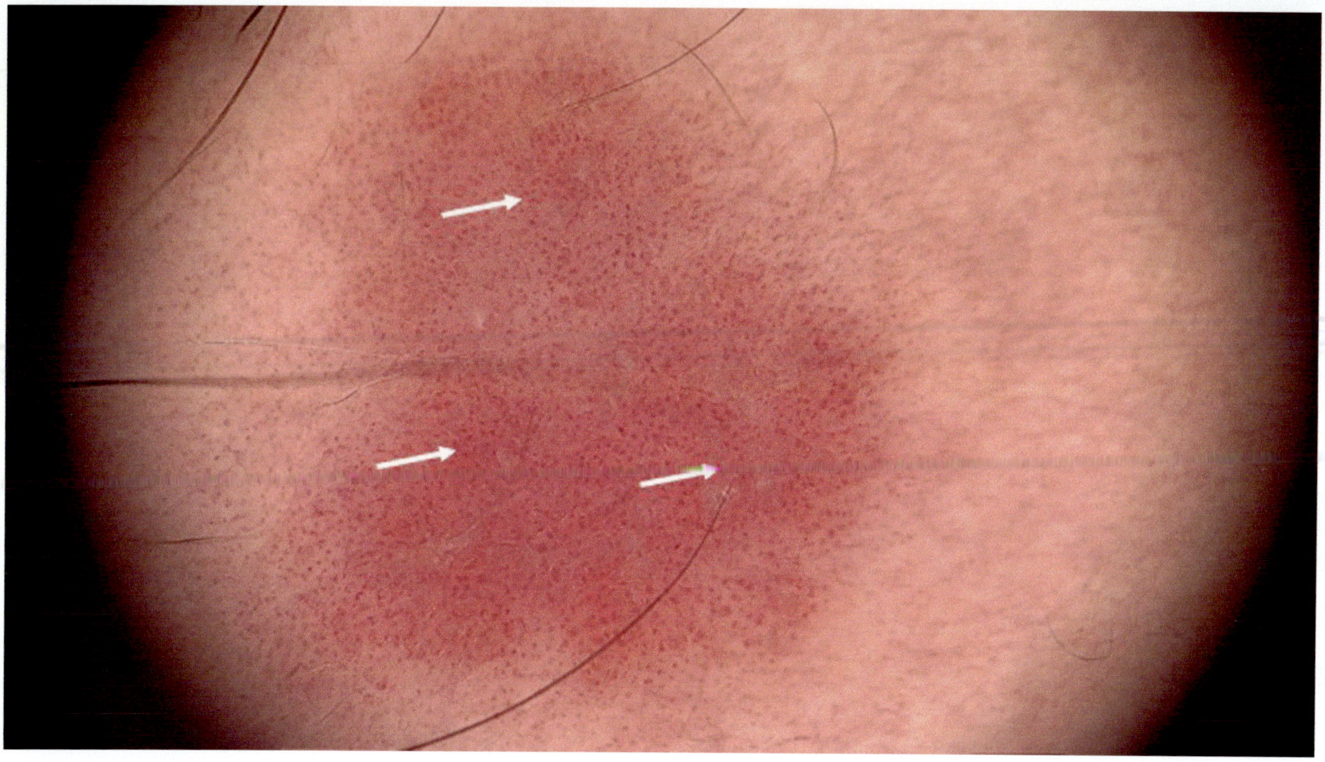

Fig. 31 Dermoscopic view under alcohol application: dotted vessels with uniform distribution throughout the lesion (white arrows)

Skin Phototype: III

Clinical diagnosis: Dermatitis vs Psoriasis

Dermoscopic findings: white scales and dotted vessels with uniform distribution throughout the lesion

Other clinical findings: None (Figs. 29, 30 and 31)

Diagnosis: Psoriasis

Key message: Dermoscopy with the examination of the vessels can differentiate dermatis (dotted vessels with with focal distribution)) from Psoriasis (dotted vessels with uniform distribution throughout the lesion)

Key message: In inflammatory diseases the morphology and distribution of the vessels are the clue in the diagnosis

Genital Area Lesions

Sgouros Dimitrios, Almpanis Zannis, Katoulis Alexander, Zoe Apalla, and Horacio Cabo

Abstract

In this chapter, some pink lesions such as eccrine spiradenoma, a plaque of psoriasis and Erythrasma clinically present some differential diagnoses, but dermoscopy is a great help in diagnosis.

Keywords

Eccrine spiroadenoma • Psoriasis • Erythrasma

Case 1

Authors: Sgouros Dimitrios, Almpanis Zannis, Katoulis Alexander

Clinical record:

Sex: Female

Age: 64 years old

Clinical description the case or the lesion: Pink-to-violaceous, lobular asymptomatic nodule arising on the lower part of the right outer labia of the vulva in a 64 years old female patient.

Body site: Genital area, vulva, right outer labia

Surface: Nodular

Maximum diameter: 1.7 cm

Duration of the lesion: Ten (10) years

History of morphologic changes: Progressively enlarging lesion

Personal history of skin cancer: None

Family history of skin cancer: None

Skin Phototype: II

Clinical diagnosis: DDx 1. BCC, 2. Bartholin's cyst, 3. Adnexal tumor

Dermoscopic findings: Lobular nodule with multifocal orange-yellowish and pink-whitish coloration. Linear irregular vessels represent the most prevalent dermatoscopic feature. White, shiny structures and a hint of a bluish nest-like formation are also detected. The lesion was excised and histopathology set the diagnosis of eccrine spiradenoma.

Other clinical findings: Clinically minor erosions (Figs. 1, 2, 3 and 4).

Diagnosis: Eccrine Spiroadenoma

Key message: Eccrine Spiradenoma is an uncommon benign adnexal tumor composed of well-demarcated nodules or lobules mostly centered within the dermis presenting usually

S. Dimitrios · K. Alexander
Second Department of Dermatology-Venereology, Medical School, "Attikon" General University Hospital, National and Kapodistrian University of Athens, 1 Rimini str, 12462 Chaidari, Athens, Greece

A. Zannis
"Pathlabs" Pathology Lab, 20 Katechaki str, 11525 Athens, Greece

Z. Apalla
Dermatology, Aristotle University of Thessaloniki, Anatolis 5, 55535 Thessaloniki, Greece

H. Cabo (✉)
Clinical Dermatology, University of Buenos Aires, Argentina, Arenales 1446 1 °C (1061) CABA, Buenos Aires, Argentina
e-mail: cabohoracio@gmail.com

H. Cabo and A. Lallas (eds.), *Dermatoscopic Atlas of Non-Pigmented Lesions*,
https://doi.org/10.1007/978-3-031-34310-0_8

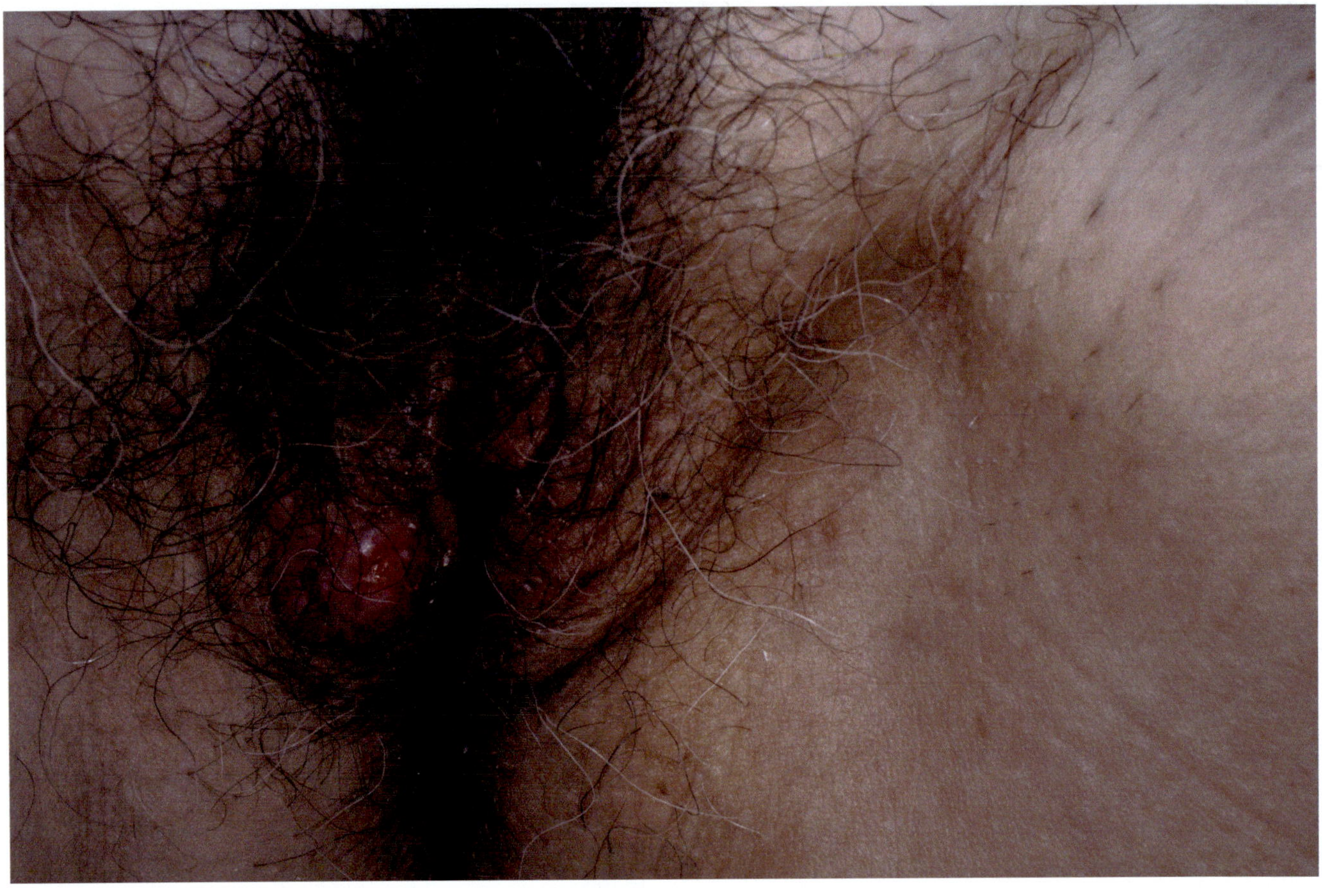

Fig. 1 **Clinical view**: Multi-lobular, pink-to-violaceous nodule on the right outer labia of the vulva

as a solitary round oval lesion. Clinically and dermatoscopically eccrine spiradenoma imitates BCC. However, a more detailed analysis of the dermatoscopic findings reveals differences between these two clinical entities. In specific, orange-yellow coloration and linear irregular vessels (either in-focused or unfocused) represent dermatoscopic characteristics which are not typically observed in BCC.

Case 2

Author: Zoe Apalla

Clinical record:

Sex: Male

Age: 56-year-old

Clinical description the case or the lesion: Erythematous plaques at the groin area, with satellite small papules at the periphery that appeared 15 days ago. Accompanied by mild pruritus. Patients' history: on treatment with cemiplimab due to penile SCC, with regional lymph node metastasis.

Body site: Groin area

Surface: Flat

Maximum diameter: Affected the groin area

Duration of the lesion: 15 days ago

History of morphologic changes: Yes, gradually enlarging

Personal history of skin cancer: Yes, penile SCC

Family history of skin cancer: No

Skin Phototype: III

Clinical diagnosis: Image strongly suggestive of candida infection

Dermoscopic findings: Images strongly suggestive of psoriasis, due to the presence of uniformly arranged dotted vessels all over the surface of the lesion.

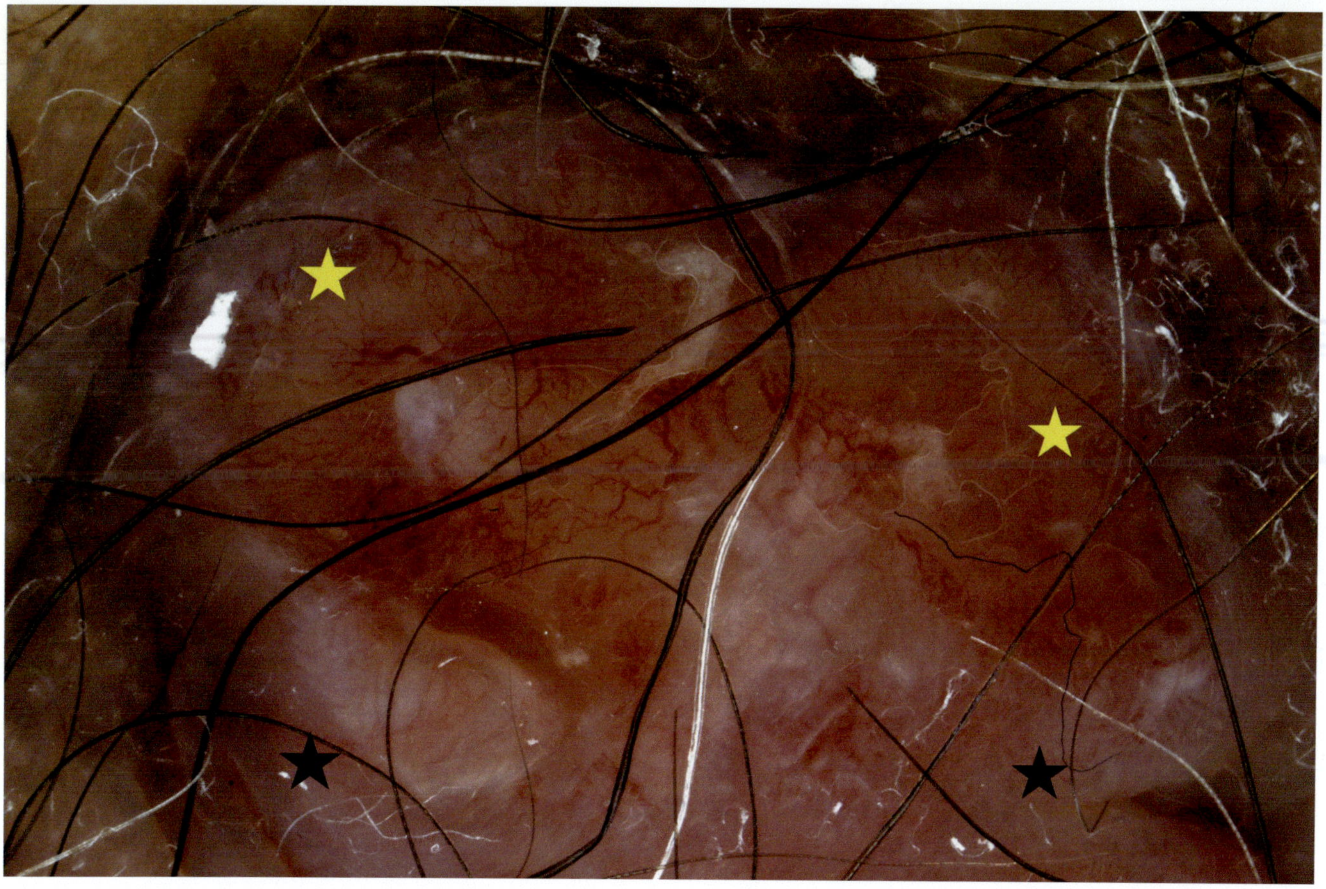

Fig. 2 **Dermoscopic view:** In-focused linear irregular vessels on top of areas with orange-to-yellowish background at the upper part of the image (yellow stars). Areas of pink-whitish coloration along with unfocused vessels and white, shiny structures are typical of the lower part of the image (black stars)

Other clinical findings: Cultures for bacteria and fungi were negative (Figs. 5 and 6).

Diagnosis: Psoriasis

Key message: Dermatoscopy is part of the clinical examination and serves to the diagnostic approach, even in cases that look easy-to-diagnose by naked-eye clinical inspection. Here our initial clinical diagnosis was candida sp. Infection; however, after performing dermatoscopy, highlighting the presence of uniformly arranged, dotted vessels, psoriasis came up as the most possible diagnosis.

Case 3

Author: Horacio Cabo

Sex: Male

Age: 45-years-old patients

Clinical description the case or the lesion: Asymptomatic erythematous squamous plaque in the groin

Body site: Groin

Surface: Flat

Duration of the lesion: More than one year

History of morphologic changes: None

Personal history of skin cancer: None

Family history of skin cancer: None

Skin Phototype: III

Clinical diagnosis: Erytrasma, Mycosis

Dermoscopic findings: Peripheral scales with uniformly distributed dotted and linear vessels.

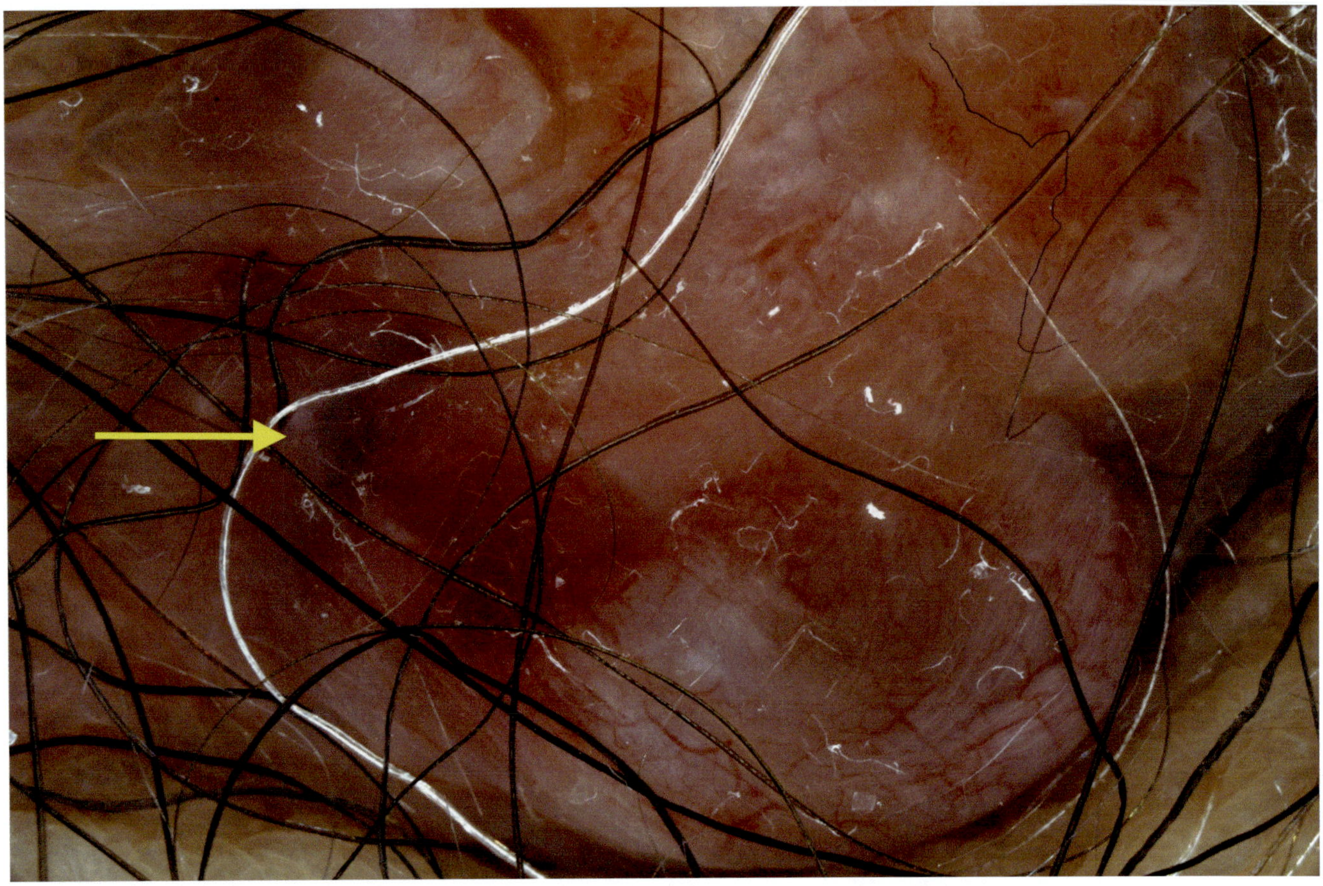

Fig. 3 **Dermoscopic view**: Alternating, lobular areas of white, shiny structures and orange-to-yellowish coloration along with linear irregular vessels. A hint of a bluish nest-like formulation is also observed (yellow arrow)

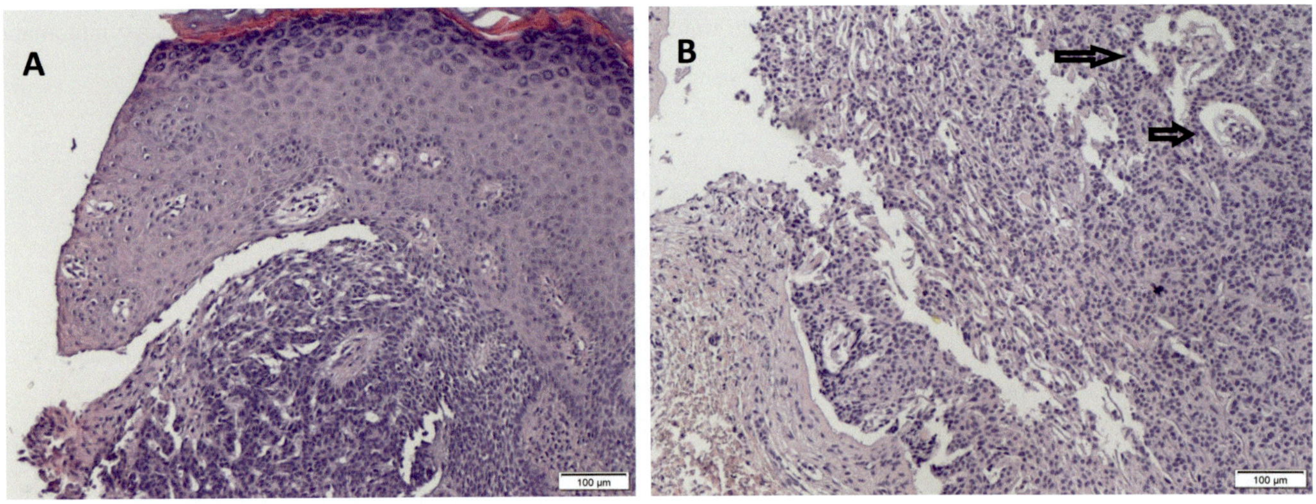

Fig. 4 **(Histopathological)**: A. Eccrine Spiradenoma characterized by a cellular basophilic lobule in the dermis (×10). B. Higher magnification of an eccrine spiradenoma shows neoplastic blue cells surrounding dilated granular lumens (×40)

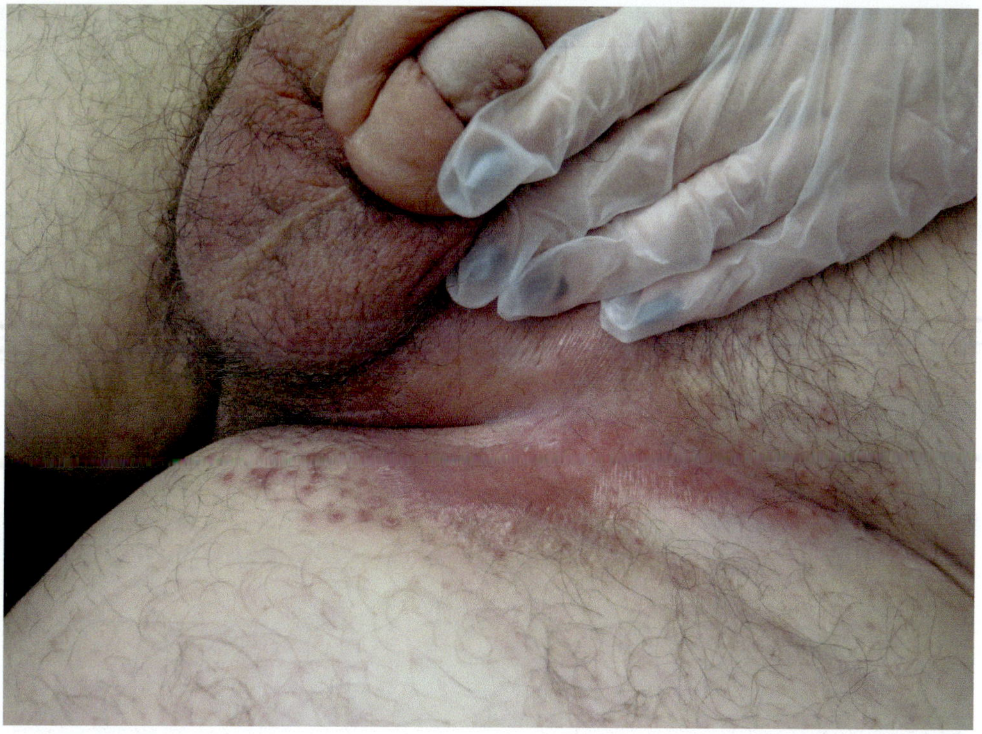

Fig. 5 Moist, erythematous plaques involving the groin area, with satellite small papules at the periphery

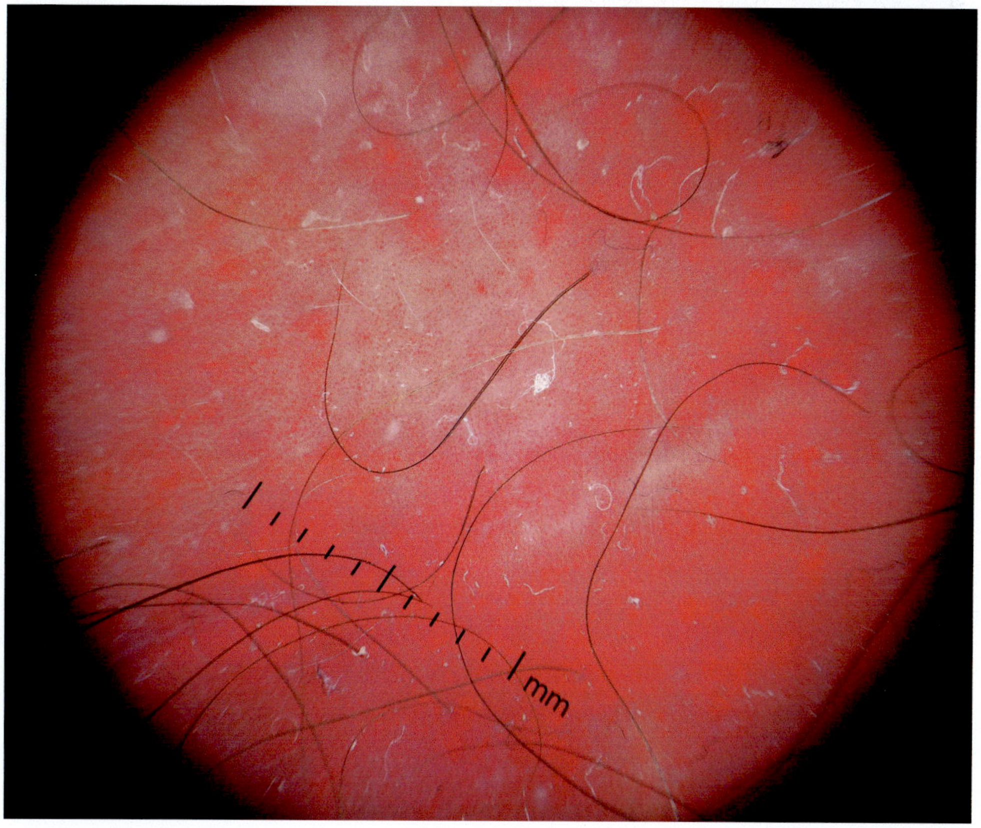

Fig. 6 Multiple dotted vessels, uniformly distributed over the surface of the lesion

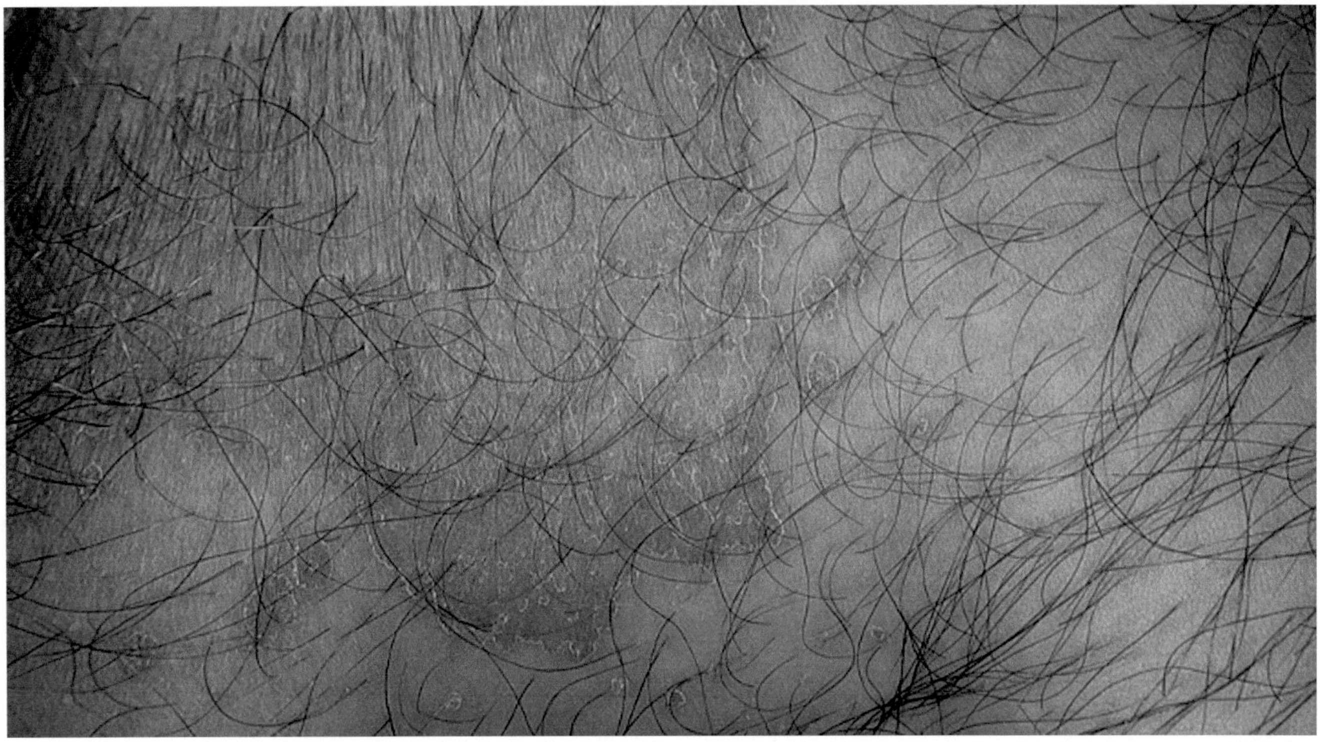

Fig. 7 Clinical view: erythematous squamous plaque in the groin

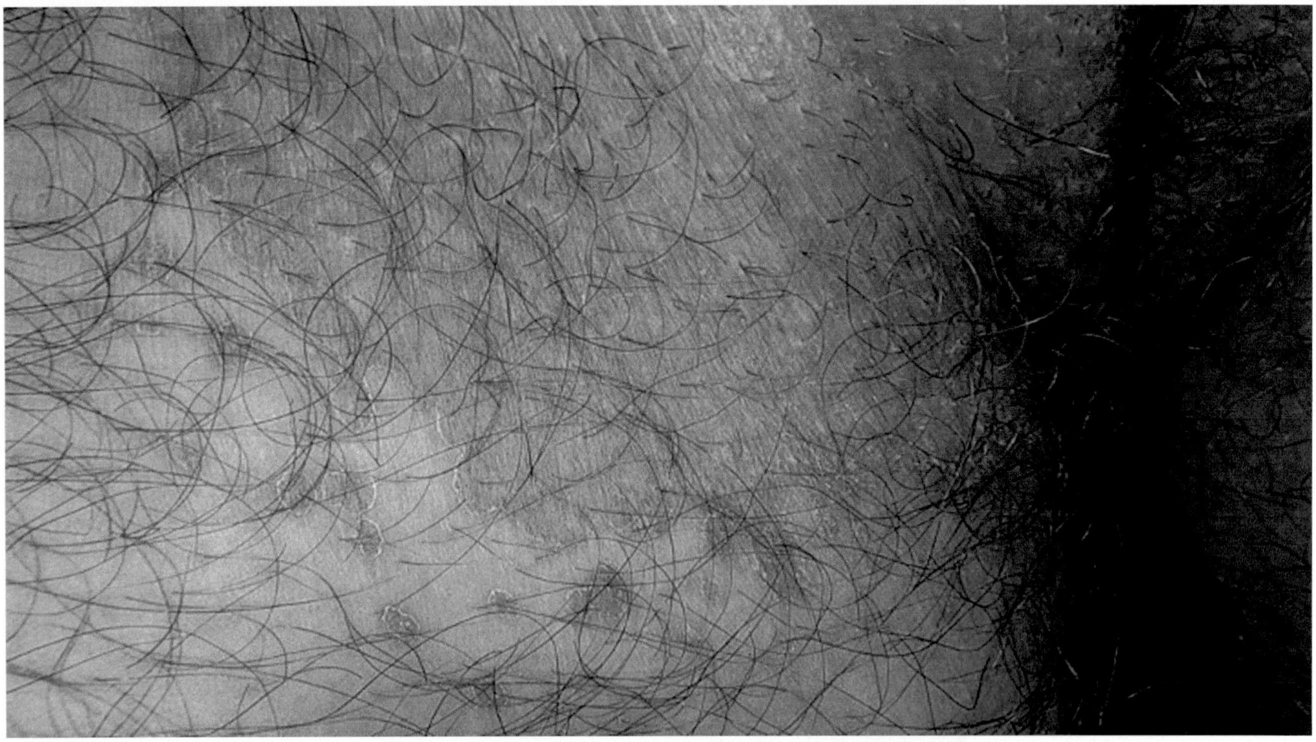

Fig. 8 Clinical view: erythematous squamous plaque in the groin

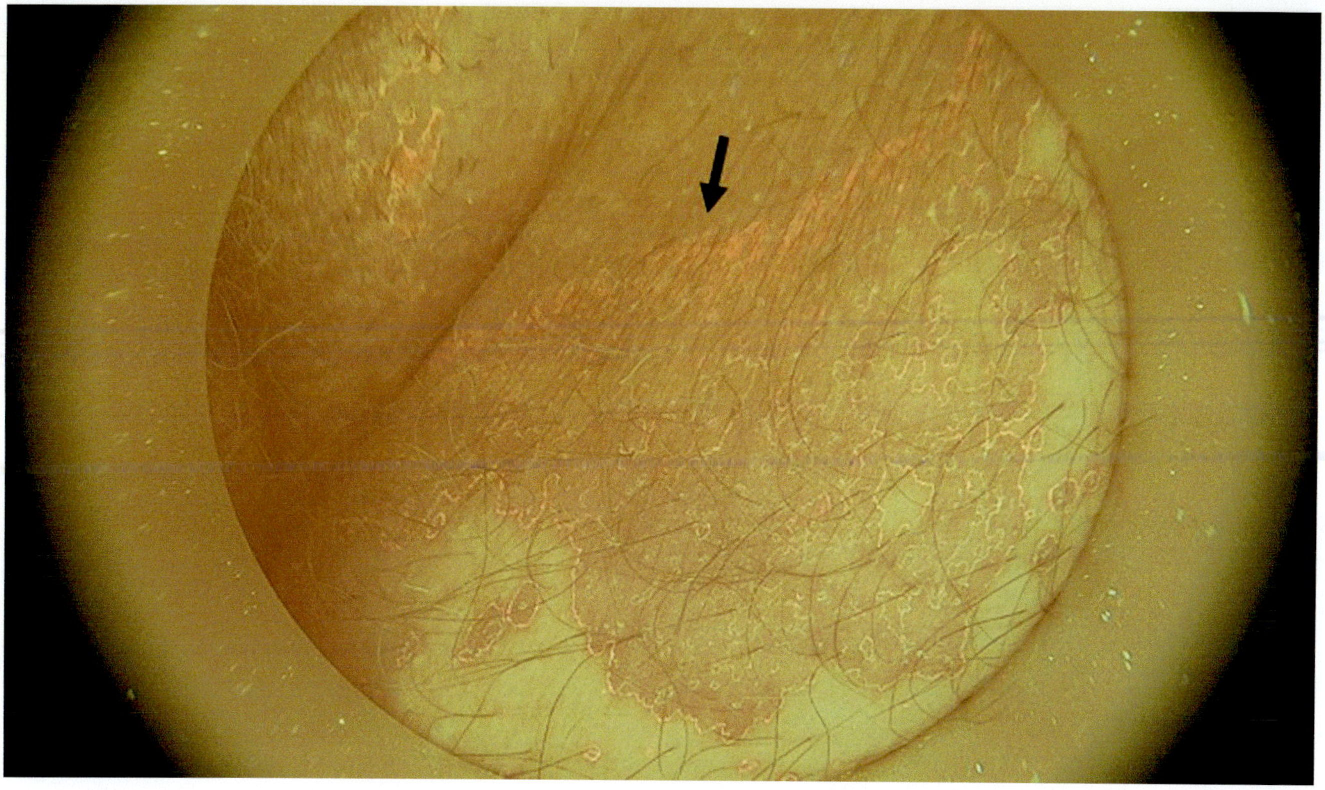

Fig. 9 Coral red fluorescence with Wood's light

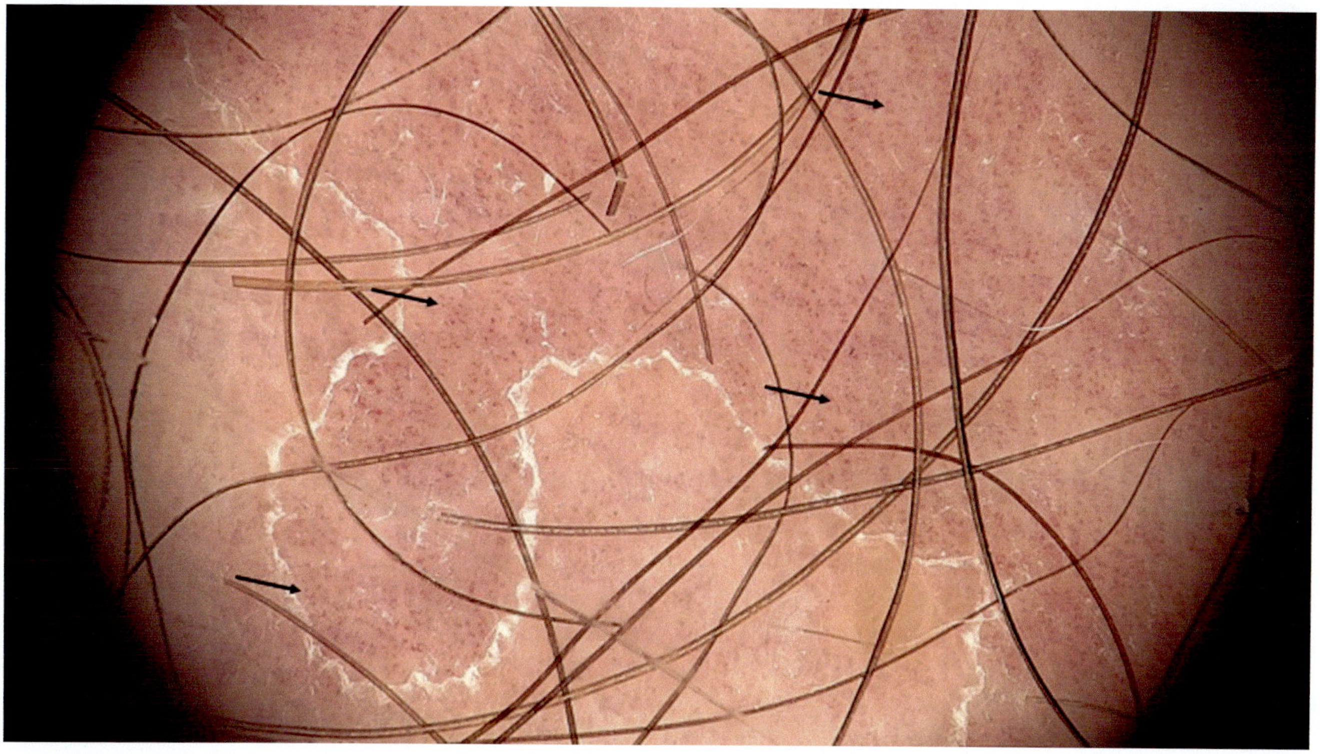

Fig. 10 Dremoscopic view: Peripheral scales with uniformly distributed dotted and linear vessels

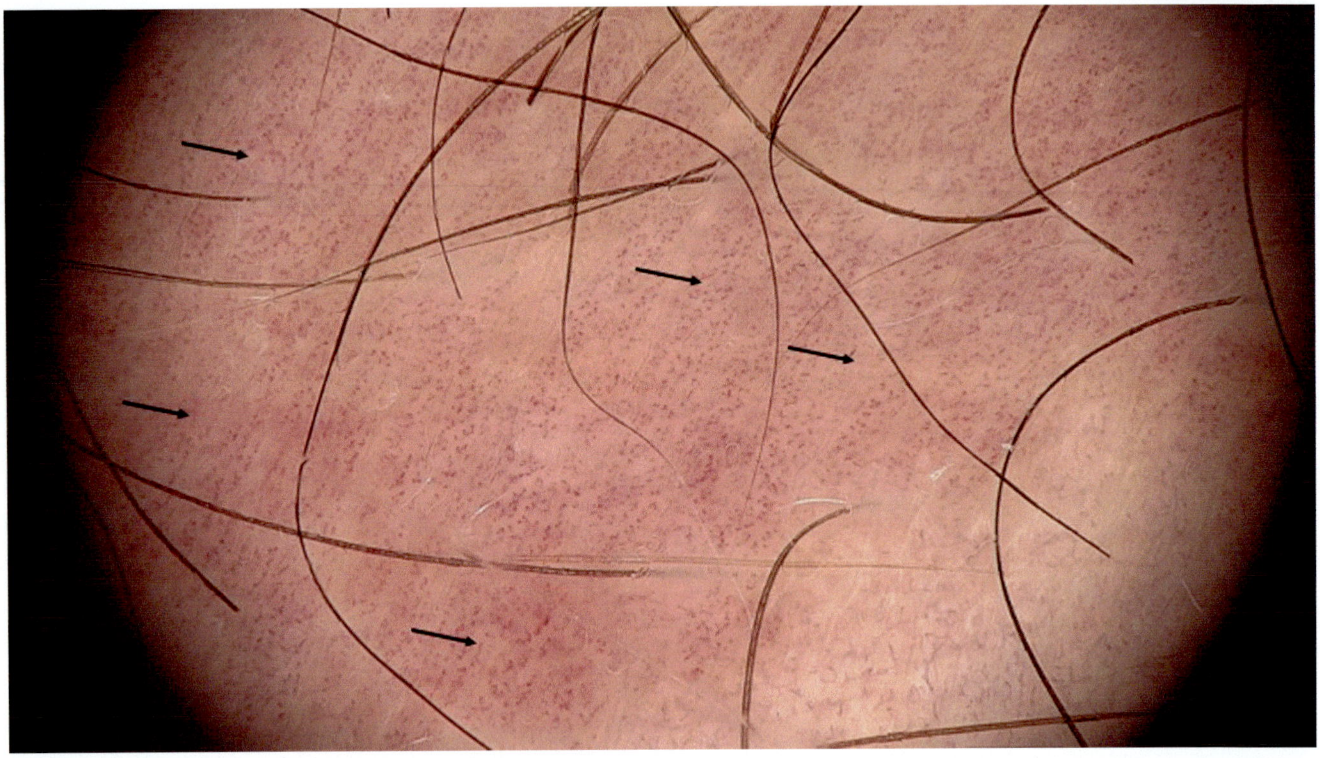

Fig. 11 Uniformly distributed dotted and linear vessels

Other clinical findings: Coral red fluorescence with Wood's light (Figs. 7, 8, 9, 10 and 11)

Diagnosis: Erytrasma

Key message: Dermoscopy is useful to distinguish mycosis of the groin (marginated eczema of Hebra-dermatitis) from Erythrasma.

Lesion on the Hands

Carlos Ortega Blanca, Jelenna Stojkovic Filipovic, Dimitrije Brasanac, and Horacio Cabo

Abstract

Keratinocytic tumor are frequently on the hands such as Bowen's Disease and Invasive Squamous cell carcinoma, both with specific dermoscopic features.

Keywords

Bowen's disease • Invasive squamous cell carcinoma

Case 1

Author: Blanca Carlos Ortega

Clinical record:

Sex: Male

Age: 87

Clinical description the case or the lesion: Irregular erythematosquamous plaque with mild itching

Body site: Back of left hand

Surface: Flat

Maximum diameter: 1 cm

Duration of the lesion: A year and a half

History of morphologic changes: Increase in size

Personal history of skin cancer: None

Family history of skin cancer: None

Skin Phototype: I

Clinical diagnosis: Actinic keratosis

Dermoscopic findings: Focal area with orthogonal white lines, structureless white central area, dotted and glomerular vessels

Other clinical findings: None (Figs. 1, 2, 3, 4 and 5)

Diagnosis: Bowen's Disease

Key message: Bowen's disease, named for John Templeton Bowen, also known as squamous cell carcinoma in situ is a type of non-melanocytic intraepidermal malignancy. It is estimated that in the general population about 3% to 5% of Bowen's disease develops into invasive squamous cell cancer. From a clinical point of view, it presents an erythematous plaque or patch with opaque yellow-white scales and erosions. The vast majority of Bowen's disease manifests itself without pigment, but in rare cases we can see its pigmented variant. The dermoscopic features of Bowen's disease were first described in 2004. Its dermoscopic pattern is characterized by glomerular vessels and scales. Glomerular vessels that are

C. O. Blanca
Clinica Privada Hospital Durango, Durango 290-706, col. Roma, del. Cuauhtémoc. CDMX, 06700 Roma, Mexico

J. S. Filipovic
Clinic of Dermatovenereology, Medical Faculty, University Clinical Center of Serbia, University of Belgrade, Pasterova 2, Belgrade, Serbia

D. Brasanac
Institute of Pathology, Medical Faculty, University of Belgrade, Doktora Subotica 1, Belgrade, Serbia
e-mail: dimitrije.brasanac@med.bg.ac.rs

H. Cabo (✉)
Clinical Dermatology, University of Buenos Aires, 1446 1 °C (1061) CABA, Buenos Aires, Arenales, Argentina
e-mail: cabohoracio@gmail.com

H. Cabo and A. Lallas (eds.), *Dermatoscopic Atlas of Non-Pigmented Lesions*,
https://doi.org/10.1007/978-3-031-34310-0_9

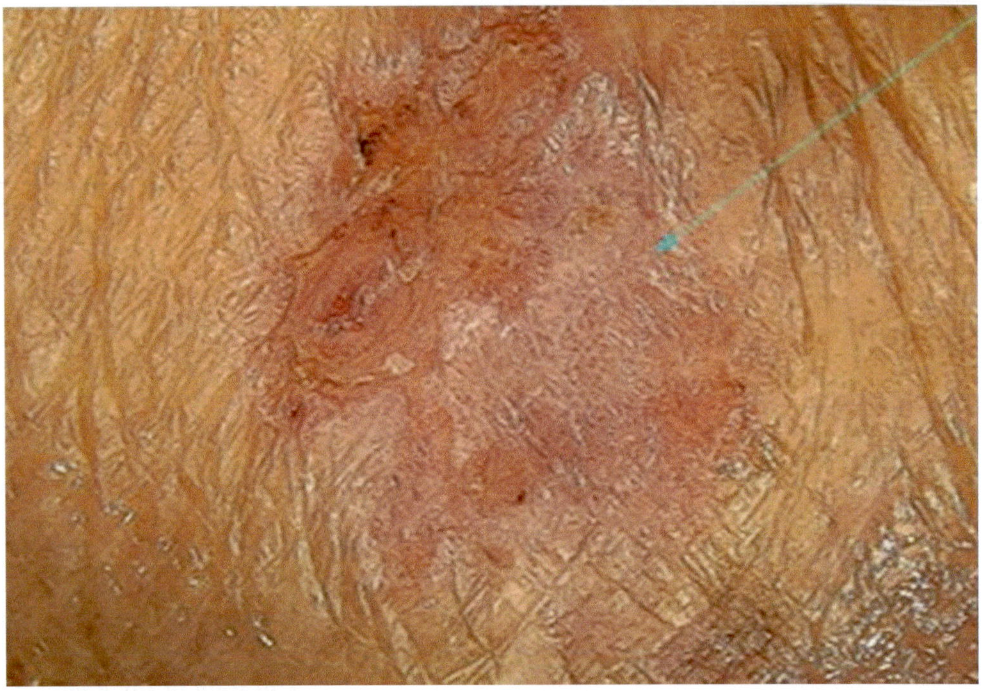

Fig. 1 Erythematous plaque (green arrow)

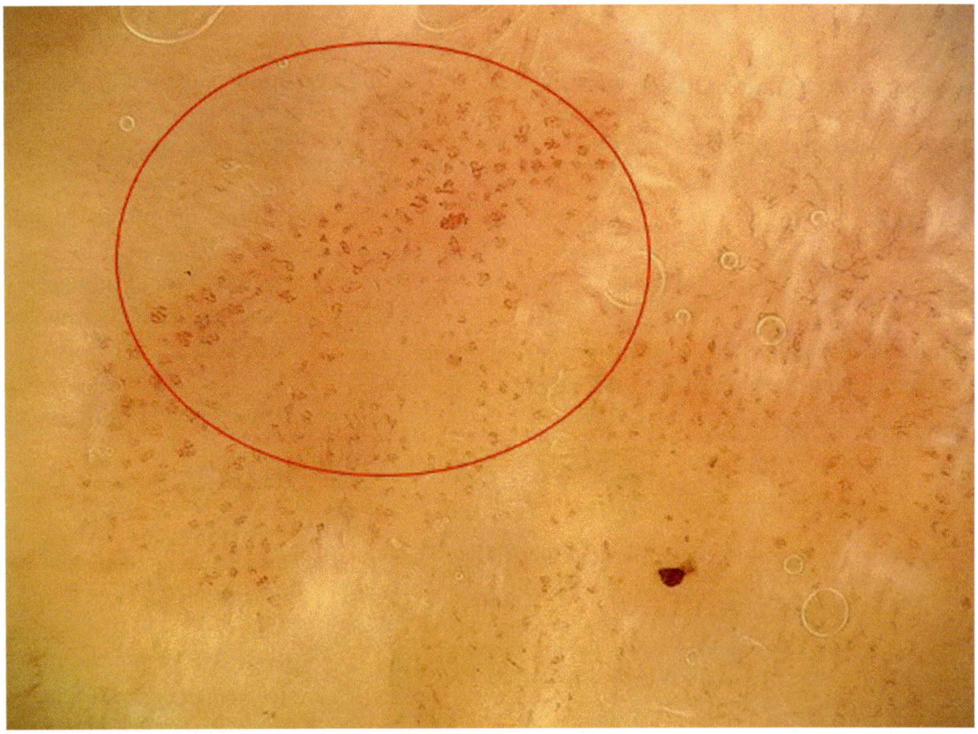

Fig. 2 Dotted and glomerular vessels (red circle)

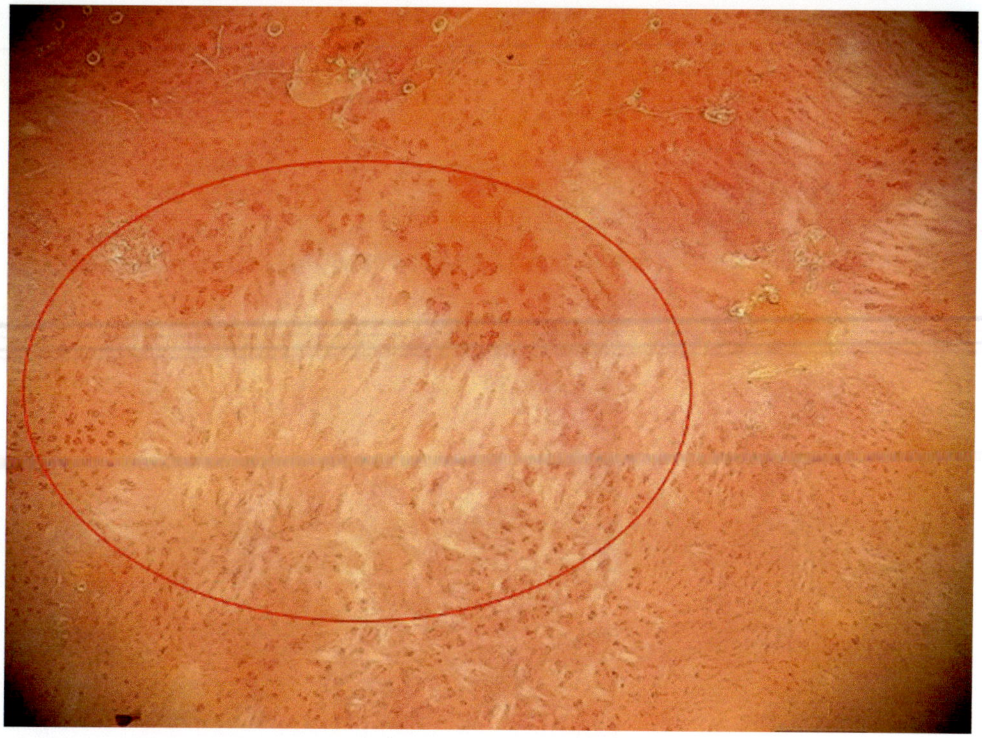

Fig. 3 Focal area with orthogonal white lines, structureless white central area, dotted and glomerular vessels (red circle)

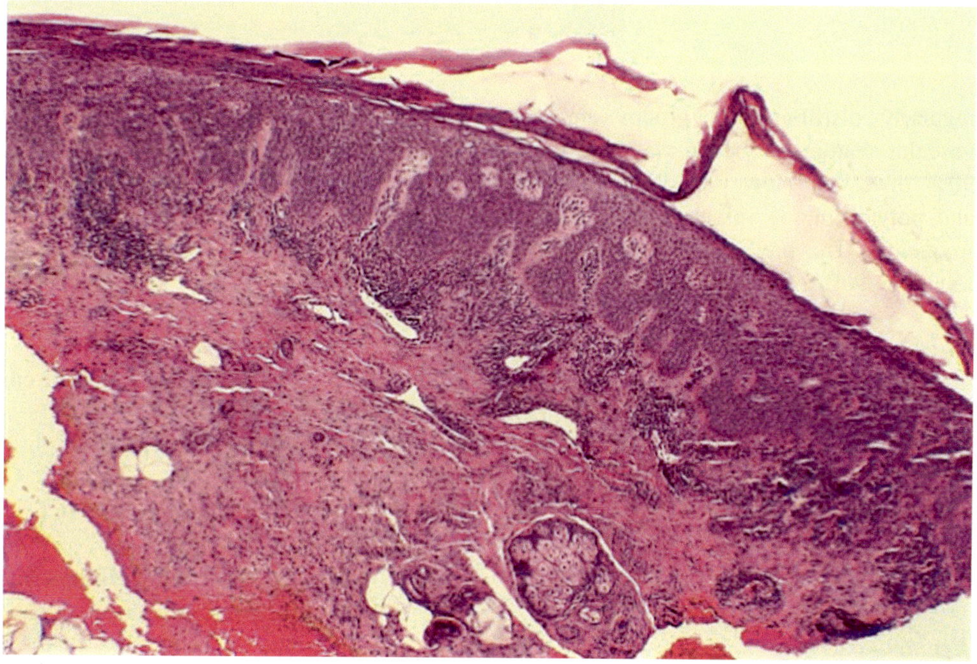

Fig. 4 Panoramic histopathological view

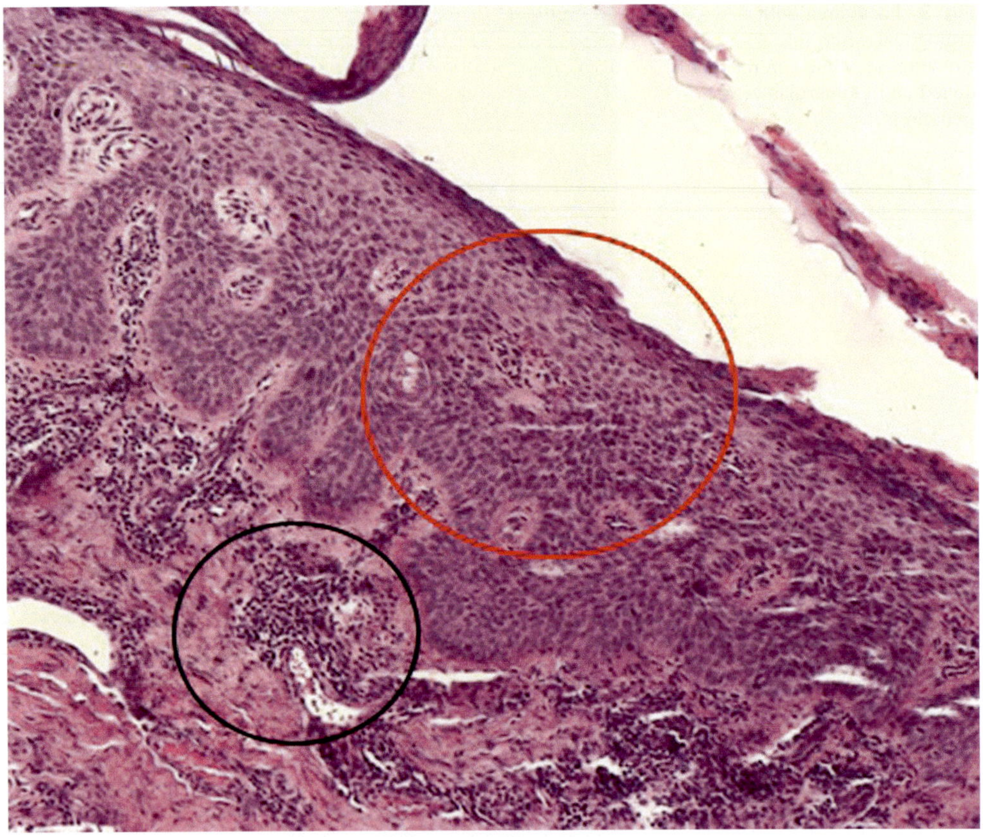

Fig. 5 Atypical keratinocytes with large, hyperchromatic nuclei and some abnormal mitosis (red circle); dermis with discrete inflammatory reaction with predominance of lymphocytes (black circle)

regularly distributed in groups are the most common vascular feature in such a way that they are identified in 90% of cases; However, dotted, hairpin, linear-irregular and polymorphous vessels can be observed although less frequently. The presence of fine white scales and are also found in 90% of cases.

Case 2

Authors: Jelena Stojkovic-Filipovic, Dimitrije Brasanac, Branislav Lekic

Clinical record:

Sex: Male

Age: 69-years-old

Clinical description the case or the lesion: Asymptomatic subungual lesion, previously treated as onychomycosis

Body site: Fourth finger of the right arm

Surface: Nodular

Maximum diameter: 1 cm

Duration of the lesion: Several years

History of morphologic changes: Slowly progressive lesion

Personal history of skin cancer: None

Family history of skin cancer: None

Skin Phototype: III

Clinical diagnosis: SCC

Dermoscopic findings: Chaotic unpigmented lesion, with eccentric structure-less pattern, eccentric red, pink and white hue. In some parts of the lesion, asymmetrically, polymorphic linear vessels (serpentine branched, curved, and coiled) of different diameters were noted. Scale, white keratin clods, erosions, ulceration, and yellow crust were also present in an asymmetrical fashion

Other clinical findings: Partial amputation of the fourth finger (Figs. 6, 7 and 8)

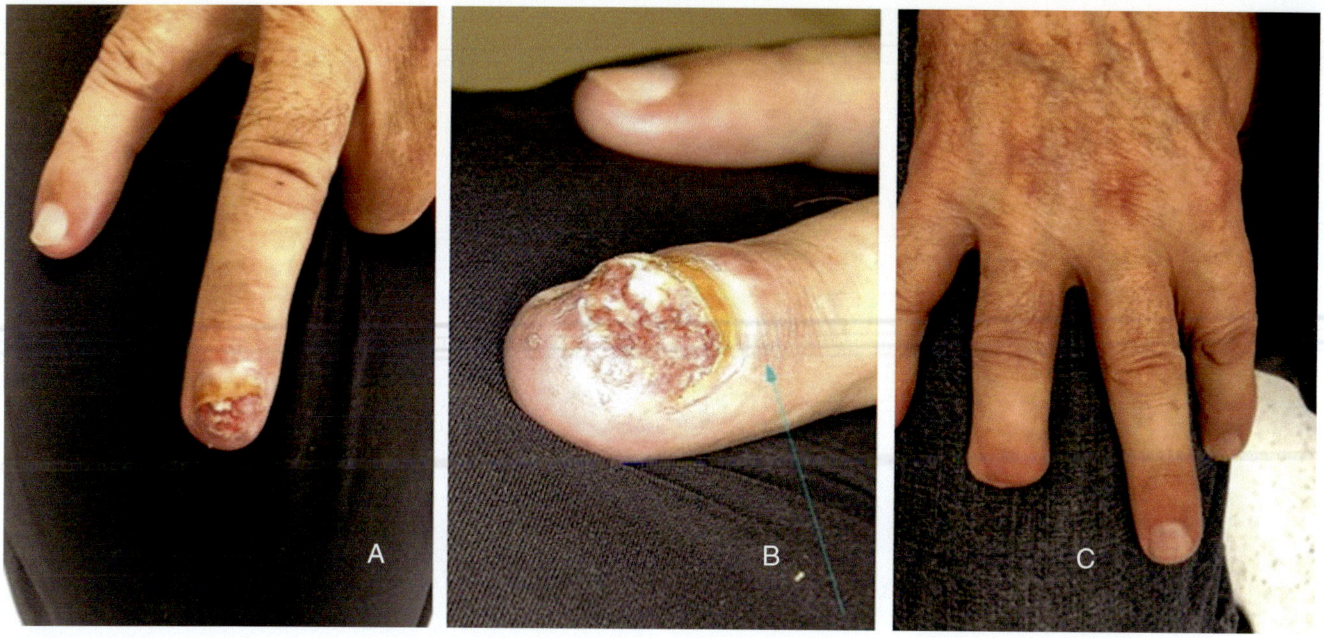

Fig. 6 A—Subungual unpigmented nodular lesion, partially destroyed yellowish nail plait; B—Periungual erythema (green arrow); C. partial amputation of distal phalanx

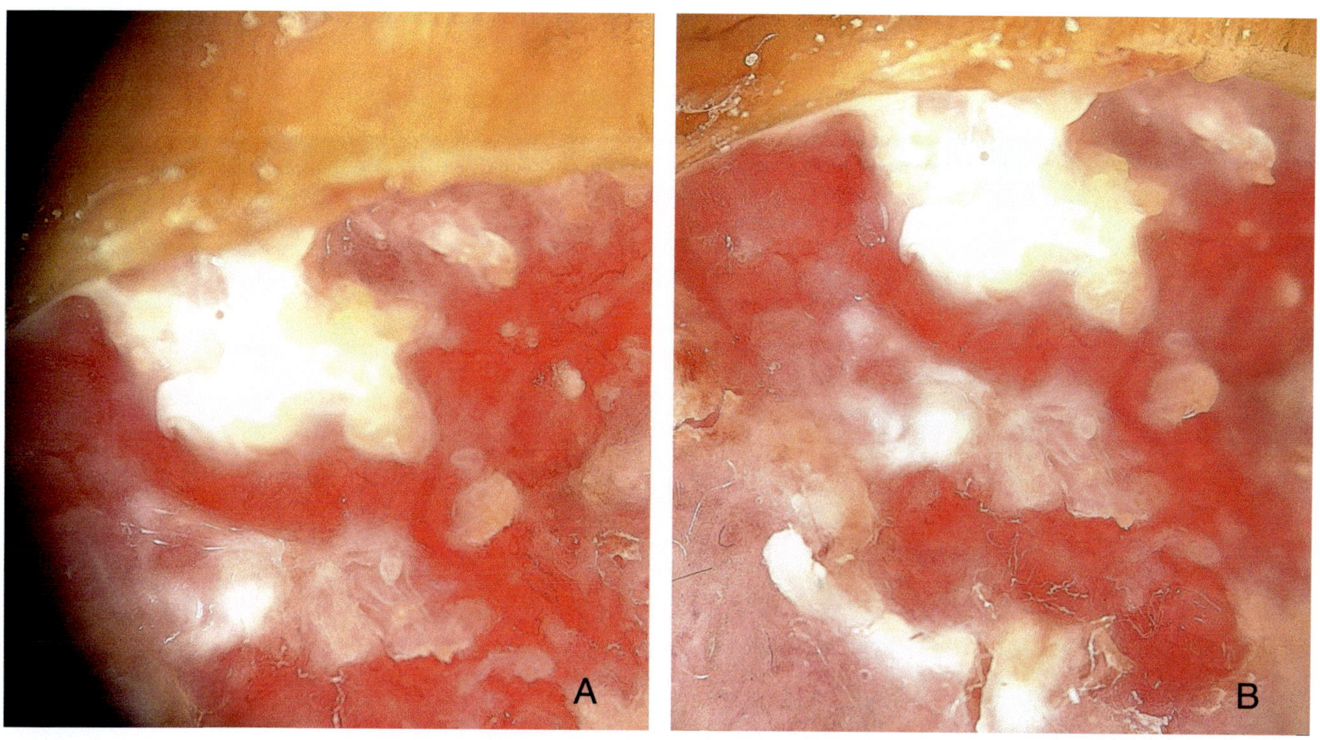

Fig. 7 A, B. a chaotic unpigmented lesion, with eccentric structureless red, pink, and white areas. Polymorphic linear vessels (serpentine branched, curved, and coiled) of different diameters. Scale, white keratin clods, erosions, ulceration, and yellow crust in an asymmetric fashion

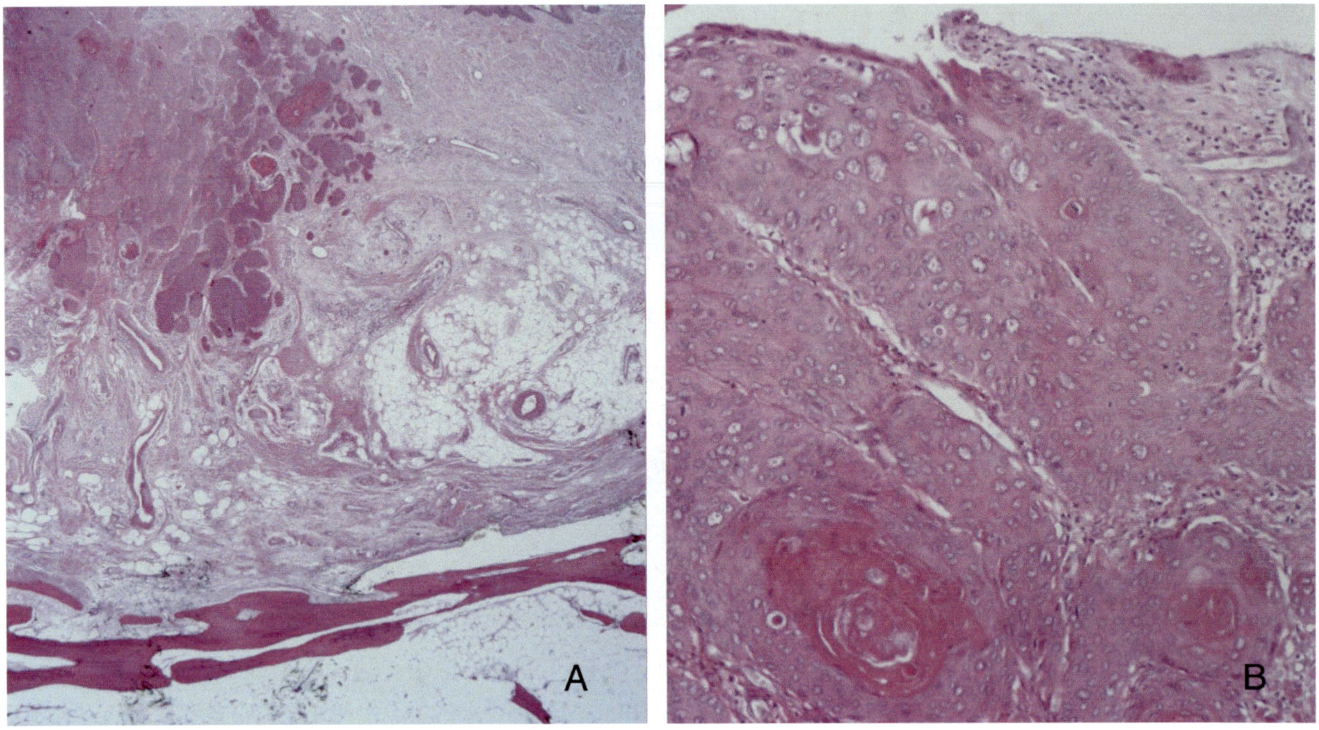

Fig. 8 A. squamous cell carcinoma originating from nail bad epithelium, infiltrating dermis and superficial fat tissue; B. superficial tumor nests with small areas of keratinization, moderate atypia and scattered mitotic figures (hematoxylin eosin stain; nests of atypical pleomorphic keratinocytes, less organized, less matured with less keratin formation (original magnification A. 12.5×, B. 100×)

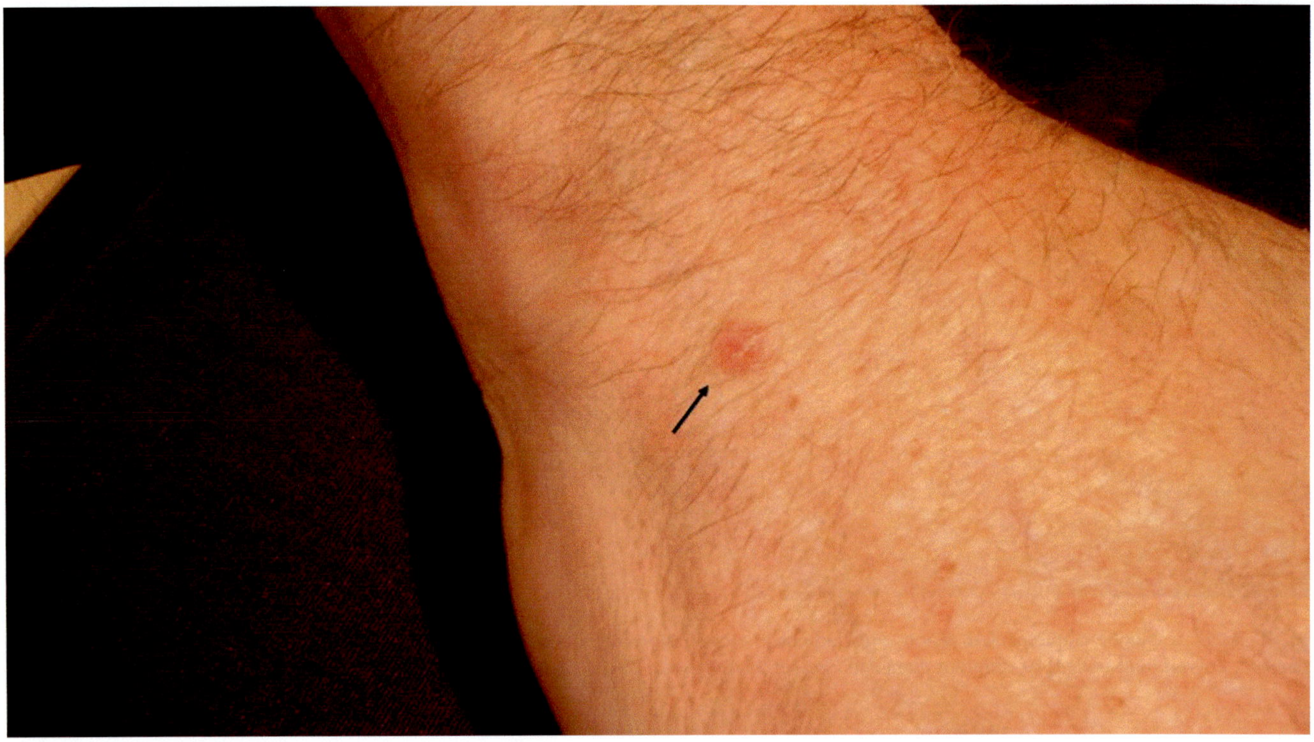

Fig. 9 Clinical view: non-pigmented lesion on the left hand (black arrow)

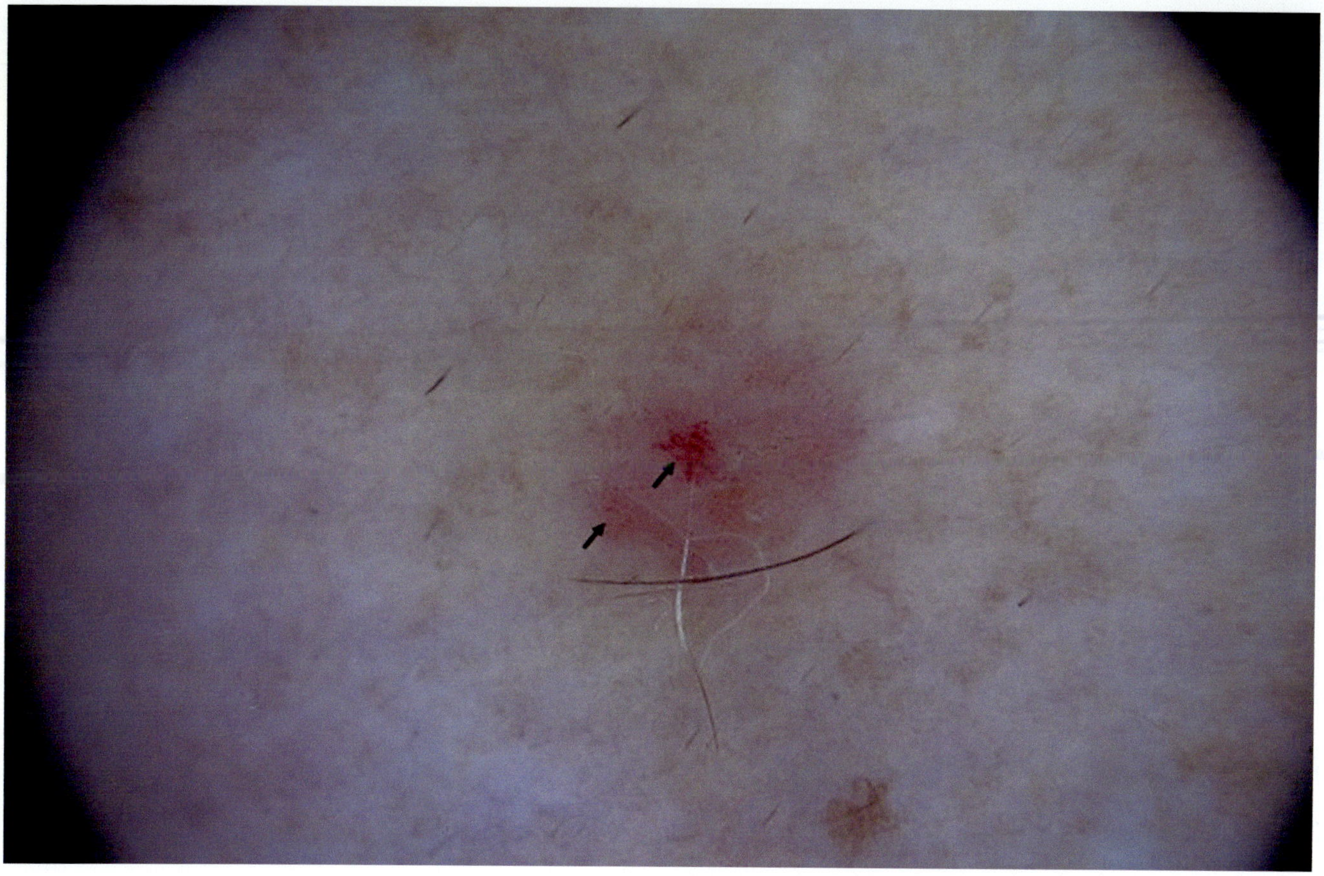

Fig. 10 Dermoscopic view: Glomerular vessels with focal distribution (black arrows)

Diagnosis: Invasive Squamous cell carcinoma

Key message: Usefulness of dermoscopy in the diagnosis of nail tumors

Case 3

Author: Horacio Cabo

Sex: Male

Age: 78-years-old patient.

Clinical description the case or the lesion: Ayntomatic non-pigmented lesion

Body site: Left hand

Surface: Flat

Maximum diameter: 9 mm

Duration of the lesion: More than one year

History of morphologic changes: Growing

Personal history of skin cancer: Basal cell Carcinomas

Family history of skin cancer: None

Skin Phototype: III

Clinical diagnosis: Basal Cell carcinoma, Actinic Keratosis, Squamous cell carcinoma

Dermoscopic findings: Glomerular vessels with focal distribution

Other clinical findings: None (Figs. 9 and 10).

Diagnosis: Invasive Squamous cell carcinoma

Key message: Vessels are the clue in pink lesions. In this casen glomerular vessels with focal distribution are the marker of Squamous cell carcinoma

Lesions on the Feet

Dominga Peirano Deck, Sebastián Vargas, Álvaro Abarzúa, Cristián Navarrete Dechent, Pablo Uribe, Leonel Hidalgo, Danica Tiodorovic, Ilut Paula Anca, Sonia Rodriguez Saa, and Horacio Cabo

Abstract

Non-pigmented lesion on the feet such as Eccrine Porome, Amelanotic Melanoma, Giant molluscum contagiosum, Acral amelanotic melanoma with their dermoscopic features are described in this chapter.

Keywords

Eccrine porome • Amelanotic melanoma • Giant molluscum contagiosum • Acral amelanotic melanoma

Case 1

Authors: Dominga Peirano Deck, Sebastián Vargas, Álvaro Abarzúa, Cristián Navarrete Dechent, Pablo Uribe

D. P. Deck · S. Vargas · Á. Abarzúa · C. Navarrete Dechent · P. Uribe · L. Hidalgo
Department of Dermatology, Escuela de Medicina, Pontificia Universidad Católica de Chile, Diagonal Paraguay 362, 6th Floor, 8330077 Santiago, Chile
e-mail: dpeirano@miuandes.cl

S. Vargas
e-mail: sivargas@uc.cl

D. Tiodorovic
Clinic of Dermatovenerology, Medical Faculty, University Clinical Center of Nis, University of Nis, Nis, Serbia

I. P. Anca
Department of Dermatology, "Iuliu Hațieganu" University of Medicine and Pharmacy, 37 Erich Bergel Street, apt 2, 400461 Cluj-Napoca, Romania

S. R. Saa
University of Mendoza, Mendoza, Argentina

H. Cabo (✉)
Clinical Dermatology, University of Buenos Aires, Arenales 1446 1 °C (1061) CABA, Buenos Aires, Argentina
e-mail: cabohoracio@gmail.com

Clinical record:

Sex: Male

Age: 67-year-old

Clinical description the case or the lesion: During a routine dermatological total body examination, a shiny erythematous papule of about 8 mm in diameter was observed in the right dorsal foot

Body site: Right dorsal foot

Surface: Palpable

Maximum diameter: 8 mm

Duration of the lesion: Unknown

History of morphologic changes: It had no signs of recent bleeding or ulceration

Personal history of skin cancer: None

Family history of skin cancer: None

Skin Phototype: II

Clinical diagnosis: Skin tumor

Dermoscopic findings: A reddish background with branched vessels with rounded endings, white interlacing areas around vessels and milky-red globules, suggestive of an eccrine porome

Other clinical findings: None (Figs. 1, 2 and 3)

Diagnosis: Eccrine Porome

H. Cabo and A. Lallas (eds.), *Dermatoscopic Atlas of Non-Pigmented Lesions*,
https://doi.org/10.1007/978-3-031-34310-0_10

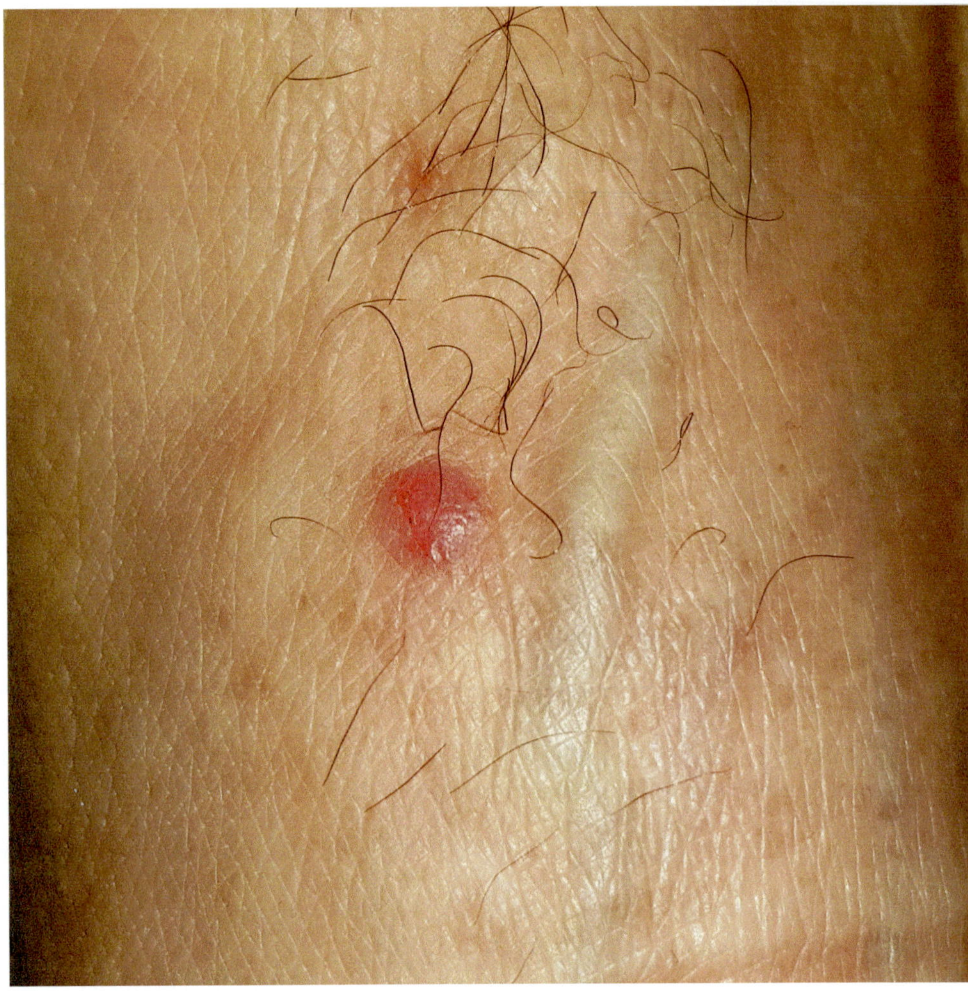

Fig. 1 A well delimited, shiny erythematous papule of about 8 mm in diameter was observed in the right dorsal foot

Key message: **Poroma** is an uncommon benign tumor derived from the ducts of eccrine or apocrine sweat glands. It usually presents as a red to pink papule, nodule, or plaque often located in the volar surfaces of the hands or feet. Poroma is easily misdiagnosed as basal cell carcinoma, pyogenic granuloma, squamous cell carcinoma and seborrheic keratosis.

Dermoscopic features associated with poroma include:

- branched vessels with rounded endings (chalice-form and cherry blossom vessels)
- white interlacing areas around vessels, yellow structureless areas
- and milky-red globules.

Additional findings common but not specific for poromas include

- polymorphous vessels
- blood spots
- erosions/ulcers,
- and milky-red areas.

Reflectance confocal microscopy (RCM), which has shown to be an important in vivo, non-invasive diagnostic technique for skin lesions.

RCM and dermoscopy may assist in the correct diagnosis of this neoplasm and help rule out some differential diagnoses. Due to about 18% of poromas will progress to porocarcinomas, early and correct diagnosis with auxiliary examination and histopathological examination are particularly important.

Case 2

Authors: Dominga Peirano Deck, Sebastián Vargas, Leonel Hidalgo, Álvaro Abarzúa, Pablo Uribe, Cristián Navarrete Dechent

Clinical record:

Sex: Female

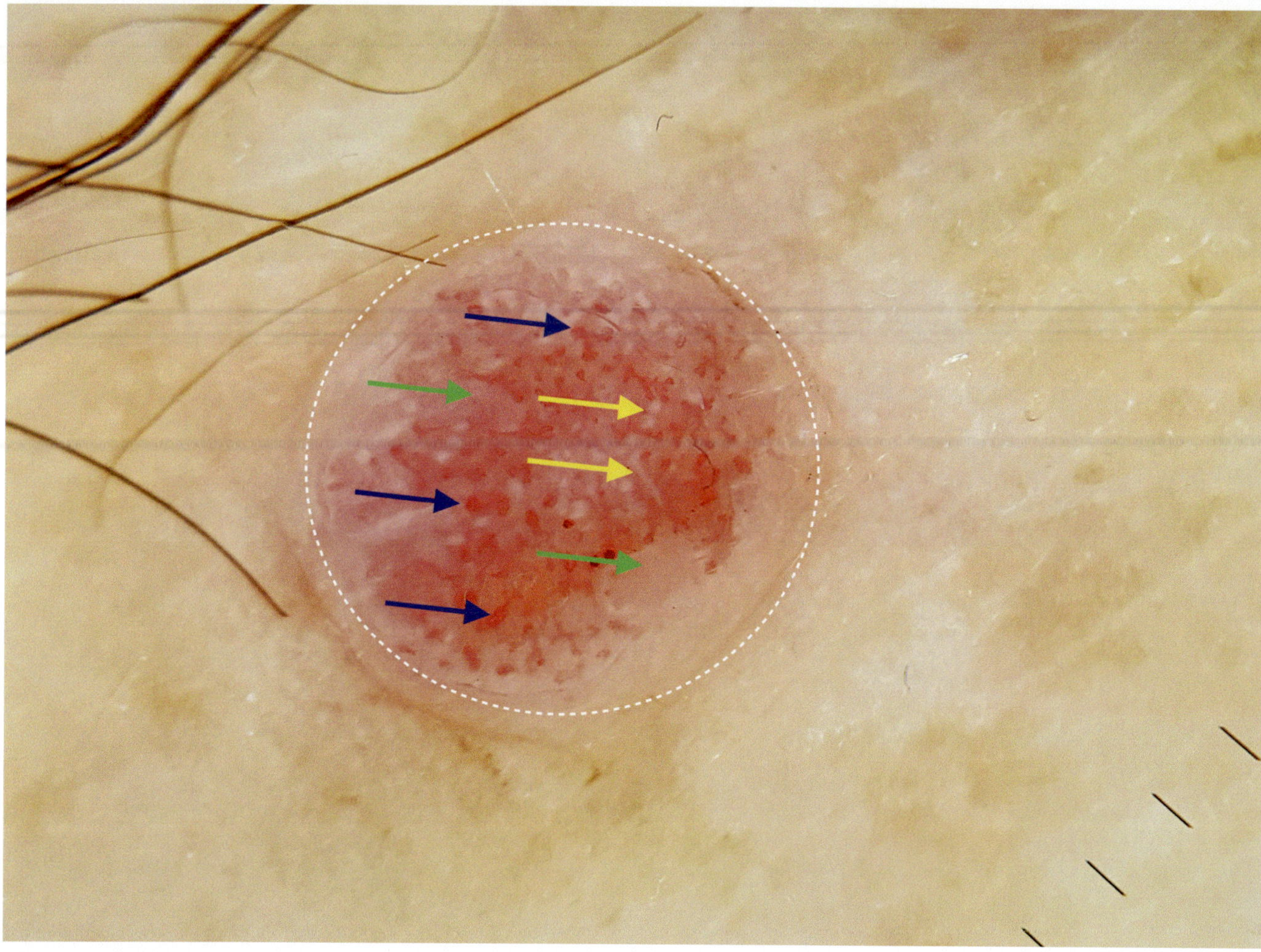

Fig. 2 **Dermoscopy image (polarized light)** A reddish background (white dotted circle) with branched vessels with rounded endings (blue arrows), white interlacing areas around vessels (yellow arrows) and milky-red globules (green arrows)

Age: 74-year-old

Clinical description the case or the lesion: An ulcerated-bleeding erythematous plaque of 15 mm in diameter in the right medial plantar foot

Body site: Right medial plantar foot

Surface: Palpable-Nodular.

Maximum diameter: 15 mm

Duration of the lesion: 3 weeks

History of morphologic changes: Ulceration and bleeding

Personal history of skin cancer: No

Family history of skin cancer: No

Skin Phototype: III

Clinical diagnosis: Amelanotic melanoma

Dermoscopic findings: The presence of polymorphous vessels, punctated vessels, milky red areas and shiny white lines using polarized light, should make us suspect an amelanotic melanoma.

Other clinical findings: (-) (Figs. 4, 5, 6)

Diagnosis: Amelanotic Melanoma

Key message: Amelanotic melanomas represent 2% of all melanoma subtypes. There is often a delay in diagnosis due

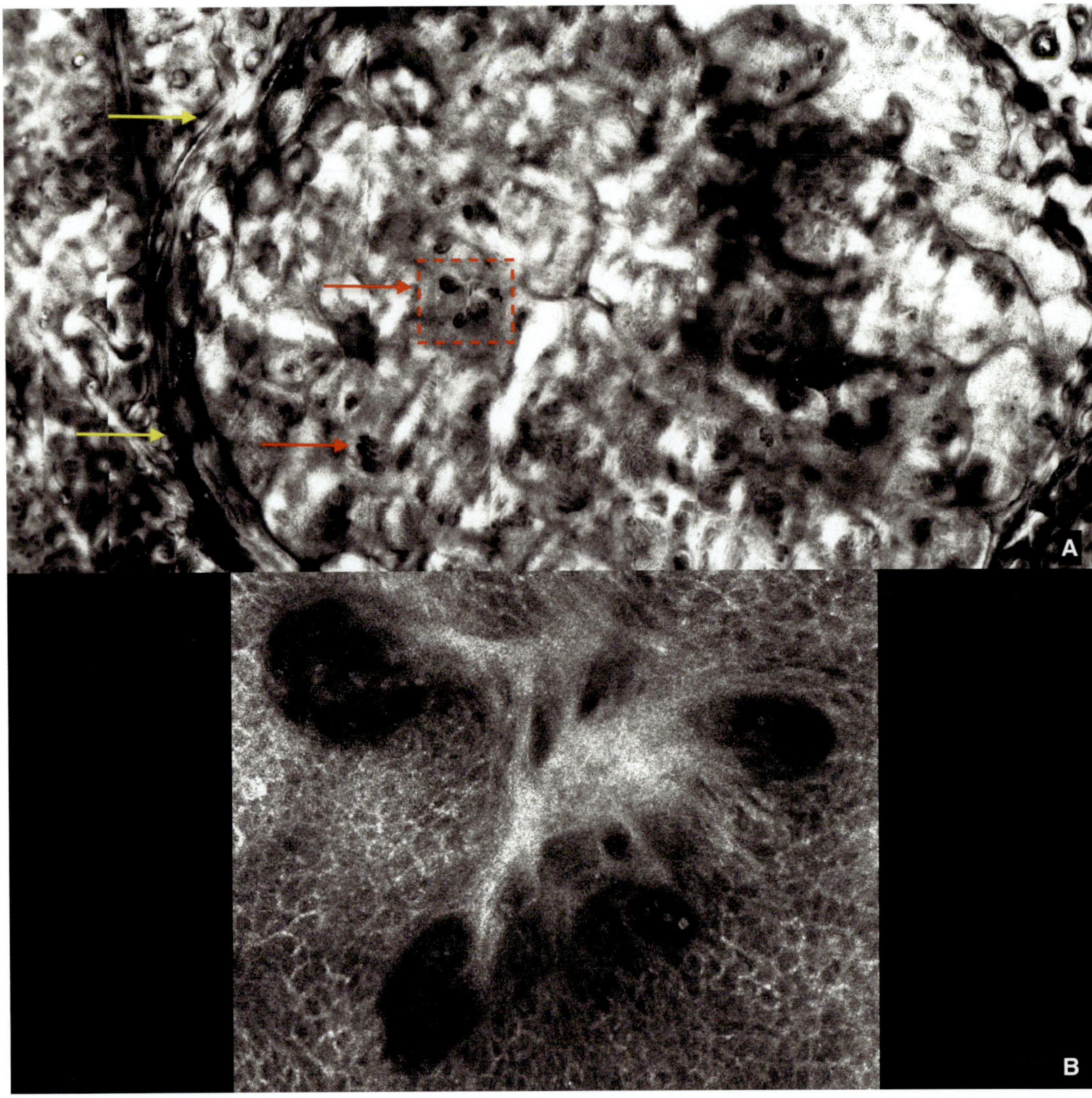

Fig. 3 **Reflectance confocal microscopy imaged. Figure A.** A well-demarcated symmetric tumor was seen (yellow arrows). At the level of the epidermis, a regular honeycomb pattern was observed. At the dermoepidermal junction, dilated vessels with a branching morphology were visualized (red arrows). **Figure B.** These vessels correlated with the branched vessels with rounded endings seen on dermoscopy. No atypical cells were seen on confocal examination

to the lack of a distinctive clinical appearance and the lack of classic ABCD features. Dermoscopy has served as an aid for the diagnosis of amelanotic melanoma. Amelanotic melanoma diagnosis should be suspected in any lesion displaying the following dermoscopic features:

- Dotted vessels
- Serpentine vessels
- Glomerular vessels
- Polymorphous vessels (combination of those described above)
- Milky red areas
- Shiny white lines
- Remnants of other pigmented melanoma specific structures in hypomelanotic melanoma (e.g. atypical network, atypical globules, etc.)

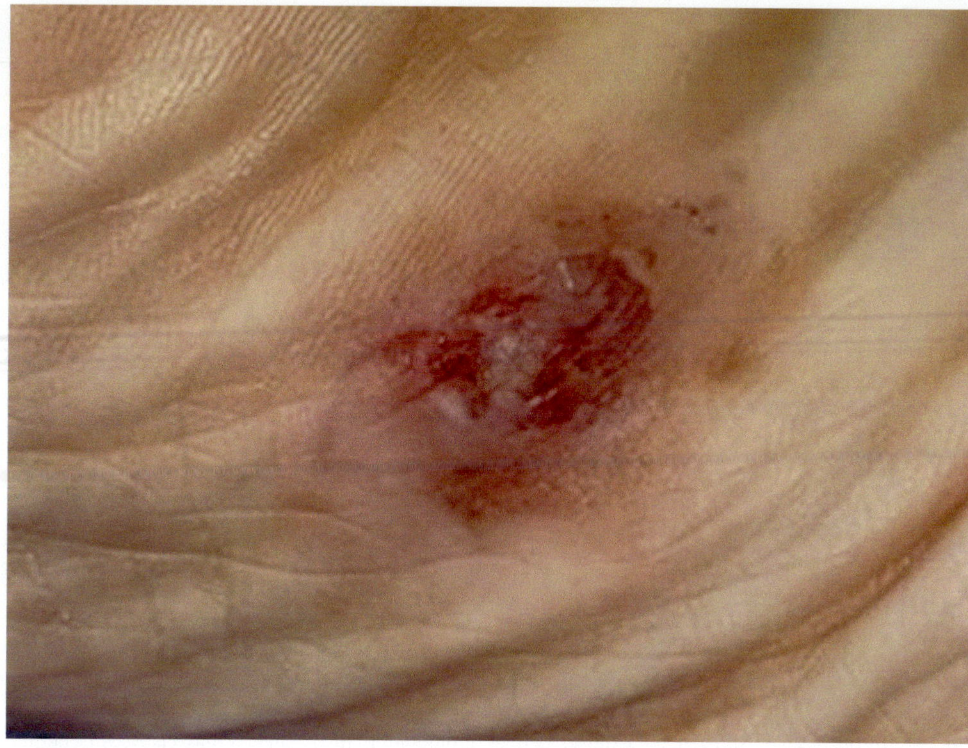

Fig. 4 A 10-mm erythematous ulcerated tumor was observed on the right medial plantar foot

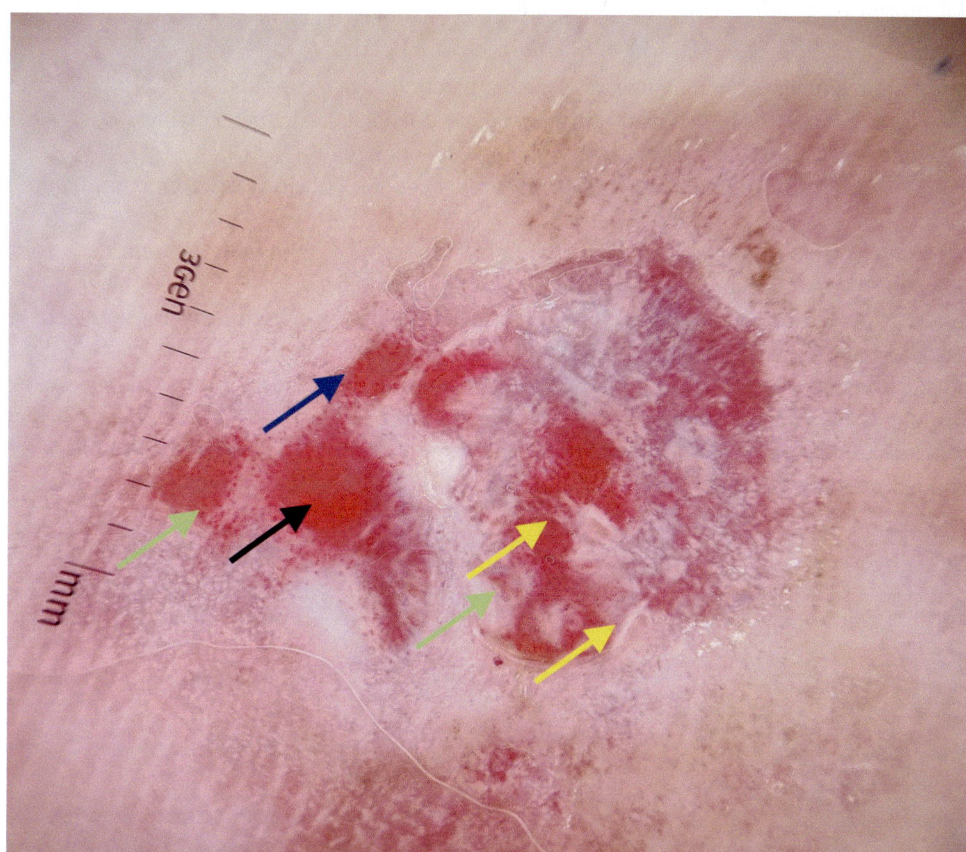

Fig. 5 **Dermoscopy (polarized light)**. The presence of polymorphous vessels (blue arrow), punctated vessels (green arrows), milky red areas (black arrow) and shiny white lines (yellow arrow) using polarized light, should make us suspect a amelanotic melanoma

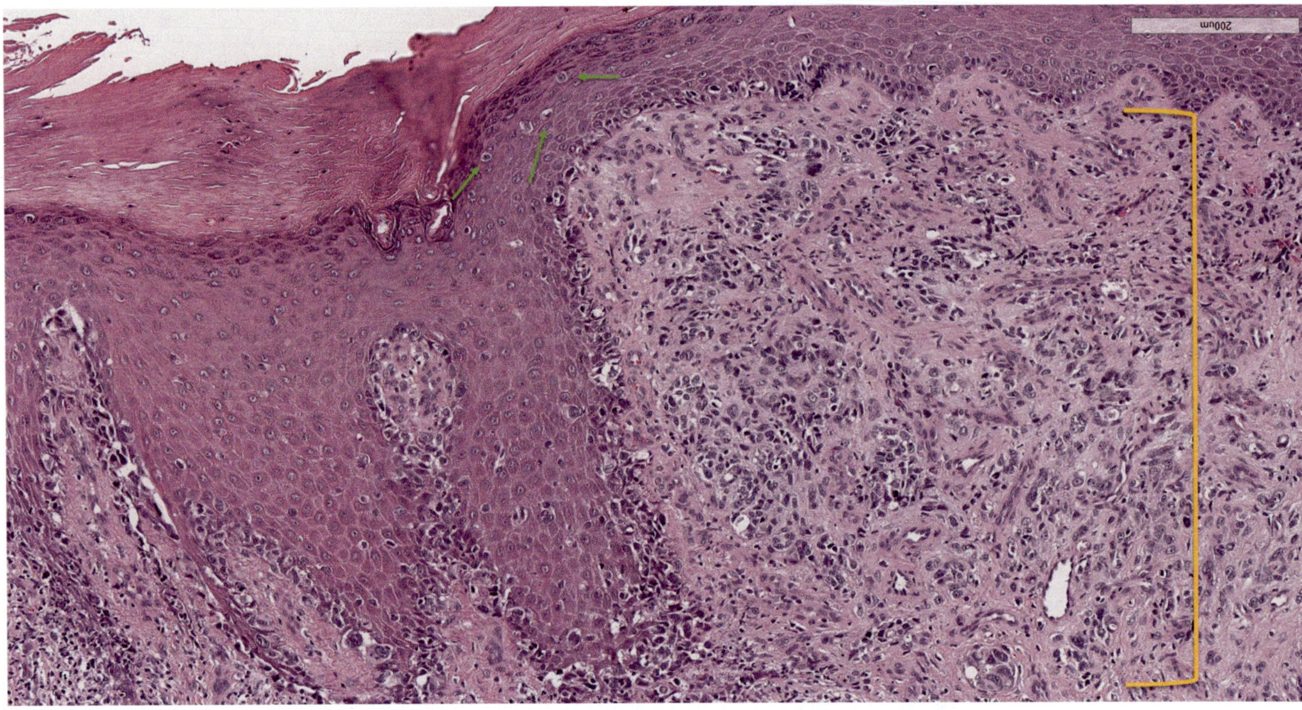

Fig. 6 Histopathology showed an extense dermal proliferation of atypical cells (yellow line) with pagetoid spread (green arrows). The final Breslow depth of this lesion was 2.3 mm. (Courtesy of Miguel Angel Villaseca, MD, Department of Pathology, Pontificia Universidad Católica de Chile)

- For acral amelanotic melanoma, a "vascular parallel ridge pattern composed of chaotically distributed red dots" has been described (in contrast to acral angioma displaying an organized linear, double-dotted ridge pattern).

Dotted vessels are considered to be the best dermoscopic indicator of the melanocytic origin of a hypopigmented tumor. It is also important to emphasize that acral melanomas also have a predilection for being amelanotic, therefore, the location of the lesion also provides clues that increase the suspicion of amelanotic melanoma. A specific sign of acral amelanotic melanomas is the vascular parallel ridge pattern with atypical red dots.

Case 3

Author: Danica Tiodorovic

Clinical record

Sex: Female

Age: 16-years-old

Clinical description of the case or the lesion: A 16-year-old girl comes to the examination accompanied by her parents due to non-pigmented nodular lesion, 18 mm in diameter, which was growing over the last year

Body site: Dorsum of the right foot

Surface: Nodular

Maximum diameter: 18 mm

Duration of the lesion: 1 year

History of morphologic changes: Occurrence one year ago and progressive increase in size

Personal history of skin cancer: None

Family history of skin cancer: None

Skin Phototype: II

Clinical diagnosis: Cutaneous adnexal tumors

Dermoscopic findings: Dermoscopy revealed multiple amorphous white-yellowish structures, crown vessels, and linear radial vessels, vessels perpendicular to the center of the lesion (Figs. 7, 8 and 9).

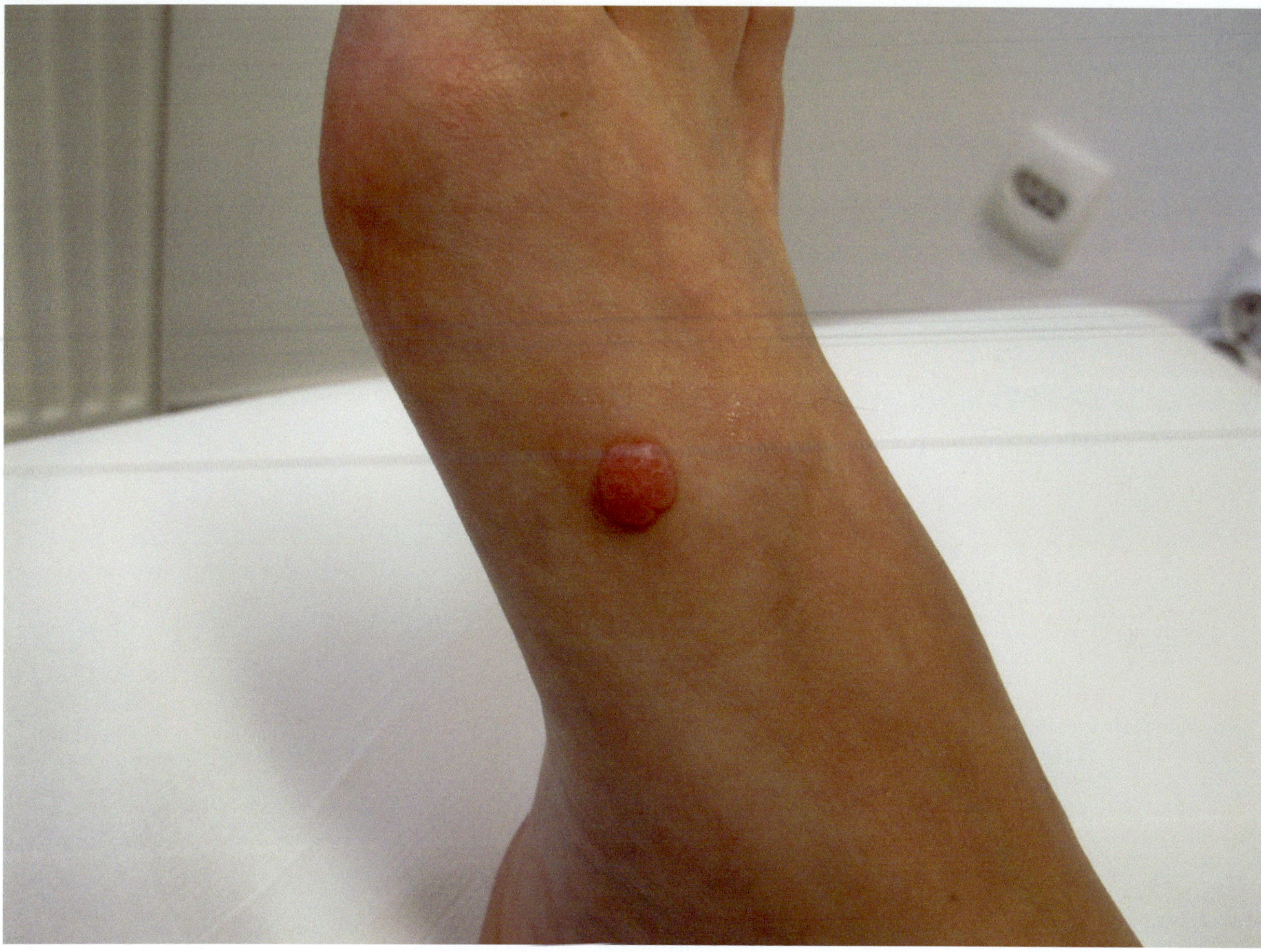

Fig. 7 Pink nodular lesion on the dorsum of the right foot

Diagnosis: Giant molluscum contagiosum

Key message: The presence of multiple amorphous white-yellowish structures accompanied by crown vessels and linear radial vessels can be observed in giant molluscum contagiosum**.** Dermoscopy can help in the proper diagnosis of this rare presentation of molluscum contagiosum.

Case 4

Author: Ilut Paula Anca

Clinical record:

Sex: Female

Age: 79-year-old

Clinical description the case or the lesion: An ulcerated nodular lesion is observed at the level of the right heel, bordered by hyperkeratotic crusts with clinical symptoms of pain and stinging

Body site: Acral-heel

Surface: Nodular

Maximum diameter: 4 cm

Duration of the lesion: 3 years

History of morphologic changes: Small nodule treated initially as a callus with keratotic substances that developed an ulceration which did not heal

Personal history of skin cancer: None

Family history of skin cancer: None

Skin Phototype: II

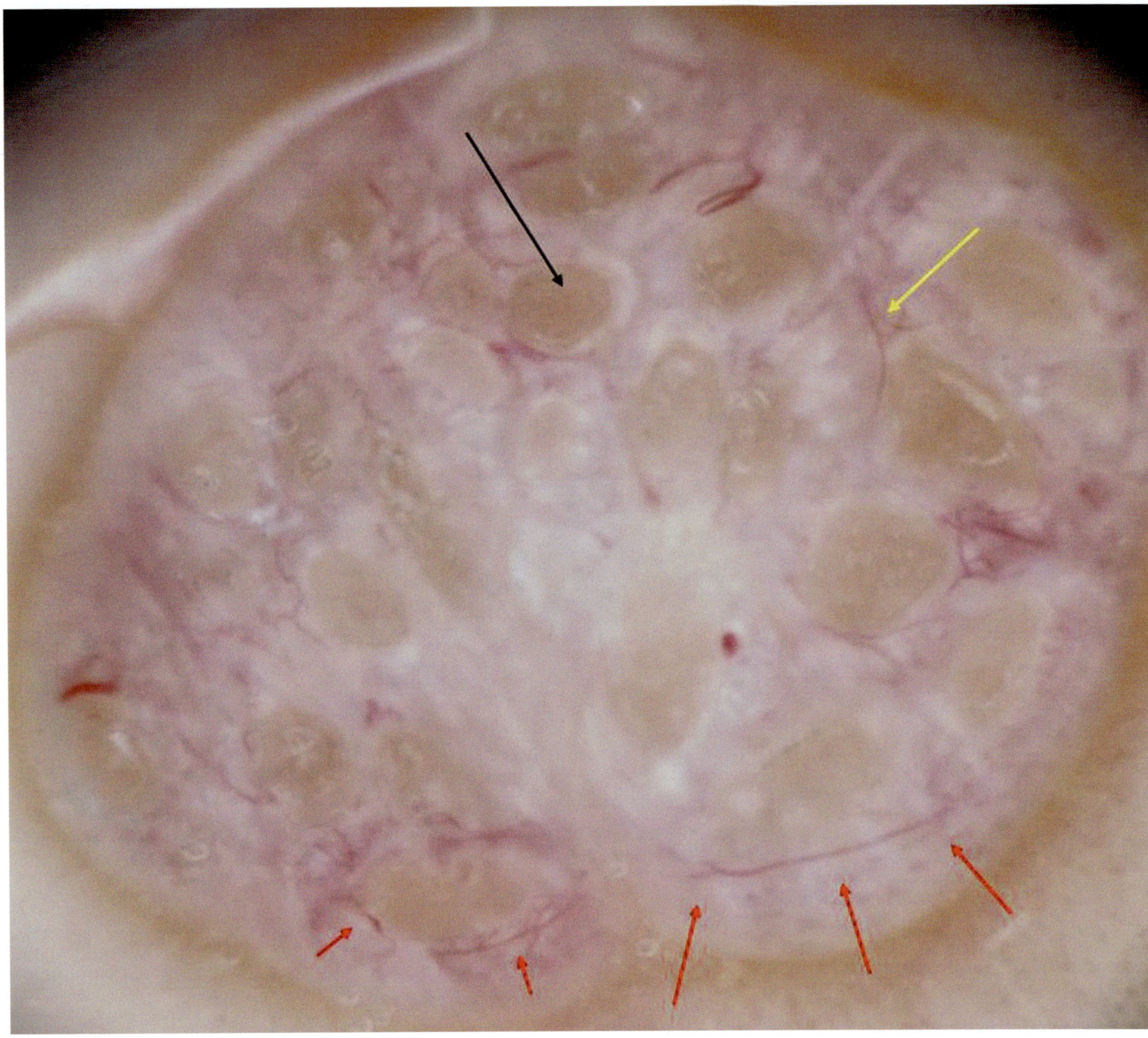

Fig. 8 Dermoscopic examination revealed multiple amorphous white-yellowish structures (black arrows), crown vessels (red arrows), and linear radial vessels (vessels perpendicular to the center of the lesion) (yellow arrow)

Clinical diagnosis: Acral amelanotic melanoma, Breslow = 9 mm

Dermoscopic findings:

- atypical vascular pattern consisting of polymorphous vessels: thick and thin linear vessels, dotted vessels, hairpin and looped vessels
- milky-red background
- ulceration
- keratin crusts/masses.

Other clinical findings: None (Figs. 10 and 11)

Diagnosis: Acral amelanotic melanoma

Key message: Acral amelanotic melanoma is a rare tumor and the absence of pigment or specific melanoma criteria makes it very difficult to diagnose. In front of a non-healing ulcerated lesion with unspecific morphology, the possibility of a melanoma should always be ruled out and at least a biopsy if not an excision should be performed.

Case 5

Author: Sonia Rodriguez Saa

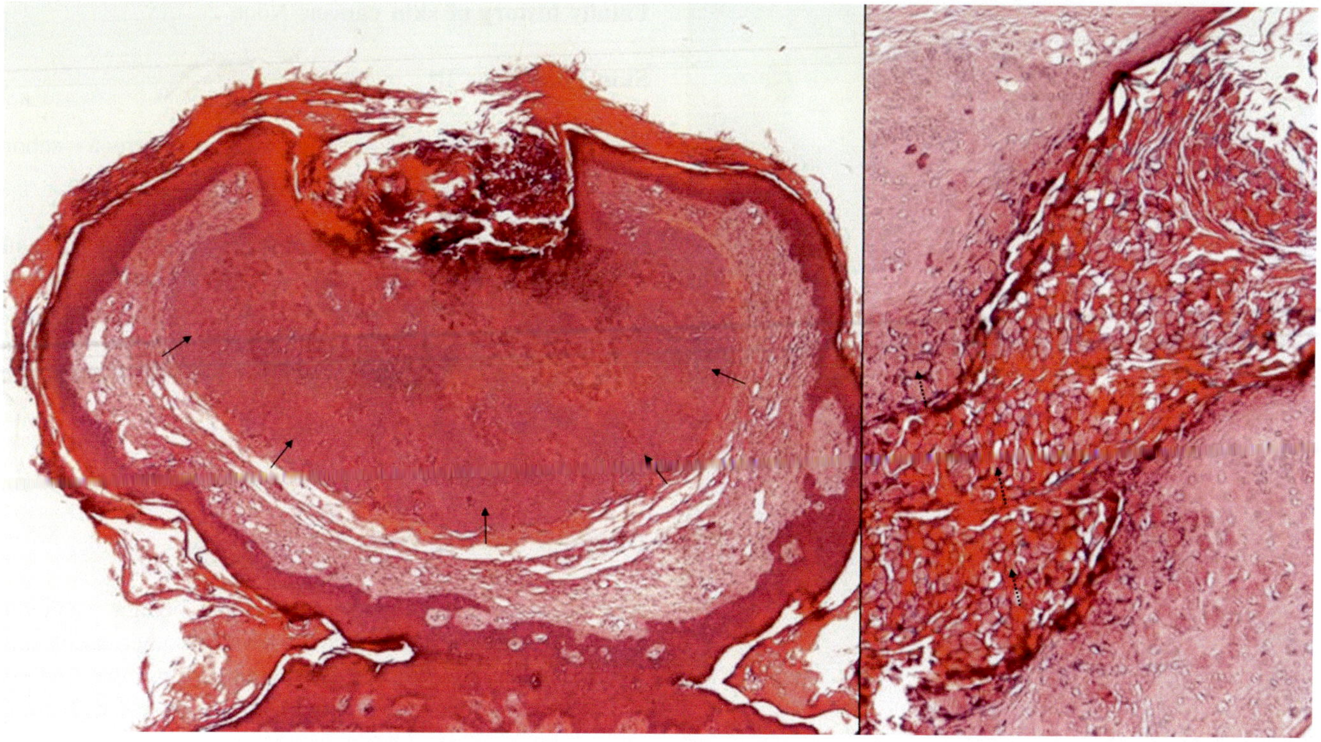

Fig. 9 Histopathology revealed inverted lobules of hyperplastic squamous epithelium (black arrows). Large intracytoplasmic eosinophilic inclusion bodies—molluscum bodies (dotted black arrows). At the granular layer, the bodies occupy the entire cell

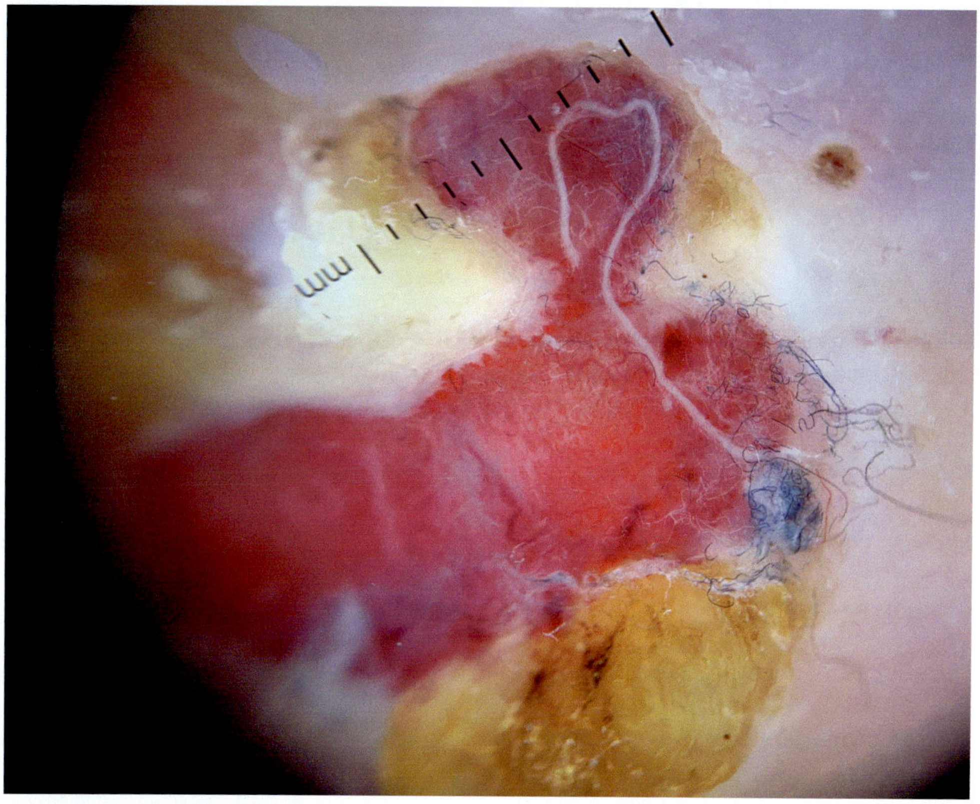

Fig. 10 A- Advanced plantar amelanotic melanoma treated previously as a plantar callus with ulceration and crusts: B - close-up

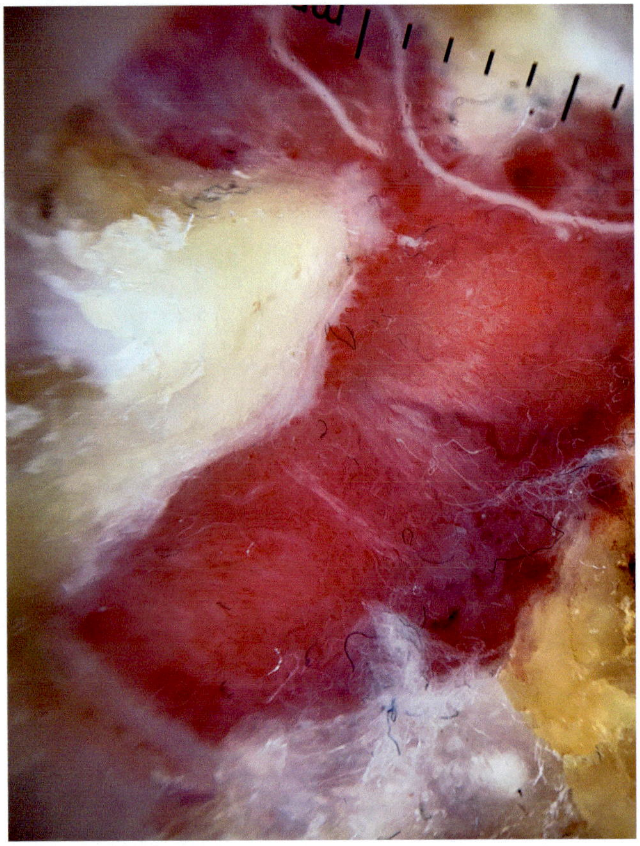

Fig. 11 Acral amelanotic melanoma: polymorphous vascular pattern consisting of atypical thick and thin linear vessels (black arrow); dotted vessels and hairpin vessels at the periphery (red arrow); keratin masses (yellow arrow) and multiple fibers stuck to the ulceration (green arrow)

Clinical record:

Sex: Female

Age: 48-years-old

Clinical description the case or the lesion: The patient received multiple treatments with topic salicylic acid without any improvement

Body site: Dorsum of the right foot

Surface: Pedunculated reddish nodule

Maximum diameter: 3 cm

Duration of the lesion: 2 years

History of morphologic changes: Slow growing

Personal history of skin cancer: None

Family history of skin cancer: None

Skin Phototype: III

Clinical diagnosis: Pyogenic granuloma—verruca—seborrheic keratosis—skin cancer

Dermoscopic findings: Polymorphic vascular pattern with multiple branched vessels with rounded endings (glomerular vessels, flower-like vessels, leef-like vessels, chalice-like vessels), milky red globules, serpentine and hairpin vessels. Also, white interlacing areas around vessels, hemorrhagic crust and keratin.

Other clinical findings: None (Figs. 12, 13 and 14)

Diagnosis: Eccrine Porome

Key message: Poromas are uncommon, benign cutaneous sweat gland tumors that clinically simulate other neoplasms. The most common poroma-associated dermoscopic findings are yellow unstructured areas, branched vessels with rounded endings, white interlacing areas around vessels, and milky-red globules.

The recognition of this dermoscopic structures might be useful for the differential diagnosis.

Case 6

Author: Horacio Cabo

Sex: Male

Age: 28-years-old patient

Clinical description the case or the lesion: Nodular pink lesion

Body site: Right foot

Surface: Nodular

Maximum diameter: 8 mm

Duration of the lesion: More than 3 months

History of morphologic changes: Growing

Personal history of skin cancer: None

Family history of skin cancer: None

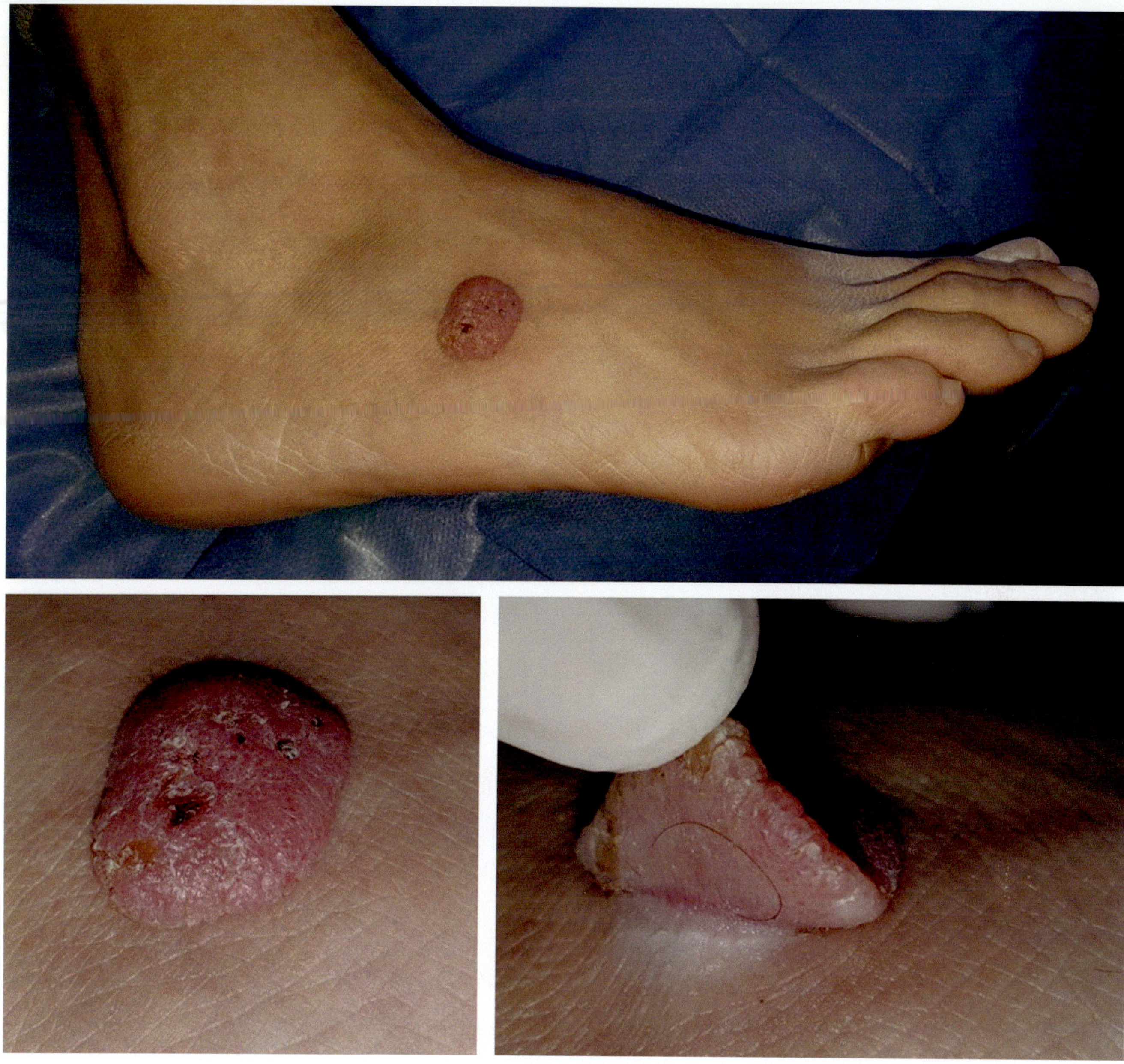

Fig. 12 Clinical view: pedunculated reddish nodule

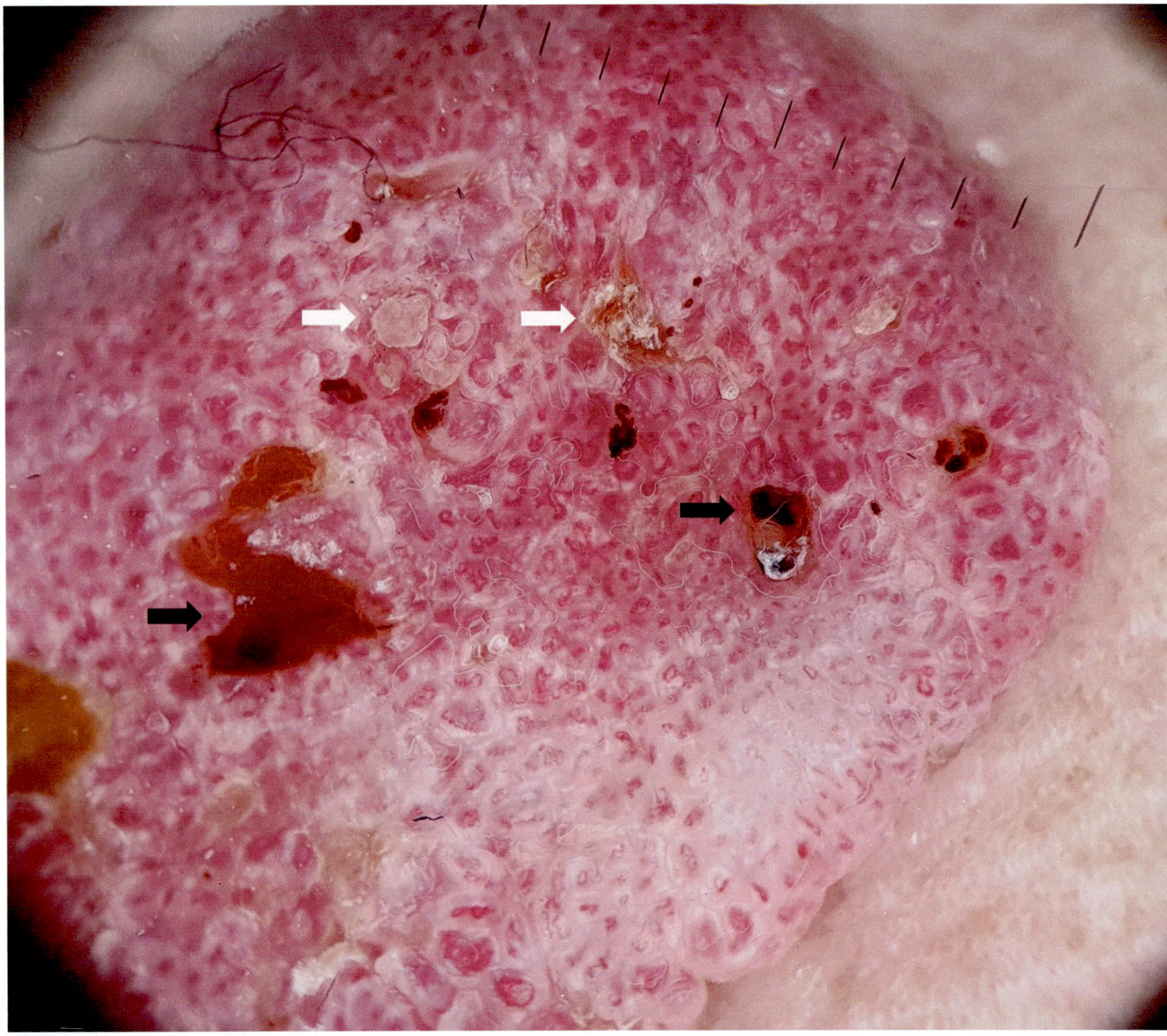

Fig. 13 On Dermoscopy, polymorphic vascular pattern, white interlacing areas around vessels, hemorrhagic crust (black arrow) and keratin (white arrow)

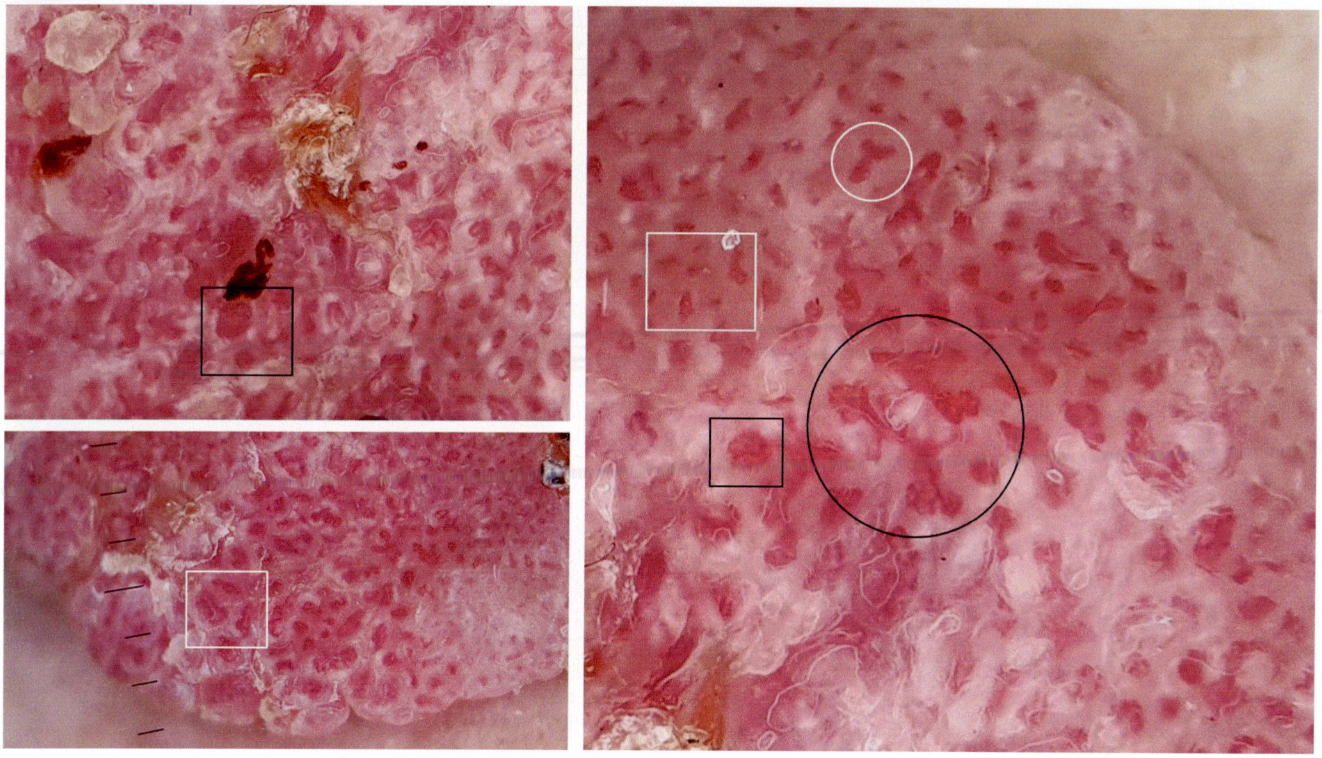

Fig. 14 More magnification shows the different vascular morphology. Multiple branched vessels with rounded endings, also known as glomerular vessels (black square), flower-like vessels (black circle) and chalice-like vessels (white circle). Serpentine and hairpin vessels (white square)

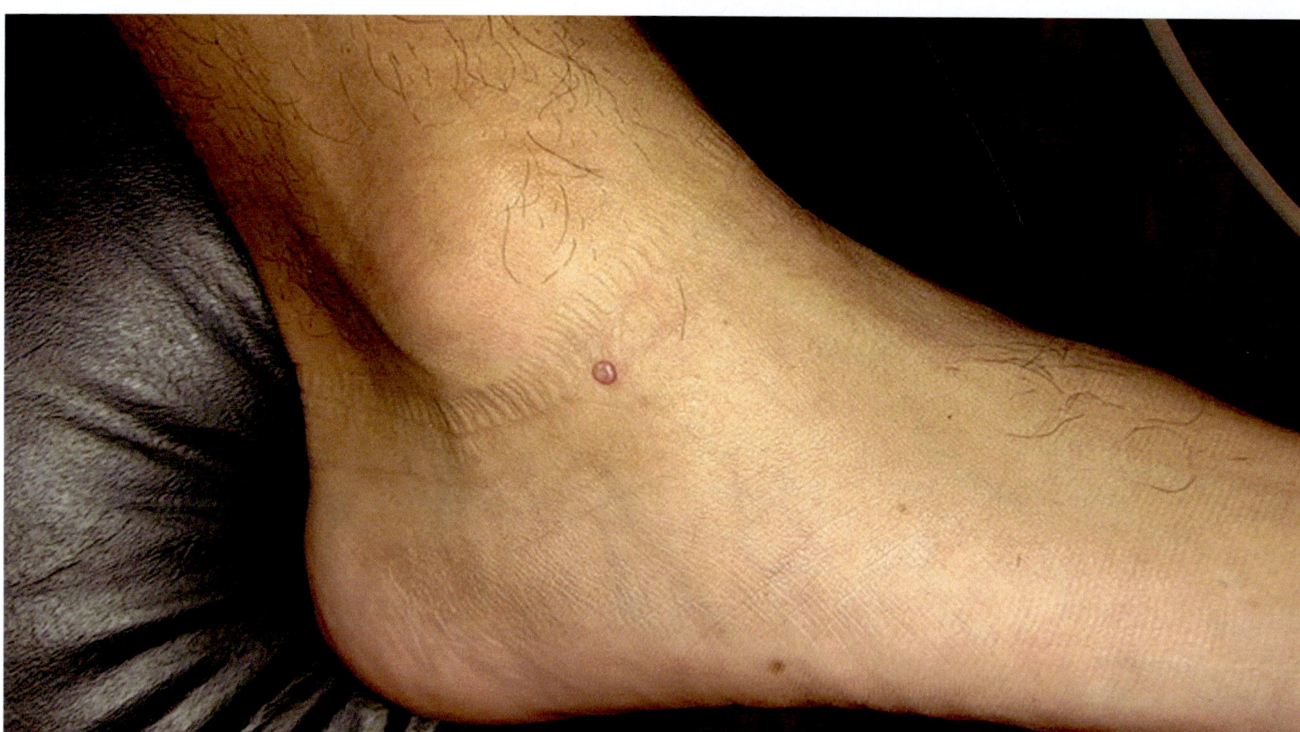

Fig. 15 Clinical view

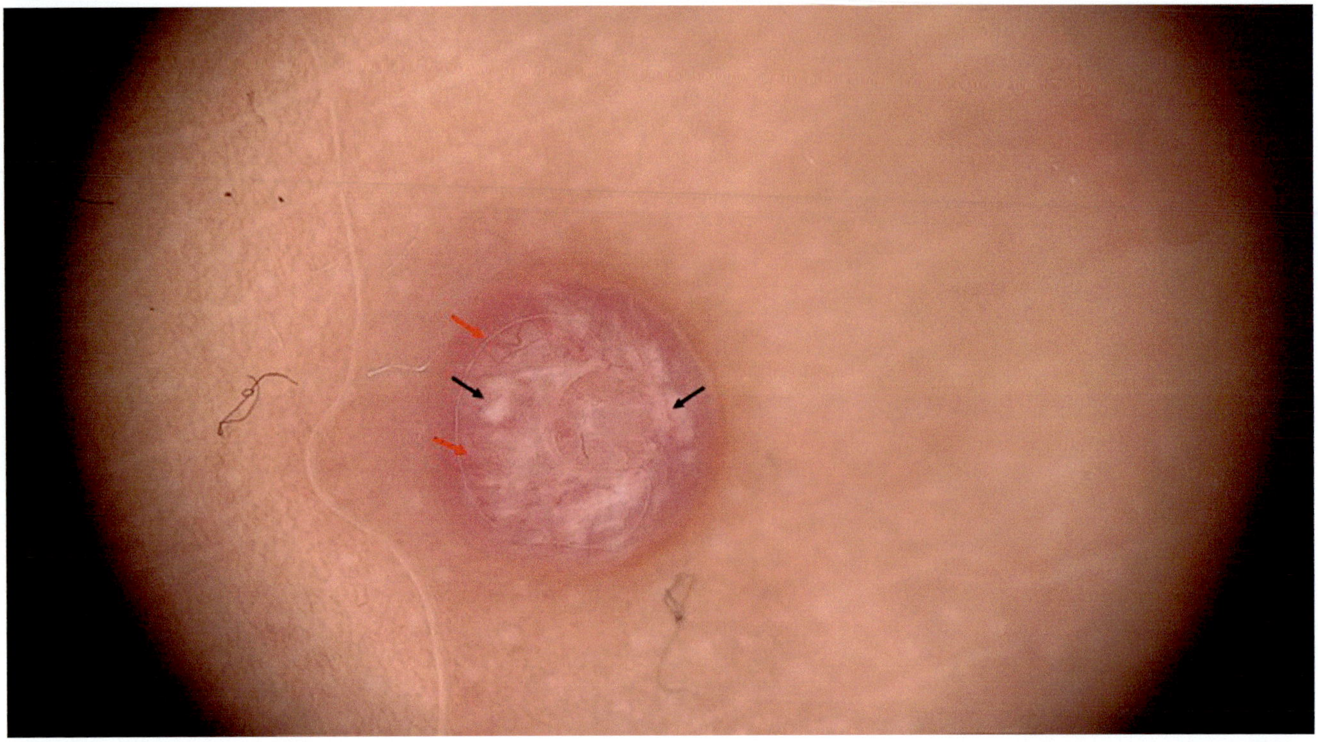

Fig. 16 Dermoscopic view: pink and white lesion with peripheral vessels (red arrows) and white round areas within (black arrows)

Skin Phototype: III

Clinical diagnosis: Wart, Molluscum contagiosum

Dermoscopic findings: Pink and white lesion with peripheral vessels and white round areas within

Other clinical findings: None (Figs. 15 and 16)

Diagnosis: Molluscum Contagiosum

Key message: Dermoscopy is useful to distinguish between warts and molluscum contagiosum

Index

H. Cabo and A. Lallas (eds.), *Dermatoscopic Atlas of Non-Pigmented Lesions*,
https://doi.org/10.1007/978-3-031-34310-0

T

V

W

MIX
Papier aus verantwortungsvollen Quellen
Paper from responsible sources
FSC® C105338

If you have any concerns about our products,
you can contact us on
ProductSafety@springernature.com

In case Publisher is established outside the EU,
the EU authorized representative is:
Springer Nature Customer Service Center GmbH
Europaplatz 3, 69115 Heidelberg, Germany

Printed by Libri Plureos GmbH
in Hamburg, Germany